The progress of experiment

This book examines the science and the politics of drug evaluation. It presents the first general history of clinical research in the United States, examining therapeutic experiments over a wide range of diseases, from syphilis and pneumonia to heart disease and diabetes. It also explores the origins of our contemporary system for judging the drugs used in battling disease, and the history of the modern clinical trial.

How do we evaluate the safety and benefit of new drugs? What tasks do we expect government to perform and which ones do we leave to the medical profession? Harry M. Marks shows that the story of modern pharmaceutical regulation is synonymous with the history of therapeutic reform – professional efforts to use science to reform the market. Accompanying this history of public policy is a detailed account of changing experimental ideals and practices. Marks outlines the history of therapeutic experimentation, from the "collective investigations" of the past century to the controlled clinical trial, which emerged after 1950 as the paradigm of scientific experimentation.

Cambridge History of Medicine

Edited by

CHARLES ROSENBERG, *Professor of History and Sociology of Science,*
University of Pennsylvania

Other titles in the series:

Continued on pages following the Index

The progress of experiment

Science and therapeutic reform in the United States, 1900–1990

HARRY M. MARKS
The Johns Hopkins University

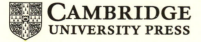

CAMBRIDGE
UNIVERSITY PRESS

PUBLISHED BY THE PRESS SYNDICATE OF THE UNIVERSITY OF CAMBRIDGE
The Pitt Building, Trumpington Street, Cambridge CB2 1RP, United Kingdom

CAMBRIDGE UNIVERSITY PRESS
THE EDINBURGH BUILDING, CAMBRIDGE CB2 2RU, United Kingdom
40 West 20th Street, New York, NY 10011-4211, USA
10 Stamford Road, Oakleigh, Melbourne 3166, Australia

First published 1997

Printed in the United States of America

Typeset in Bembo

Library of Congress Cataloging-in-Publication Data
Marks, Harry M., 1947–
    The progress of experiment : science and therapeutic reform
in the United States, 1900–1990 / Harry M. Marks.
        p.   cm. – (Cambridge history of medicine)
    Includes bibliographical references.
    ISBN 0-521-58142-7
    1. Therapeutics – United States – History – 20th century.
    2. Clinical drug trials – United States – History – 20th century.
    3. Drugs – Law and legislation – United States – History – 20th century.
    I. Title.   II. Series.
    RM47.U6M37   1997
    615.5′0973′0904—dc21   96-38997
                                          CIP

*A catalog record for this book is available from
the British Library.*

ISBN 0-521-58142-7 hardback

*To Barbara Gutmann Rosenkrantz
and to the memory of Edward T. Gargan,
teachers, mentors, and friends*

CONTENTS

ACKNOWLEDGMENTS

This book and its author have had several homes over the past decade, each of which welcomed us more than we had any reason to expect. The project began at the Harvard School of Public Health where Howard Frazier, Fred Mosteller, and Marc J. Roberts encouraged a young historian with some heretical ideas about controlled clinical trials. Leon Eisenberg invited me to spend more of my time at the Department of Social Medicine at Harvard Medical School and generously arranged my obligations so that I had time to take an occasional class across the river at MIT, where Harvey Sapolsky allowed me to pass this enterprise off as a thesis in political science. While I doubt that any of them agreed with what I was saying, much less with my approach to studying statistics, policy, or history, each was generous with support, both moral and material. Only in America, as my grandparents might have said, and, even then, perhaps only at Harvard!

Since leaving Cambridge, I have been in the company of fellow historians: Diana Long and Janet Golden at the Wood Institute of the College of Physicians of Philadelphia, and Gert Brieger, who welcomed me to the (then) Institute of the History of Medicine at The Johns Hopkins University as a Harvey Fellow, and then as Assistant Professor, the Elizabeth Treide and A. McGehee Harvey Professorship in the History of Medicine, in the new Department of the History of Science, Medicine and Technology. My colleagues here, Dan Todes, Ed Morman, Mary Fissell, and Bill Leslie, have made my return to doing full-time history easy and a delight.

Writing what turned out to be contemporary history of science does wonders in teaching one about all the things one doesn't know. My understanding of post-1950 developments in the world of clinical trials has been greatly enriched by the willingness of participants to share their thoughts, their time, and, in several cases, the invaluable contents of their file drawers. I am especially grateful for the cooperation of the late Dr. Thomas C. Chalmers, Dr. Jerome Green, Paul Meier, Sam Greenhouse, Marvin Zelen, Paul Canner, the late Dr. Christian Klimt, Dr. Angela Bowen, Dr. Robert Reeves, and Dr. Robert Bradley. Likewise, numerous colleagues and participants have given me the benefit of commenting on earlier drafts of this material: Dr. Ancel Keys, Dr. Jerome Green, Dr. Thomas C.

Chalmers, Dr. Louis Lasagna, Dr. W. Bruce Fye, Fredrick L. Holmes, Dr. Jesse Roth, John Harley Warner, John Patrick Swann, and James Harvey Young. Curt Meinert and John C. Bailar III, current and former colleagues, took time out from their busy schedules to read and criticize several chapters in the book, while Bill Leslie took on the heroic task of reading a late draft of the complete manuscript.

To Steve Thomas, who led a European-oriented intellectual back to his native shores, I am greatly indebted. An exemplar as well as an advocate of the importance of friendship in civil (and civic) life, Steve introduced me to contemporary Anglo-American political theory well before the fall of the Berlin Wall. My intellectual obligations to Peter Buck and Art Goldhammer, if less readily identifiable, are no less important to me, as is their friendship. Charles Rosenberg is, as others no doubt know, an exemplary editor, replete with smart advice and well supplied with the appropriate amounts of encouragement and guilt-enhancement, and the wisdom to know when each is best applied. Two thoughtful reviewers for Cambridge University Press made crucial observations about the history of statistics which significantly affected the final manuscript. The Press's Brian MacDonald dutifully corrected my unfailingly incorrect use of "which" for "that" and saved me from numerous other embarrassments.

A book like the present could not be written without the assistance of the curators who helped me find my way to the materials I most urgently needed. I am among those fortunate historians who know that Dick Wolfe will always answer their inquiries, or drag down yet another box of uncataloged papers from the attic of the Rare Books and Manuscripts collection of the Francis A. Countway Library of Medicine, Harvard Medical School. I have been no less dependent on the help of Janice Goldblum at the National Academy of Sciences, Beth Carroll-Horrocks and Marty Levitt at the American Philosophical Society, Ms. Maguerite Falucco at the American Medical Association, Tom Rosenbaum at the Rockefeller Archive Center, Gerard Shorb and Nancy McCall at the Alan Mason Chesney Archives here at Hopkins, Aloha South and Marjorie Ciarlante at the National Archives, and especially John Swann, Suzanne White, and Gerry Deighton at the U.S. Food and Drug Administration, who never complained when I asked them to dredge another shipload of cartons out of the Suitland repository.

For aid in getting to the archives and time to write about what I found there, I acknowledge the support of the National Center for Health Services Research [HS 05151] and the Health Services Improvement Fund, Inc., of New York for the dissertation version of this project. The Rockefeller Foundation sustained a postdoctoral year of research, writing, and job hunting at the Francis Wood Institute of the College of Physicians of Philadelphia. At Hopkins, I am especially indebted to Dr. A. McGehee Harvey and Mrs. Elizabeth Treide Harvey and their friends for their generous support in endowing the fellowship and professorship which made it possible for me to complete this book. To Dr. Harvey I am personally thankful for encouraging an outsider to the world of clinical research to write about its history, a topic he had "written the book" on long before I became aware of its fascinations.

For permission to quote from the Commonwealth Fund records, I would like to thank the Rockefeller Archive Center. The University of Pennsylvania Press has graciously allowed me to use portions of my article, "Notes from the Underground: The Social Organization of Therapeutic Research," in Russell Maulitz and Diana Long, eds., *Grand Rounds: One Hundred Years of Internal Medicine.* Michael Bliss generously gave his permission for me to make use of his description of Elizabeth Hughes's bout with diabetes, from *The Discovery of Insulin* (University of Chicago Press, 1982).

I cannot measure nor describe all I owe to JoAnne Brown, as colleague and life companion – much more than this mere book, though I doubt I could have finished it without her. To Irina, thanks for the new title and for the daily delights of her company. I would like to dedicate the book to two friends and teachers who taught me about the practice of history while helping me understand that we are always living in it: to Barbara Gutmann Rosenkrantz and to the memory of the late Edward T. Gargan.

ABBREVIATIONS

Ann Int Med	*Annals of Internal Medicine*
Ann NY Acad Sci	*Annals of the New York Academy of Sciences*
AJPH	*American Journal of Public Health*
APS	Library of the American Philosophical Society, Philadelphia
BHM	*Bulletin of the History of Medicine*
BMSJ	*Boston Medical and Surgical Journal*
Bulletin	*Bulletin of the American Medical Association,* Council on Pharmacy and Chemistry, AMA Archives, Chicago
Bull NY Acad Med	*Bulletin of the New York Academy of Medicine*
Chesney Archives	Alan Mason Chesney Archives, The Johns Hopkins Medical Institutions, Baltimore
Countway Library	Archives, Francis M. Countway Library of Medicine, Harvard Medical School, Boston
JAMA	*Journal of the American Medical Association*
JCD	*Journal of Chronic Diseases*
JHM	*Journal of the History of Medicine and Allied Sciences*
NA	National Archives, College Park, MD
NAS	National Academy of Sciences Archives, Washington, DC
NEJM	*New England Journal of Medicine*
NLM	National Library of Medicine, Bethesda, MD
OD, NIH	Records of the Office of the Director, National Institutes of Health, Bethesda, MD
RAC	Rockefeller Archives Center, Pocantico Hills, NY
W-NRC	Washington-National Records Center, Suitland, MD

Introduction

Medicine has for long possessed the qualities necessary to make a science.[1]

Bensalem will have an intellectual history consisting of the progress of science. It will have a social history consisting of the impact of science. It will, however, have no political history.[2]

"Modern" medicine, "scientific" medicine: the terms are virtually synonymous. The modernity of twentieth-century medicine consists of its reliance on the physical and biological sciences. Yet the association is deceptive, so familiar that it passes without further investigation. What does it mean, what should it mean, to call medicine a science? Is medicine dependent on science for its tools, its knowledge, or its methods? Is medicine scientific because physicians use an advanced technology, the x-ray, because they rely on a knowledge of pathology and radiology to interpret the image produced by the machine, or because of the rigor with which the technology and knowledge are used to arrive at clinical decisions?

From the seventeenth-century iatrochemist van Helmont through the twentieth-century educational reformer Abraham Flexner, it was generally believed that establishing medicine as a science meant grounding medical practices in one or more of the laboratory-based disciplines which study the functioning of biological organisms – biochemistry, physiology, genetics, immunology – disciplines which in turn were to be based on the sciences of physics and chemistry. Scientific medicine was a matter of applying at the bedside knowledge produced elsewhere, a conception of medical science that still thrives today.[3]

1 "Tradition in Medicine," in *Hippocratic Writings*, ed. G. E. R. Lloyd (New York: Penguin Books, 1983), p. 71.
2 Samuel H. Beer, "Two Models of Public Opinion: Bacon's 'New Logic' and Diotima's 'Tale of Love,' " *Political Theory* (May 1974), 166.
3 Claude Bernard's *An Introduction to the Study of Experimental Medicine* (New York: Dover Publications, 1957), as introduced by L. J. Henderson in 1927, provides the locus classicus for twentieth-century proponents of this view. For a contemporary example, see George K. Radda, "The Use of NMR Spectroscopy for the Understanding of Disease," *Science* 223 (August 8, 1986), 640. (The author is aptly titled Professor of Molecular Cardiology at the University of Oxford.) On the tensions among

Historians of medicine have followed medical researchers in focusing on the laboratory sciences of the nineteenth and twentieth centuries: their practices, their organization, and their political ideals.[4] Meanwhile, in this century, another interpretation of the project has been put forth: clinical medicine was, or could be, every bit as scientific as the research laboratory, if "scientific method" were directly applied to judging the results of medical treatment. Paramount among the means for placing medical practice on a scientific basis has been the controlled experiment.

This book examines the beliefs and activities of a disparate group whom I have labeled "therapeutic reformers," individuals who sought to use the science of controlled experiments to direct medical practice. They range from the pharmacologist Torald Sollman, who for fifty-five years guided the American Medical Association's Council on Pharmacy and Chemistry as it reviewed the claims drug manufacturers made for their products, to the gastroenterologist Thomas C. Chalmers, who once advocated that the very first patient to be treated with an experimental drug should be enrolled in a randomized controlled trial.[5] This community of reformers includes individuals trained in the laboratory disciplines of pharmacology and physiology, clinical specialists whose interests range from the infectious diseases of syphilis and pneumonia to the chronic conditions of diabetes and heart disease, physicians and nonphysicians from the quantitative disciplines of statistics and epidemiology, practicing clinicians, government officials, and journal editors.

Historians of science and medicine are accustomed to studying groups bound by professional training and circumstance: the discipline of biochemistry, or the medical specialty of cardiology.[6] This is not a history of clinical pharmacology or of biostatistics, although clinical pharmacologists and statisticians figure prominently in this story. Rather, the therapeutic reformers discussed here constitute a *political* community, a group joined by their belief in the power of science to unite

---

the laboratory sciences, see William Coleman, "The Cognitive Basis of the Discipline: Claude Bernard on Physiology," *Isis* 76 (March 1985), 49–70.

4 Charles E. Rosenberg and Morris J. Vogel, eds., *The Therapeutic Revolution: Essays in the Social History of American Medicine* (Philadelphia: University of Pennsylvania Press, 1979); William Coleman and Frederick Holmes, eds., *The Investigative Enterprise: Experimental Physiology in Nineteenth-Century Medicine* (Berkeley: University of California Press, 1988); John Harley Warner, "Ideals of Science and Their Discontents in Late Nineteenth-Century American Medicine," *Isis* 82 (September 1991), 454–478; Andrew Cunningham and Perry Williams, eds., *The Laboratory Revolution in Medicine* (Cambridge: Cambridge University Press, 1992); Adele Clarke and Joan H. Fujimura, eds., *The Right Tools for the Job: At Work in the Twentieth-Century Life Sciences* (Princeton: Princeton University Press, 1992).

5 Thomas C. Chalmers, "Randomization of the First Patient," *Medical Clinics of North America* 59 (July 1975), 1035–1038.

6 See Robert E. Kohler, *From Medical Chemistry to Biochemistry: The Making of a Biomedical Discipline* (Cambridge: Cambridge University Press, 1992); W. Bruce Fye, *American Cardiology: The History of a Specialty and Its College* (Baltimore: Johns Hopkins University Press, 1996). For a study that takes the research group and research animal as the basis unit of analysis, see Robert E. Kohler, *Lords of the Fly: Drosophila Genetics and the Experimental Life* (Chicago: University of Chicago Press, 1994).

both medical researchers and practitioners *despite* obvious differences of training and circumstance.[7] Although connected in some cases by the accidents of personal biography, what binds reformers is the shared belief that better knowledge about the effects and uses of drugs will lead directly to better therapeutic practice.

My aim in the book is twofold. First, I wish to examine the changing character of reformers' efforts to direct clinical therapeutic practice. In the first half of the century, reformers depended on the integrity and expertise of individual researchers to produce reliable, untainted, knowledge about the effects of medical treatment. They relied on an organization of experienced researchers, the Council on Pharmacy and Chemistry, to sift and weigh the claims manufacturers offered about the effects of specific therapies on disease. U.S. Food and Drug Administration officials adopted the council's approach to judging the benefits and risks of treatment in their efforts to regulate the safety of new drugs during the 1930s and 1940s.

Reformers in the second half of the century abandoned their predecessors' trust in the judgment of experienced clinicians. In its place, they offered an impersonal standard of scientific integrity: the double-blind, randomized, controlled clinical trial. Yet despite obvious differences in their ideas about experiments, evidence, and clinical judgment, "methodological reformers" shared their predecessors' conviction that elevating the scientific standards of drug evaluation would lead directly to improvements in clinical practice.

Reformers' trust in the powers of science went hand in hand with a suspicion of the motives of business. Throughout the century, reformers have regarded evidence from corporate sponsored research as guilty until proven innocent. Early in the century, Progressive-era reformers warned that only an independent science of drug evaluation, securely controlled by the medical profession, could resist corporate impulses to "debauch our medical journals" and "taint our textbooks."[8] In less colorful language, reformers' suspicions persist today, embodied in proposals that researchers identify any business interests in the products they study.[9]

---

7 For a related use of the notion of political identity, see John Harley Warner, "Remembering Paris: Memory and the American Disciples of French Medicine in the Nineteenth Century," *BHM* 65 (1991), 312–315.

8 George H. Simmons, "The Commercial Domination of Therapeutics and the Movement for Reform," *JAMA* 48 (May 18, 1907), 1645.

9 International Committee of Medical Journal Editors, "Conflict of Interest," *Ann Int Med* 118 (April 15, 1993), 646–647; "American Federation for Clinical Research Guidelines for Avoiding Conflict of Interest," *Clinical Research* 38 (April 1990), 39–40. For a survey of conflict of interest policies, see M. D. Witt and L. O. Gostin, "Conflict of Interest Dilemmas in Biomedical Research," *JAMA* 271 (February 16, 1994), 547–551. See also R. A. Davidson, "Source of Funding and Outcome of Clinical Trials," *Journal of General Internal Medicine* 1 (May–June 1986), 155–158; Paula A. Rochon, Jerry H. Gurwitz, Robert W. Simms, Paul R. Fortin, David T. Felson, Kenneth L. Minaker, and Thomas C. Chalmers, "A Study of Manufacturer-Supported Trials of Nonsteroidal Anti-inflammatory Drugs in the Treatment of Arthritis," *Archives of Internal Medicine* 154 (January 24, 1994), 157–163. On the history of corporate involvement in university drug research, see John P. Swann, *Academic Scientists and the Pharmaceutical Industry: Cooperative Research in Twentieth-Century America* (Baltimore: Johns Hopkins University Press, 1988).

Reformers' appeals for an independent science of drug evaluation were integral to their political vision of the medical profession as a body united through science. Medicine's contemporary critics take the profession's scientific aspirations as both illusory and delusive: medicine is not, they argue, a science and its claims in this regard are chimerical.[10] What such demystifying criticisms ignore is the role such visions of science have played within the profession itself.

Medical practitioners have always been divided by differences in formal training and professional opportunity. In the present century, the rapid pace of technological and scientific change has aggravated existing inequalities in the profession, between hospital-based physicians and community-based doctors, between specialists and general practitioners, between metropolitan and rural physicians.[11] Operating from the islands of academic medicine, therapeutic reformers offered practitioners the vision of a profession united by a faith in science which transcended all accidental differences of training and technological sophistication.[12]

Reformers' pursuit of a profession unified by science came at a price. Reformers believed that they need only provide physicians with a scientifically grounded knowledge of drugs' uses and effects to improve therapeutic practice. Until very recently, reformers have sidestepped the question of what to do about physicians who do not use drugs appropriately or prudently.[13] Nor were reformers often successful in transcending the differences that divided researchers of diverse disciplinary backgrounds or between doctors who practiced under different material circumstances.

Reformers' need to create a "republic of science" continues to haunt contemporary efforts at therapeutic reform. Physicians dispute the relative merits of statistical and clinical expertise in evaluating medical treatments, while reformers find it difficult to define the point at which reasonable disagreement about

10 See E. Richard Brown, *Rockefeller Medicine Men: Medicine and Capitalism in America* (Berkeley: University of California Press, 1979); John Ehrenreich, "Introduction," in John Ehrenreich, ed., *The Cultural Crisis of Modern Medicine* (New York: Monthly Review Press, 1978), pp. 1–38.

11 On the role of the nineteenth-century and early twentieth-century hospital in medical careers, see Charles E. Rosenberg, *The Care of Strangers: The Rise of America's Hospital System* (New York: Basic Books, 1987), pp. 58–68, 166–189. On divisions in the professional order and efforts to overcome them in the present century, see Rosemary Stevens, "The Curious Career of Internal Medicine: Functional Ambivalence, Social Success," in Russell C. Maulitz and Diana E. Long, eds., *Grand Rounds: One Hundred Years of Internal Medicine* (Philadelphia: University of Pennsylvania Press, 1988), pp. 339–364; idem, *In Sickness and in Wealth: American Hospitals in the Twentieth Century* (New York: Basic Books, 1989).

12 The notion of science provides the basis for what Benedict Anderson calls, in the political context of modern nationalism, an "imagined" community. See his *Imagined Communities: Reflections on the Origin and Spread of Nationalism* (London: Verso Books, 1983). For an argument that the notion of a scientific community is a mid-twentieth-century invention, see David A. Hollinger, "Free Enterprise and Free Inquiry: The Emergence of Laissez-Faire Communitarianism in the Ideology of Science in the United States," *New Literary History* 21 (1990), 897–919. I am grateful to Bill Leslie for calling my attention to Hollinger's essay.

13 Jerry Avorn, "Drug Regulation and Drug Information – Who Should Do What to Whom?," *AJPH* 85 (January 1995), 18–19; Peter Temin, *Taking Your Medicine: Drug Regulation in the United States* (Cambridge: Harvard University Press, 1980).

therapeutic merit becomes irrational dissent from a scientific standard of practice.[14] Should physicians be allowed to prescribe human growth hormone for children who are growing more slowly than their peers, but who show no signs of hormonal deficiency? What kinds of evidence are needed before physicians conclude that the use of calcium channel blockers for treating hypertension is unsafe? When should patients with HIV disease be allowed to take still experimental drugs?[15]

Invariably, such discussions involve questions of political values as well as scientific merit. Although the project of reforming professional therapeutic practice has always been a problem of political order as well as of science, reformers seem incapable of addressing matters of science and politics in the same breath. Part of my reason for writing this book is to suggest that the science and politics of therapeutic reform need not be as inimical as contemporary reformers sometimes suggest.

My second aim in the book is to chart the changing intellectual and social history of therapeutic experiments, from the early 1900s when the laboratory sciences provided the standard of the "well-controlled" experiment to the latter half of the century when the clinically based randomized controlled trial offered a new standard of scientific excellence. The controlled clinical trial has a history that, in the public health tradition, dates backs at least to James Lind's controlled test of lemons for scurvy prevention in the British Navy of the 1740s.[16] Generally, physicians have focused their attention on a series of celebrated examples ranging

14 Alvan R. Feinstein, "An Additional Basic Science for Clinical Medicine. Parts I–IV," *Ann Int Med* 99 (1983), 393–397, 554–550, 705–712, 843–848. On clinical controversies, see the discussion in Chapters 7 and 8.

15 On human growth hormone, see David B. Allen, C. G. D. Brook, N. A. Bridges, P. C. Hindmarsh, Harvey J. Guyda, and Douglas Frazier, "Therapeutic Controversies: Growth Hormone (GH) Treatment of Non-GH Deficient Subjects," *Journal of Clinical Endocrinology and Metabolism* 79 (1995), 1239–1248; E. Kirk Neeley and Ron G. Rosenfeld, "Use and Abuse of Human Growth Hormone," *Annual Review of Medicine* 45 (1994), 407–420. On calcium channel blockers, see Bruce M. Psaty, Susan R. Heckbert, Thomas D. Koepsell, et al., "The Risk of Myocardial Infarction Associated with Antihypertensive Drug Therapies," *JAMA* 274 (August 23–30, 1995), 620–625; Curt D. Furberg, Bruce M. Patsy, and Jeffrey V. Meyer, "Nifedipine: Dose-Related Increase in Mortality in Patients with Coronary Heart Disease," *Circulation* 92 (1995), 1326–1331; Lionel H. Opie and Franz H. Messerli, "Nifedipine and Mortality: Grave Defects in the Dossier," ibid., 1068–1073; Salim Yusuf, "Calcium Antagonists in Coronary Heart Disease and Hypertension: Time for Reevaluation?" ibid., 1079–1082. On AIDS therapies, see Jeffrey Levi, "Unproven AIDS Therapies: The Food and Drug Administration and ddI," in Committee to Study Biomedical Decision Making, Institute of Medicine, *Biomedical Politics* (Washington, DC: National Academy Press, 1991), pp. 9–37; Paul D. Stolley and Tamar Lasky, "Shortcuts in Drug Evaluation," *Clinical Pharmacology and Therapeutics* 52 (July 1992), 1–3. See also the discussion in John Lantos, "How Can We Distinguish Clinical Research from Innovative Therapy," *American Journal of Pediatric Hematology/Oncology* 16 (1994), 72–75.

16 For an account of Lind's work which places it into context, see Ulrich Tröhler, *Quantification in British Medicine and Surgery 1750–1830, with Special Reference to Its Introduction into Therapeutics* (Ph.D. thesis, University of London, 1978), pp. 198–220. See also Alice Henderson Smith, "The Relative Content of Anti-scorbutic Principle in Limes and Lemons. B. Historical Inquiry," *Lancet* ii (1918), 737–738. Earlier episodes of "controlled" tests sometimes cited seem to me to have far more to do with biblical traditions of trial by lots or, as in Ambroise Paré's case, with the contemporary

from Lind's field trial through the introduction of the "numerical method" in the Paris Clinic of the nineteenth century to the Medical Research Council's controlled trial of streptomycin for tuberculosis treatment in post–World War II Britain. These disparate episodes are then linked in a transhistorical narrative of antecedents deemed to constitute the history of the present-day randomized controlled trial.[17] In turn, historians William Coleman, Ulrich Tröhler and George Weisz have treated several of these episodes in greater detail, without assuming the burden of a transhistorical narrative.[18]

My approach has been to focus on the activities, circumstances, and ideas of clinical researchers in situ, ignoring European (and American) antecedents except where they can be shown to have a direct influence on the practices and ideals of twentieth-century reformers active in the United States.[19] The resulting account differs from earlier historical narratives in at least three ways. First, I have emphasized the changing meanings that researchers attached to terms such as experimental "controls" or "randomized" experiments. Second, I have given greater attention to the material circumstances under which researchers of successive generations worked, and to the effects of these circumstances on their ideas of experimentation. Successive approaches for producing and weighing evidence about the effects of drug therapies incorporated different assumptions about which group was best suited to perform such assessments: community-based physicians in the "collective investigations" of the preceding century, university-based specialists in the "cooperative studies" of the 1930s and 1940s, and the indispensable statisticians in the randomized clinical trials of the 1950s and beyond. The historical pathway to the latter was neither as smooth nor as direct as previous accounts suggest.

Third, this is quintessentially an American story. While the controlled clinical trial may be an international scientific accomplishment, the ways in which trials were organized and understood mark them as belonging to a particular place as

---

rhetoric of empirical versus learned medicine, than with subsequent developments of controlled experimentation in the nineteenth and twentieth centuries.

17 See, for example, J. P. Bull, "The Historical Development of Clinical Therapeutic Trials," *JCD* 10 (1959), 218–248; Abraham Lilienfeld, "Ceteris Paribus: The Evolution of the Clinical Trial," *BHM* 56 (1982), 1–18. The recent study by the historian J. Rosser Matthews, while adding both new episodes and considerable new detail to the canonical narratives of Bull and Lilienfeld, employs a similar approach. See *Quantification and the Quest for Medical Certainty* (Princeton: Princeton University Press, 1995).

18 See, in particular, Tröhler, *Quantification in British Medicine and Surgery* (n. 16); George Weisz, "Academic Debate and Therapeutic Reasoning in Mid-19th Century France," in Ilana Löwy, Olga Amsterdamska, John Pickstone, and Patrice Pinell, eds., *Medicine and Change: Historical and Sociological Studies in Medical Innovation* (Paris: INSERM, 1993), pp. 287–315; William Coleman, "Experimental Physiology and Statistical Inference: The Therapeutic Trial in Nineteenth-Century Germany," in Lorenz Krüger, Gerd Gigerenzer, and Mary S. Morgan, eds., *The Probabilistic Revolution* (Cambridge: MIT Press, 1987), vol. 2, pp. 201–208. See also William A. Silverman's exemplary case study of clinical evidence and clinical trials in post–World War II neonatology: *Retrolental Fibroplasia: A Modern Parable* (New York: Grune and Stratton, 1980).

19 I discuss the historical literature on the nineteenth-century U.S. traditions in Chapters 1 and 2.

well as time.[20] Historians of the United States will easily recognize the conviction of Progressive-era therapeutic reformers that science is a moral as well as an intellectual activity; the insistence of researchers in the 1920s and 1930s that new organizations were needed to conduct adequate studies of new drugs; and the almost paranoid obsession of researchers in the 1950s with purging subjectivity from controlled experiments. Other familiar features of the story include the influence of private organizations (the Council of Pharmacy and Chemistry) on public policy, and the enduring faith that the social and political obstacles to a rational therapeutics can be solved by better and more science.[21]

If I have anything to add to the conventional wisdom on twentieth-century U.S. history, it comes from my conviction that reformers were influenced less by the writings of public intellectuals or the irresistible forces of bureaucratization and professionalization than by intellectual traditions and circumstances particular to the local world of academic medicine. To paraphrase Marx, men make their own history but not under the circumstances described in the prefaces to history books. Perhaps that is why my scientists seem far more hostile to corporate America than prevailing historiography would predict; why their organizations are far less effective and enduring than proponents of the "organizational" synthesis might expect; and why my postwar bureaucratic state is far less heavy-handed (or effective) in furthering the cause of a rational therapeutics than neoliberal critics of the regulatory state might allow.[22]

20 For analyses in a similar vein of comparable developments in Great Britain, see the forthcoming dissertations by Desiree Cox-Maximov, *The Making of the Clinical Trial in Britain, 1900–1950: A Cultural History* (Cambridge University), and Alan Yoshioka, *British Clinical Trials of Streptomycin: 1946–1951* (Imperial College).

21 On science, morality, and politics, see Charles Rosenberg's *No Other Gods: On Science and American Social Thought* (Baltimore: Johns Hopkins University Press, 1978), pp. 1–21; David A. Hollinger, "Inquiry and Uplift: Late Nineteenth-Century American Academics and the Moral Efficacy of Scientific Practice," in Thomas L. Haskell, ed., *The Authority of Experts: Studies in History and Theory* (Bloomington: Indiana University Press, 1984), pp. 142–156; Dorothy Ross, *The Origins of American Social Science* (Cambridge: Cambridge University Press, 1991). On organizations, see Louis Galambos, "The Emerging Organizational Synthesis in Modern American History," *Business History Review* 44 (Autumn 1970), 279–290; idem, "Technology, Political Economy and Professionalization: Central Themes of the Organizational Synthesis," *Business History Review* 57 (Winter 1983), 471–493. On private organizations and public policy, see the classic works of Grant McConnell, *The Decline of Agrarian Democracy* (Berkeley: University of California Press, 1953), and Philip Selznick, *TVA and the Grass Roots: A Study in the Sociology of Formal Organization* (Berkeley: University of California Press, 1949). For more recent work in this tradition, see J. David Greenstone, ed., *Public Values and Private Power in American Politics* (Chicago: University of Chicago Press, 1982). On objectivity in American social science after World War II, see Peter Novick, *That Noble Dream: The "Objectivity Question" and the American Historical Profession* (Cambridge: Cambridge University Press, 1988), pp. 281–360.

22 On science and the corporation, David F. Noble's pathbreaking *America by Design: Science, Technology and the Rise of Corporate Capitalism* (New York: Alfred A. Knopf, 1977) remains unsurpassed. On organizations, see Louis Galambos, "The Emerging Organizational Synthesis" (n. 21), and Brian Balogh, "Reorganizing the Organizational Synthesis: Federal-Professional Relations in Modern America," *Studies in American Political Development* 5 (Spring 1991), 119–172. Contrast Matthew E. Crenson's and Francis E. Rourke's views of the "inevitability" of postwar bureaucracy with Barry Karl's views of the fragility of the prewar state. Crenson and Rourke, "By Way of Conclusion:

My interest in the history of therapeutic reform dates to the late 1970s, when I was working with a group of statisticians, economists, and physicians at the Harvard School of Public Health. My colleagues were puzzled by the seeming indifference, if not hostility, of many clinicians to randomized controlled trials. I, in turn, was intrigued by the strength of my colleagues' belief in the power of evidence to transform clinical practice. Yet I would not have been able to follow up on the story had it not been for the emergence at that time of a new sociology of science, whose practitioners insisted that even orthodox science was fair game for social and historical inquiry, by researchers using the same tools in studying the "failed" sciences of the past, phlogiston and phrenology, as in investigating the "false" science of the present – cold fusion and the mysterious molecules of Dr. Benveniste.[23]

From the study of scientific controversies, the new sociologists of science went on to inquire into the domain of scientific practice: the nature and organization of scientific work in different settings, the role of social conventions in stabilizing agreement about observed phenomenon, the diverse repertoire of resources scientists use in pursuing their work.[24] Each of these developments has left its mark on this book. Yet sociologists have focused almost exclusively on science's heartland, the laboratory, largely ignoring the domain of the clinic where the social character of the science conducted is perhaps too obvious to merit their attention.[25]

Readers acquainted with the complex and sophisticated body of sociological

American Bureaucracy since World War II," in Louis Galambos, ed., *The New American State: Bureaucracies and Policies since World War II* (Baltimore: Johns Hopkins University Press, 1987), pp. 137–177; Barry D. Karl, *The Uneasy State: The United States from 1915 to 1945* (Chicago: University of Chicago Press, 1983).

23 For those who do not recall the incident, Benveniste and his colleagues found an immunological reaction even after diluting an antibody 10^{60} times. See E. Davenas, F. Bauvais, J. Amara, M. Oberbaum, B. Robinzon, A. Miadonna, A. Tedeschi, B. Pomeranz, P. Fortner, P. Belon, J. Sainte-Laudy, B. Poitevin, and J. Benveniste, "Human Basophil Degranulation Triggered by Very Dilute Antiserum against IgE," *Nature* 333 (June 30, 1988), 816–818. On cold fusion, see Thomas F. Gieryn, "The Ballad of Pons and Fleischmann: Experiment and Narrative in the (Un)Making of Cold Fusion," in Ernan McMullin, ed., *The Social Dimensions of Science* (Notre Dame, IN: University of Notre Dame Press, 1992), pp. 217–243. On symmetry in explaining "true" and "false" science, see G. Nigel Gilbert and Michael Mulkay, "Warranting Scientific Belief," *Social Studies of Science* 12 (1982), 383–408.

24 See especially Bruno Latour, *Laboratory Life: The Social Construction of Scientific Facts* (Beverly Hills, CA: Sage Publications, 1979); Peter Galison, "Bubble Chambers and the Experimental Workplace," in Peter Achinstein and Owen Hannaway, eds., *Observation, Experiment and Hypothesis in Modern Physical Science* (Cambridge: MIT Press, 1985); Karin Knorr-Cetina, *The Manufacture of Knowledge: An Essay on the Constructivist and Contextual Nature of Science* (Oxford: Pergamon Press, 1981). More recent work can be sampled in Andrew Pickering, ed., *Science as Practice and Culture* (Chicago: University of Chicago Press, 1992); David Gooding, Trevor Pinch, and Simon Schaffer, *The Uses of Experiment: Studies in the Natural Sciences* (Cambridge: Cambridge University Press, 1989).

25 See, however, the forthcoming work by Ilana Löwy, *Between Bench and Bedside: Science, Healing and Interleukin 2 in a Cancer Ward* (Cambridge: Harvard University Press, 1996); and the pioneering work of Leigh Star: Susan Leigh Star, "Simplification in Scientific Work: An Example from Neuroscience Research," *Social Studies of Science* 13 (May 1983), 205–229; idem, "Triangulating Clinical and Basic Research: British Localizationists, 1870–1906," *History of Science* 24 (1986), 29–48.

study on contemporary science may wonder what a historian has to add.[26] First is a greater awareness of the historical character of scientific inquiry. Sociologists have been at great pains to emphasize as well as analyze the social character of scientific knowledge. Yet for the historian, the notion that science is "social" is a truism: we are more interested in the different kinds of societies in which scientists work, the different forms of power and influence available to them, or in the fates of different sciences within a given society.

For example, clinical researchers in the 1930s and 1940s relied on inquiries they termed "cooperative investigations," intended to transcend the limitations of isolated researchers in studying medical treatments. In the early 1930s, researchers emphasized the power of cooperative investigations to transcend the methodological vulnerability of individually conducted research, the use of idiosyncratic definitions of disease and treatment, and a reliance on small case series whose conclusions were easily affected by the ordinary cycles of spontaneous recoveries and remissions. During World War II, in contrast, researchers emphasized the greater efficiency of centrally planned cooperative investigations: their ability to quickly provide urgently needed answers to questions about the uses of new drugs. In two successive decades, contemporaries invested the same scientific activity with two very distinct meanings. Similarly, just as the resources available to cooperative investigations expanded enormously during World War II, as soon as the war was over, researchers resumed their search for new funding (and new justifications) for their research. It is difficult to understand the social character of cooperative investigations in either decade without exploring these differences in historical circumstances and meaning.[27]

Contemporary sociological studies also invest science with great power. In one recent influential account, science is a "golem," a powerful creature capable of running amuck. In another, it is a lever capable of lifting the world.[28] By contrast,

26 For a historian's overview of recent work in the sociology of science, see Jan Golinski, "The Theory of Practice and the Practice of Theory: Sociological Approaches in the History of Science," *Isis* 81 (September 1990), 492–505. For further discussion of the issues addressed here, see Harry M. Marks, "Other Voices: A Reply to Labinger," *Social Studies of Science* 25 (1995), 329–334; idem, *Local Knowledge: Experimental Communities and Experimental Practices, 1918–1950,* a paper presented at the conference on Twentieth Century Health Sciences: Problems and Interpretations, University of California, San Francisco, May 1988.

27 For a thoughtful discussion of the limits of such historicizing, see Steven Shapin, "Discipline and Bounding: The History and Sociology of Science As Seen through the Externalism–Internalism Debate," *History of Science* 30 (1992), 347–355.

28 Harry Collins and Trevor Pinch, *The Golem: What Everyone Should Know about Science* (Cambridge: Cambridge University Press, 1994); Bruno Latour, "Give Me a Laboratory and I Will Raise the World," in Karin D. Knorr-Cetina and Michael Mulkay, eds., *Science Observed: Perspectives on the Social Study of Science* (London: Sage Publications, 1983), pp. 141–170. In his account of Louis Pasteur's anthrax vaccine, Bruno Latour appears to recognize the significance of social engineering, when he notes that Pasteur's vaccine never seemed to work outside the boundaries of the Francophone world. Yet within France, Latour makes Pasteur's social engineering look so easy that a careless reader may easily come away with the wrong impression. For a critical discussion of Latour's work emphasizing these issues, see Simon Schaffer, "The Eighteenth Brumaire of Bruno Latour," *Studies in the History and Philosophy of Science* 22 (1991), 175–192.

the sciences discussed in this book are weak, incapable of transforming the world of clinical practice as easily as reformers hope. The kind of social engineering that science requires to transform the world is, as sociologists *should* know, a far more difficult task in scale and complexity than physicists' no less ambitious efforts to measure gravity.

Since World War II, the organization and conduct of clinical experiments have been radically transformed by medicine's encounter with the discipline of statistics. When I began work on this project, the history of statistics after 1750 was best pursued by reading old statistical journals.[29] Now, the historian has a wealth of perspectives to chose from in seeking to understand the theory and practice of statistics in historical context. Nonetheless, there remain few historical guides to statistics after 1900, regardless of whether one is interested in debates among the high priests of statistical inference (R. A. Fisher, Jerzy Neyman, L. J. Savage) or the more mundane details of statistical practice in business, agriculture, or medicine.[30]

I therefore chose a very narrow focus: to examine the ways in which ideas about randomized experiments and statistical analysis were introduced into clinical medicine, and the role professional statisticians played as allies of therapeutic reformers. My approach is premised on the convictions that ideas can best be studied in context, and that the administrative memo can reveal as much about the intellectual history of an era as the more formal treatises sometimes favored by intellectual historians.[31] Other versions of the story can and hopefully will be written that give greater attention to statistics in other domains – the laboratory, the factory and the classroom – and other disciplines.

I have divided the book into two parts, corresponding to the two eras of therapeutic reform discussed above. Chapters 1 through 4 deal with the era of organizational reforms; Chapters 5 through 8 cover the era of methodological

29 In addition to the classic works of Westergaard and Todhunter, the collection of articles by Egon Pearson and Maurice Kendall was very useful: E. S. Pearson and Maurice Kendall, eds., *Studies in the History of Statistics and Probability* (London: C. Griffin, 1970), 2 vols. For seventeenth-century studies, see Ian Hacking, *The Emergence of Probability: A Philosophical Study of Early Ideas about Probability, Induction and Statistical Inference* (Cambridge: Cambridge University Press, 1975); Peter Buck, "Seventeenth-Century Political Arithmetic: Civil Strife and Vital Statistics," *Isis* 68 (1977), 67–84.

30 On statistics prior to 1900, see especially Stephen M. Stigler, *The History of Statistics: The Measurement of Uncertainty before 1900* (Cambridge: Harvard University Press, 1986); Lorraine J. Daston, *Classical Probability in the Enlightenment* (Princeton: Princeton University Press, 1988); Ian Hacking, *The Taming of Chance* (Cambridge: Cambridge University Press, 1990); Theodore M. Porter, *The Rise of Statistical Thinking, 1820–1900* (Princeton: Princeton University Press, 1986). For twentieth-century statistics, see the pioneering synthesis by Gerd Gigerenzer, Zeno Swijtink, Theodore Porter, Lorraine Daston, John Beatty, and Lorenz Krüger, *The Empire of Chance: How Probability Changed Science and Everyday Life* (Cambridge: Cambridge University Press, 1989).

31 If anyone should find this proposition disconcerting, I refer to the authority of Antonio Gramsci, for my therapeutic reformers certainly are among Gramsci's organic intellectuals, and to the historian William Bouswma, "From History of Ideas to History of Meaning," in idem, *A Usable Past: Essays in European Cultural History* (Berkeley: University of California Press, 1990), pp. 336–347.

reformers. A brief introduction to Part II provides an overview of the second half of the book, and of the transformations in experimental theory and research practice enabled by statisticians and their ideas.

My narrative begins in 1906, when the American Medical Association created the Council on Pharmacy and Chemistry to judge the claims of drug manufacturers for their products. The council, an assemblage of pharmacologists and clinicians from medical schools around the country, weekly exchanged evidence and views on drugs submitted by firms, publishing the results of their deliberations in the *Journal of the American Medical Association*. The council attempted to dominate the two central institutions of modern therapeutics – the laboratory and the market – by regulating the information practitioners received about new drugs. In Chapter 1, I describe the council's activities between 1906 and 1930 in organizing a system of consultants to gather and winnow evidence on new drugs, and thereby direct the profession's clinical practice.

The council's standards of drug evaluation and system of consultants were taken up by the U.S. Food and Drug Administration (FDA) officials charged with administering the 1938 Federal Food, Drug and Cosmetic Act, a development I discuss in Chapter 3. Like the Council on Pharmacy and Chemistry, FDA officials consulted extensively with academic specialists about their experiences with the drugs companies wished to place on the market. Similarly, FDA officials negotiated with companies over the claims and warnings they could put on their products before issuing them to physicians. And, like the council, the FDA refrained from more direct interference with practitioners' right to ignore what science had to say about the uses of drugs.

In Chapter 2, I describe the efforts of early twentieth-century researchers to link laboratory studies of drug action with clinical investigations of their value in treating disease. While many researchers followed the traditional path of discovering and testing new compounds in the laboratory, therapeutic reformers were interested in studies that would assess the clinical merit of widely used drugs. In the late 1920s, researchers introduced the "cooperative investigation," an organized collaboration intended to replace the observations of individual experts with a standardized evaluation of therapeutic results in hundreds of patients.

I describe the activities of one such study, the Cooperative Clinical Group, a collaboration of researchers from a half-dozen university clinics to evaluate standard methods of treating syphilis. The complex and hazardous regimen of arsenical treatments preferred by the group's university specialists ultimately proved irrelevant to community practitioners who relied on newer, less potent versions of the drugs. The contemporary efforts by the Commonwealth Fund to transfer the technology of serum treatments for pneumonia from the well-staffed, well-equipped environment of the university hospital to the rural practitioner's office met a similar fate, also analyzed in this chapter.

Cooperative investigations were revived, financially and intellectually, by the desire of medical researchers during World War II to gather large amounts of data about the effects of penicillin quickly and efficiently. Civilian supplies of penicillin, available in only limited quantities, were centrally allocated by the wartime Committee on Medical Research of the Office of Scientific Development and Research to researchers who agreed to follow a planned protocol for studying the drug. After the war, Veterans Administration researchers emulated these efforts in a series of centrally planned studies of streptomycin treatments for tuberculosis. These wartime and postwar initiatives are the subject of Chapter 4.

The bureaucracies of cooperative studies ultimately proved unable to discipline participating researchers into following a fixed protocol for selecting patients and measuring treatment effects. After the war, researchers turned to a new impersonal device for treatment evaluation – the randomized experiment – which reformers promoted as a means for controlling physicians' enthusiasm for new treatments. The statisticians who introduced randomization into medical research soon became the indispensable allies of therapeutic reformers.

In Chapter 5, I examine the intellectual and social alliance of statisticians with clinical researchers in the 1950s, while Chapters 6 and 7 examine the fate of two ambitious clinical trials of the 1960s: the Diet-Heart Study and the University Group Diabetes Program. The Diet-Heart study, a proposed ten-year investigation into the effects of lowering cholesterol on heart disease, ran headlong into the doubts of some researchers about the possibility of successfully altering diets, and the fears of others that the study would consume more than its fair share of the National Institutes of Health budget. The University Group Diabetes Program, a study of alternate treatments for adult-onset diabetes, was plunged into a decade-long controversy when investigators reported that patients receiving one of the drugs studied were dying of heart disease at higher rates than patients in the control group. The stories of these two studies illustrate the difficulties of getting physicians and laboratory researchers to believe in and support the randomized clinical trial.

It takes considerable *chutzpah* to undertake a history of therapeutic experimentation in the twentieth century. While historians have generally abandoned all pretenses to be comprehensive, in this case I am well aware of how much of the story remains unknown. The topic itself is immense and uncharted, and not an area of great professional interest to historians of science or the social history of medicine.[32]

Like the fourteenth-century European mariner, the best a historian of

---

32 As of 1990, the authors represented in two collections constituted a fairly comprehensive selection of historians interested in the history of clinical research in the United States for the present century: Rosenberg and Vogel, *The Therapeutic Revolution* (n. 4); Maulitz and Long, *Grand Rounds* (n. 11). More recent work shows signs of a welcome change in this direction. See Keith Wailoo, " 'A Disease *sui generis*': The Origins of Sickle Cell Anemia and the Emergence of Modern Clinical Research, 1904–1929," *BHM* 65 (Summer 1991), 185–209, and especially Marcia Lynn Meldrum, *Departures from the Design: The Randomized Clinical Trial in Historical Context, 1946–1970* (Ph.D. thesis, State University of New York at Stony Brook, 1994). I am grateful to Dr. Meldrum for making a copy of her thesis available to me.

twentieth-century medical research can manage is to know where the gaps and edges of his map lie. Fortunately, a decade's worth of historical scholarship has made it easier for me to identify the more obvious holes in my account. To begin with, this is not a history of the experimental subject, the patient, without whom there would be nothing for medical researchers (or historians) to write about. I have yet to encounter a source that would tell me much about patients, other than as researchers imagined them; even medical sociologists, who have somewhat more ready access to patients than historians, have not written much about the individual research subject.[33] Whether one can meaningfully write about professional order and therapeutic research without writing about the patient is a judgment I leave to readers.

Individual readers will no doubt have their own personal list of clinical domains and research studies that should have been discussed. My own list would include the program in cancer chemotherapy launched by the National Cancer Institute in the 1950s; the 1954 field trials of the Salk polio vaccine; and the developments in clinical trials for AIDS in the 1980s. Fortunately, Ilana Löwy and Steven Gary Epstein have begun writing about the first and last of these, respectively, while Marcia Meldrum and Sydney Halpern are working on the history of antipolio vaccines.[34] Despite their role in popularizing the notion of a controlled experiment, the 1954 field trials of polio vaccine arguably belong to the distinct tradition of public health trials of vaccines and antitoxins, the subject for yet another book.

History does not end conveniently for the historian, at the point at which his book concludes. Historians who choose to write about contemporary topics must bear the risk that future developments will reveal to all the fragility of their analyses of the past. In the 1980s and 1990s, clinical research was transformed by consumer activists seeking a greater say in the planning and conduct of clinical research. In response, some clinical investigators charged that activists were introducing politics into a realm where only science should prevail.

Like its historical predecessors, I will argue, the contemporary clinical trial should be understood as a social institution, intended to achieve the goal of therapeutic reformers: to see that physicians use the best possible therapies available. Whether clinical trials are the best (or only) instrument for achieving this goal is a political question, as is the question of how important we think this goal

33 On patients in clinical research, see Susan E. Lederer, *Subjected to Science: Human Experimentation in America before the Second World War* (Baltimore: Johns Hopkins University Press, 1995); Ann Oakley, "Who's Afraid of the Randomized Controlled Trial? Some Dilemmas of the Scientific Method and 'Good' Research Practice," *Women and Health* 15 (1989), 25–59.

34 Löwy, *Between Bench and Bedside* (n. 25); Steven Gary Epstein, *Impure Science: AIDS, Activism and the Politics of Knowledge* (Ph.D. thesis, University of California at Berkeley, 1993). On the Salk vaccine trials, see Paul Meier, "The Biggest Public Health Experiment Ever: The 1954 Field Trial of the Salk Polio Vaccine," in Judith M. Tanur, ed., *Statistics: A Guide to the Unknown* (San Francisco: Holden-Day, 1972), pp. 2–13. For a more detailed examination, see Meldrum, *Departures from the Design* (n. 32), pp. 45–172. Sydney Halpern examines the history of earlier vaccine trials in "Local Moralities in Medical Sciences," a paper presented at the American Association for the History of Medicine, May 1994, New York.

is.[35] Presumably, all of us would like our doctors to use the best possible means in caring for our ills. Therapeutic reformers have long argued that determining the value of medical treatments is a scientific question, best determined by experts "qualified by scientific training and experience to evaluate the effectiveness" of the treatment in question.[36] That experts – clinical investigators and statisticians – have a good deal of value to say about the means and ends of evaluating therapies is a claim I have no wish to challenge. That they alone should be the guardians of clinical care I have reasons to doubt. In the concluding chapter, I examine these contemporary controversies about the role of science and politics in clinical trials and drug regulation. But first, some history about the aims and means of therapeutic reform.

35 The general point was long ago made by the statistician Paul Meier and the lawyer Charles Fried, both of whom argued that the contemporary clinical trial presumes a prior political agreement about the social importance of obtaining reliable therapeutic knowledge. Paul Meier, "Statistics and Medical Experimentation," *Biometrics* 31 (June 1975), 525–527; Charles Fried, *Medical Experimentation: Personal Integrity and Social Policy* (New York: American Elsevier, 1974). I read Professor Fried's book in the mid-1980s, when this project was well underway; had I read his prescient analysis any earlier, I might never have undertaken the project.
36 The language is that of the FDA's regulations for new drug testing. *Code of Federal Regulations,* Title 21, chap. 1, 130.4b (1967).

PART I

Of institutions and character:
The era of organizational reform

1

A rational therapeutics

On August 15, 1922, Elizabeth Hughes arrived at the Toronto clinic of Fred Banting. A fourteen-year-old diabetic being treated with a starvation diet of 900 calories, Hughes had been losing weight steadily all spring. On arrival, she weighed forty-five pounds and had all the signs of terminal diabetes: "hair brittle and thin, abdomen prominent, shoulders drooped, muscles extremely wasted, subcutaneous tissues almost completely absorbed. She was scarcely able to walk on account of weakness." Banting immediately began treatment with an experimental drug. Within two weeks, she was able to tolerate a normal diet and, by November, she returned home to resume a normal life. Elizabeth Hughes died on April 15, 1981, at the age of seventy-three.[1]

Banting's experimental drug was insulin, the means for rescuing thousands of diabetics from almost certain death. Along with diphtheria antitoxin, insulin was arguably the most successful accomplishment of what historian Charles Rosenberg has termed a "therapeutic revolution": the introduction of a seemingly interminable series of potent therapeutic agents.[2] From the antipyretic chemical compounds of the 1880s, to the serums and vaccines of the 1890s and early 1900s, and the purified hormones of the 1920s and 1930s, physicians encountered an increasing number and variety of innovative treatments. Diphtheria antitoxin aside, few of these products were as effective as Banting and Best's insulin and few recoveries as dramatic as Elizabeth Hughes's resurrection. Physicians glancing backward from the late twentieth century regard these decades as a therapeutic dark ages, in which their predecessors were helpless, if no longer so ignorant. But however

1 The account of Hughes's condition, and that of other diabetics treated with Banting and Best's wonder drug, comes from Michael Bliss, *The Discovery of Insulin* (Chicago: University of Chicago Press, 1982), pp. 144, 151–165, 244.
2 Charles Rosenberg, "The Therapeutic Revolution: Medicine, Meaning and Social Change in Nineteenth Century America," in Morris J. Vogel and Charles E. Rosenberg, eds., *The Therapeutic Revolution: Essays in the Social History of American Medicine* (Philadelphia: University of Pennsylvania Press, 1979), pp. 3–25. On the complexities of evaluating insulin's impact, see James Wright Presley, *A History of Diabetes Mellitus in the United States, 1880–1990*. (Ph.D. thesis, University of Texas at Austin, 1991), pp. 288–308. Prior to insulin, diphtheria antitoxin represented both the symbol and substance of the therapeutic revolution. See Evelyn Maxine Hammonds, *The Search for Perfect Control: A Social History of Diphtheria, 1880–1930* (Ph.D. thesis, Harvard University, 1993).

puny and inconsequential their weapons seem in retrospect, contemporary physicians found themselves armed for the first time with the means to treat even terminally ill patients with success.[3]

The new therapeutics was a product of two institutions: the laboratory and the market. Many physicians readily recognized the laboratory's contribution, material vindication of medicine's growing faith in laboratory science. Each new class of treatments saw first life in a laboratory. Antipyretics were engineered in the chemical laboratories of German pharmaceutical firms. Serums and vaccines were manufactured in the bacteriological laboratories of European research institutes and United States public health departments. Animal extracts such as insulin were devised in the university laboratories of Canada, Britain, and the United States.[4] But regardless of where each product was first conceived, drug firms controlled its manufacturing and promotion, fashioning its attributes once in the factory and then again in the market.[5]

3 For a useful overview of therapeutic practices and advances for infectious diseases in the present century, see Harry Dowling, *Fighting Infection: Conquests of the Twentieth Century* (Cambridge: Harvard University Press, 1977). For two perspectives on these "advances" from the 1970s, see Lewis Thomas, *The Youngest Science: Notes of a Medicine Watcher* (New York: Viking Press, 1983), pp. 12–18, 40–43, and Paul Beeson, "Changes in Medical Therapy during the Past Half Century," *Medicine* 59 (1980), 79–99.

4 For a quick sketch of the new antipyretics, see Charles C. Mann and Mark L. Plummer, *The Aspirin Wars: Money, Medicine, and 100 Years of Rampant Competition* (New York: Alfred A. Knopf, 1991), pp. 21–28, and, on their use in practice (alongside older fever treatments), see John Harley Warner, *The Therapeutic Perspective: Medical Practice, Knowledge, and Identity in America, 1820–1885* (Cambridge: Harvard University Press, 1986), pp. 101, 157, 269.

  On serums and vaccines, generally, see Dowling, *Fighting Infection* (n. 3), pp. 22–54. On the production and use of diphtheria antitoxin, see David Blancher, *Workshops of the Bacteriological Revolution: A History of the Laboratories of the New York City Department of Health, 1892–1912* (Ph.D. thesis, City University of New York, 1979), pp. 107–110, 112–118, 206–208, 212–217; Barbara Gutmann Rosenkrantz, *Public Health and the State: Changing Views in Massachusetts, 1842–1936* (Cambridge: Harvard University Press, 1972), pp. 112–127; Edward T. Morman, *Scientific Medicine Comes to Philadelphia: Public Health Transformed* (Ph.D. thesis, University of Pennsylvania, 1986), pp. 159–163, 168–169, 171–172, 222–227; Jonathan M. Liebenau, "Public Health and the Production and Use of Diphtheria Antitoxin in Philadelphia," *BHM* 61 (1987), 216–236; Hammonds, *The Search for Perfect Control* (n. 2).

  On insulin, see Bliss, *Discovery of Insulin* (n. 1); Jonathan Liebenau, "The MRC and the Pharmaceutical Industry: The Model of Insulin," in Joan Austoker and Linda Bryder, eds., *Historical Perspectives on the Role of the MRC: Essays on the History of the Medical Research Council of the United Kingdom* (Oxford: Oxford University Press, 1989), pp. 163–180; John Patrick Swann, *Academic Scientists and the Pharmaceutical Industry: Cooperative Research in Twentieth-Century America* (Baltimore: Johns Hopkins University Press, 1988), pp. 122–149.

5 Recent historiography has emphasized the links between academic scientists and corporate researchers in drug development. See Timothy Lenoir, "A Magic Bullet: Research for Profit and the Growth of Knowledge in Germany around 1900," *Minerva* 26 (Spring 1988), 66–88; Jonathan Liebenau, *Medical Science and Medical Industry: The Formation of the American Pharmaceutical Industry* (Baltimore: Johns Hopkins University Press, 1987); idem, "The MRC and the Pharmaceutical Industry" (n. 4), pp. 163–180; idem, "Paul Ehrlich As a Commercial Scientist and Research Administrator," *Medical History* 34 (1990), 65–78; Swann, *Academic Scientists* (n. 4). On the development of the modern drug industry, see Mann and Plummer, *The Aspirin Wars* (n. 4); Louis Galambos with Jane Eliot Sewell, *Networks of Innovation: Vaccine Development at Merck, Sharpe & Dohme, and Mulford, 1895–1995* (Cambridge: Cambridge University Press, 1995).

From the eighteenth century on, the drug trade had not lacked for manufactured products. Firms produced proprietary versions of the traditional materia medica as well as the elixirs and pills of medicine-show fame. In the last decades of the nineteenth century, so-called proprietary compounds appropriated an increasing share of the U.S. drug market, from 28 percent of all drugs produced in 1880 to a high of 72 percent in 1900.[6] Like the nostrums traditionally marketed by patent medicine manufacturers, the composition of such compounds was kept secret. Some consisted principally of colored water, others contained large quantities of alcohol or codeine, while yet others concealed ingenious combinations of the new chemical compounds manufactured in Germany. In marketing, such distinctions were readily erased. Firms promoted the inert product as vigorously as the one with active ingredients; they invoked laboratory science in promotions to lay audiences and physician consumers alike.[7]

In discussing therapeutic reform at the turn of this century, historians have followed the lead of contemporary reformers in emphasizing the excesses of drug advertising aimed at lay audiences. The drug industry pioneered in relying heavily on newspapers and the nascent advertising trade to promote its wares. Coincident with the development of national marketing of consumer goods, drug advertisers sought to bypass the physician as a source of therapeutic information and authority. The colorful images and accompanying puffery used in these promotions have attracted considerable scholarly attention.[8] Yet the same techniques were increasingly aimed at physicians as well. Among therapeutic reformers, the gullible

6 On the early drug trade and its connections with commercial culture, see Roy Porter, "The Language of Quackery in England, 1660–1800," in Peter Burke and Roy Porter, eds., *The Social History of Language* (Cambridge: Cambridge University Press, 1987), pp. 73–103. On the nineteenth-century trade, see James Harvey Young, "Patent Medicines: An Element in Southern Distinctiveness?," in Todd L. Savitt and James Harvey Young, eds., *Disease and Distinctiveness in the American South* (Knoxville: University of Tennessee Press, 1988), pp. 154–193; James Harvey Young, *The Medical Messiahs: A Social History of Health Quackery in Twentieth-Century America* (Princeton: Princeton University Press, 1967), pp. 13–29. Value of drug products sold taken from U.S. Census Office, *Report on the Manufactures of the United States* . . . (Washington, DC: Government Printing Office, 1882), pp. 34, 63; idem, *Manufactures* (Washington, DC: Government Printing Office, 1902), part I, pp. 180–191, 340–341.

7 Young, *Medical Messiahs* (n. 6), pp. 5–6, 26–27; Jan R. McTavish, "Aspirin in Germany: The Pharmaceutical Industry and the Pharmaceutical Profession," *Pharmacy in History* 29 (1987), 103–115; idem, "What's in a Name? Aspirin and the American Medical Association," *BHM* 61 (1987), 353–354; Rima D. Apple, " 'To Be Used Only under the Direction of a Physician': Commercial Infant Feeding and Medical Practice, 1870–1940," *BHM* 54 (1980), 402–417; idem, " 'Advertised by Our Loving Friends': The Infant Formula Industry and the Creation of New Pharmaceutical Markets," *JHM* 41 (1986), 3–23; J. Worth Estes, "Public Pharmacology: Modes of Action of Nineteenth-Century 'Patent' Medicines," *Medical Heritage* 2 (1986), 218–228; Robert Hessler, "A Study of Reprints and Clinical Reports on Proprietary Medicines," *American Medicine* 9 (June 10, 1905), 951–954.

8 On the links between advertising and patent medicines, see Sidney A. Sherman, "Advertising in the United States," *Quarterly Publications of the American Statistical Association* 7 (December 1900), 135–136, insert; Daniel Pope, *The Making of Modern Advertising* (New York: Basic Books, 1983), pp. 37, 42–45; Young, *Medical Messiahs* (n. 6), pp. 21–23. On the links to national marketing, see Pope, *Making of Modern Advertising,* and Susan Strasser, *Satisfaction Guaranteed: The Making of the American Mass Market* (New York: Pantheon Books, 1989).

physician soon vied with the ignorant layman as a symbol of the corrupt state of therapeutics.[9]

Over the course of the nineteenth century, medical educators and researchers had engaged in a series of efforts at therapeutic reform, which earned for them the epithet of "therapeutic nihilists."[10] By the early twentieth century, the medical profession's scientific leadership faced a novel intellectual and political problem: how best to harvest the riches of the laboratory while protecting medicine from the incursions of the market? Whereas earlier generations of therapeutic reformers had sought to dampen unwarranted enthusiasm for useless nostrums and ineffective treatments, the new generation had the difficult task of ensuring that only effective drugs were chosen from the diverse repertoire of products being touted. In their quest for effective drugs, reformers also sought to ensure that physicians would use drugs effectively and appropriately, which meant purging professional therapeutics of commercial influences.[11] For these tasks, the radical therapeutic

The historical literature on therapeutic reform similarly stresses attacks on the promotion of drugs to lay audiences. See David L. Dykstra, "The Medical Profession and Patent and Proprietary Medicines during the Nineteenth Century," *BHM* 29 (1955), 401–419; Peter Temin, *Taking Your Medicine: Drug Regulation in the United States* (Cambridge: Harvard University Press, 1980), pp. 30–31. But cf. Young, *Medical Messiahs* (n. 6), p. 26, who notes the increasing use of promotions targeted at physicians.

9 William J. Robinson, "The Composition of Some So-called Ethical Synthetics and 'Ethical' Nostrums," *JAMA* 41 (April 16, 1904), 1016–1017; Julius Noer, "Practical Medicinal Therapeutics As It Appears from the Prescription File," *Wisconsin Medical Journal* 3 (1904), 274–275; E. L. Boothby, "Regarding the Lack of Progress in Scientific Therapeutics," *Wisconsin Medical Journal* 3 (1904), 270; H. W. Wiley, "The Ethics of Pharmacy," *JAMA* 45 (July 15, 1905), 182; N. S. Davis, "Effect of Proprietary Literature on Medical Men," *JAMA* 46 (May 5, 1906), 1339; Reid Hunt, "What the Individual Physician Can Do to Improve the Materia Medica," *JAMA* 53 (August 14, 1909), 497–499; Charles Wallis Edmunds, "Therapeutic Progress," *JAMA* 52 (February 13, 1909), 522; R. A. Hatcher, "The Sufficiency of Standard Remedies for Therapeutic Needs," *New York State Journal of Medicine* 9 (August 1909), 312; George Blumer, "The Need of Reorganization in the Methods and Teaching of Therapeutics," *BMSJ* 169 (1913), 261–266.

10 For discussions of organized efforts to evaluate drugs prior to the nineteenth century, see Matthew Ramsey, "Traditional Medicine and Medical Enlightenment: The Regulation of Secret Remedies in the Ancien Regime," *Historical Reflections/Réflexions historiques* 9 (Spring–Summer 1982), 216–232; M. Bouvet, "Sur l'essai des médicaments en France avant 1789," *Revue d'histoire de la pharmacie* 149 (June 1956), 305–326. I am indebted to Matt Ramsey for calling my attention to Bouvet's article.

For a general introduction to the views of early nineteenth-century therapeutic reformers in the United States, and some examples of their work on specific therapies, see James H. Cassedy, *American Medicine and Statistical Thinking, 1800–1860* (Cambridge: Harvard University Press, 1984), pp. 60–91, esp. 73–77. For a fuller account, which explores the political dilemmas faced by therapeutic "skeptics," see John Harley Warner, " 'The Nature-Trusting Heresy': American Physicians and the Concept of the Healing Power of Nature," *Perspectives in American History* 11 (1977–1978), 291–324; and idem, "The Selective Transport of Medical Knowledge: Antebellum American Physicians and Parisian Medical Therapeutics," *BHM* 59 (Summer 1985), 213–231. For an account that implicitly minimizes the differences between mid-nineteenth-century reformers and later generations, see Martin S. Pernick, *A Calculus of Suffering: Pain, Professionalism and Anesthesia in Nineteenth-Century America* (New York: Columbia University Press, 1985), esp. pp. 21–31, 93–124.

11 C. Skinner, "Proprietary Medicines," *Louisville Monthly Journal of Medicine and Surgery* 9 (1902–1903), 291–292; Noer, "Practical Medicinal Therapeutics" (n. 9), 274–277; Horatio C. Wood Jr.,

skepticism of an earlier era was deemed unsuitable: "an overskeptical mind is as undesired as an overcredulous one."[12] Circumstances called for a new attitude to replace the purported "therapeutic nihilism" of early nineteenth-century skeptics: "rational therapeutics."

The intellectual program for a rational therapeutics originated in the late 1860s and 1870s among medical school professors inspired by the internationally renowned physiologist Claude Bernard. As John Harley Warner has written, men such as Horatio Wood, professor of materia medica and pharmacology at the University of Pennsylvania, and Roberts Bartholow, professor of materia medica and therapeutics at Jefferson Medical College, gathered under the banner of "physiological therapeutics" to insist that the laboratory study of drug action was the engine of future therapeutic progress. Initially one among several reform currents, the movement for an experimentally based therapeutics was reinforced by the late nineteenth-century achievements of laboratory science, and by the increasing influence of German laboratory medicine on American medical educators.[13] By 1900, a younger generation imbued with these ideals had absorbed "physiological therapeutics" into their own campaign for therapeutic reform.[14]

In the opening decades of the present century the notion of a rational therapeutics referred first to the use of therapeutic agents whose mechanisms of action were scientifically established prior to their introduction into clinical practice. A rational, as opposed to an empirical remedy, was one whose effects were demonstrable in the laboratory and ideally one that acted on the cause, not the symptoms, of disease. Where no specific cure existed, however, symptomatic treatment was

"Proprietary Therapeutics," *Columbus Medical Journal* 29 (1905), 328–334; Hunt, "What the Individual Physician Can Do" (n. 9), 497–502; George H. Simmons, "Proprietary Medicines: Some General Considerations," *JAMA* 46 (May 5, 1906), 1333–1337; M. L. Stevens, "The Physician and the Manufacturer of Pharmaceutical Preparations: Ethics of Their Relation," *Charlotte Medical Journal* 17 (1900), 15–21; H. Bert Ellis, "Necessity for a National Bureau of Medicines and Foods," and T. D. Davis, "Discussion," both in *Bulletin of the American Academy of Medicine* 6 (December 1903), 486–494 and 495–496.

12 James P. Herrick, "The Relation of the Association to Therapeutics," *Transactions of the Association of American Physicians* 38 (1923), 5. See also Boothby, "Regarding the Lack of Progress in Scientific Therapeutics" (n. 9), 266–272; Lewellys F. Barker, "On the Present Status of Therapy and Its Future," *Bulletin of the Johns Hopkins Hospital* 11 (July–August 1900), 149–155; Morris Fishbein, "Scientific Therapy and Pharmaceutic Research," *JAMA* 84 (May 16, 1925), 1518.

13 Warner, *Therapeutic Perspective* (n. 4), pp. 235–257; John Harley Warner, "Ideals of Science and Their Discontents in Late Nineteenth-Century American Medicine," *Isis* 82 (1991), 454–478. As Warner notes (459), the laboratory deserved and received credit for the introduction of antipyrine and chloral hydrate prior to the 1890s development of diphtheria antitoxin.

    Interestingly, by 1910 Wood himself thought the pendulum had swung too far in the laboratory's direction, and was deriding the laboratory pharmacologist who lacked clinical experience. See H. C. Wood, "Reflections upon the Teaching of Therapeutics, Based upon Forty Years Experience," *Transactions of the College of Physicians of Philadelphia* 33 (1911), esp. 103–110.

14 Among the other late nineteenth-century currents for reform discussed by Warner, both hygienic therapeutics (which stressed rest and diet over drugs) and preventive medicine were alive and flourishing in the early twentieth century. See Barker, "On the Present Status of Therapy" (n. 12), 154; Blumer, "Need for Reorganization" (n. 9), 264–265. It would be useful to have a more systematic account of nondrug therapeutics in this period.

accepted as "rational," provided researchers were able to demonstrate and justify symptomatic relief.[15]

At the same time, rational therapeutics referred to the conduct of clinical practice. In rational practice, the dosage and uses of a drug were in accordance with what was known about its pharmacological activity and effects. It made no sense to use even an effective drug at doses that were subtherapeutic or in clinical circumstances where it could not possibly benefit the patient.[16]

Reformers accordingly pursued two related goals in the name of rational therapeutics. On the one hand, they sought to control the introduction and promotion of new drugs. On the other, they attempted to foster a scientific and critical attitude toward therapeutics in the medical profession itself. The two reforms were interdependent. Restricting the number of drugs to a handful of proven remedies would lessen practitioners' confusion and thereby contribute to more "rational" therapeutic practice. At the same time, successful efforts to reform the industry depended upon the support of a reformed profession, one capable of recognizing the merits of using only carefully screened products.

The intellectual program for a rational therapeutics was widely shared among clinical scientists, medical educators and those they inspired.[17] The program took specific institutional form in the American Medical Association's (AMA) Council on Pharmacy and Chemistry. Established by the AMA's Board of Trustees in 1905,

---

15 See Henry Hurd, "Laboratories and Hospital Work," *Bulletin of the American Academy of Medicine* 2 (August 1896), 485–490; Solomon Solis-Cohen, "Progress in Therapeutics," *Procceedings of the Philadelphia Country Medical Society* 21 (March 1900), 119–120; A. Jacobi, "Phases in the Development of Therapy," *Yale Medical Journal* 41 (1905–1906), 490–492; Richard C. Cabot, "Therapeutics Based on Pathological Physiology," *BMSJ* 155 (July 19, 1906), 57–59; S. J. Meltzer, "The Present Status of Therapeutics and the Significance of Salvarsan," *JAMA* 56 (June 10, 1911), 1709–1711. On "rational" symptomatic treatment, see Solis-Cohen, 123; Joseph I. Miller, "The Value of Symptomatic Treatment," *Transactions of the Association of American Physicians* 30 (1915), 516–518; J. H. Means and A. L. Barach, "The Symptomatic Treatment of Pneumonia," *JAMA* 77 (October 15, 1921), 1217. For a useful case study of a drug neglected due to rational therapeutics, see James S. Goodwin and Jean M. Goodwin, "Failure to Recognize Efficacious Treatments: A History of Salicylate Therapy in Rheumatoid Arthritis," *Perspectives in Biology and Medicine* 25 (Autumn 1981), 78–92.

16 Both aspects are clearly identified in N. S. Davis, "Need of Much More Accurate Knowledge concerning Both the Immediate and Remote Effects of the Remedial Agents in General Use . . .," *JAMA* 38 (May 31, 1902), 1415–1416; Solis-Cohen, "Progress in Therapeutics" (n. 15), 118–123; Robert A. Hatcher, "The Duty of the Medical Profession toward the Council on Pharmacy and Chemistry," *JAMA* 67 (November 14, 1916), 1340; Jacob Diner, "Rational Drug Therapy," *JAMA* 72 (January 25, 1919), 264–265; L. G. Rowntree, "The Role and Development of Drug Therapy," *JAMA* 77 (October 1, 1921), 1061–1065; Harry Gold, "Recent Advances in Drug Therapy," *International Clinics* (December 1930), 89–90; and Theodore Koppanyi, "Applied Pharmacodynamics: Rational Therapeutics," *Medical Annals of the District of Columbia* 4 (May 1935), 127–132. Pharmacologically oriented writers were somewhat more inclined to stress the importance of understanding a drug's metabolic fate; some reformers were skeptical that the average practitioner could or would acquire "a full scientific appreciation of the mode of [a] drug's action." Fishbein, "Scientific Therapy and Pharmaceutic Research" (n. 12), 1519.

17 See, in addition to the sources cited in notes 15 and 16, E. A. Landman, "Rational Medical Treatment," *Transactions of the New Hampshire Medical Society* (1911), 171–188; George M. Dock, "The Movement for Exact Treatment," *Journal of the Iowa State Medical Society* 2 (August 15, 1912), 91–94; Blumer, "Need of Reorganization" (n. 9), 261–63.

the council assumed the task of ensuring that the therapeutic potential of new laboratory products would be realized at the bedside. The remainder of this chapter describes the council's efforts in the early decades of the century to inculcate a critical attitude among practicing physicians toward the use of new drugs.

REFORMING THE PROFESSION

From the AMA's founding in 1847, its leaders had been interested in therapeutic reform. The promotion of patent medicines, the appropriate use of therapeutic innovations, and the elimination of so-called sectarian schools of therapeutics, such as homeopathy, were all objects of AMA concern. Yet the fledgling organization lacked both the political resources and the cultural authority to direct therapeutic practices in a divided profession. A regional organization heavily weighted toward academic and hospital physicians, the AMA had limited influence outside the urban northeast. To steer clear of divisions of opinion within its own membership, the AMA refrained from taking an official position on the merits of nineteenth-century innovations such as anesthesia. Although proposals for reforming therapeutics surfaced periodically during the remainder of the century, it was not until the first decade of the twentieth century that the organization began to act.[18]

Physician and medical journalist George H. Simmons came to the AMA in 1899 from Lincoln, Nebraska, where he was secretary of the State Medical Society and editor of the *Western Medical Review*. As secretary to the AMA's Board of Trustees, Simmons aided President Charles McCormack in reinventing the AMA as a mass-based organization, where his dual role as editor of the *Journal of the American Medical Association* (*JAMA*) and general manager of the reorganized AMA gave him considerable influence with its leadership.[19]

Along with other reformers, Simmons thought that the evaluation of new medical products was properly a job for the federal government. According to James Burrow, when "efforts to secure federal control failed," Simmons and others

18 On the social bases of the nineteenth-century AMA, and its subsequent reorganization, see William G. Rothstein, *American Physicians in the Nineteenth Century: From Sects to Science* (Baltimore: Johns Hopkins University Press, 1972), pp. 212, 316–320; James G. Burrow, *Organized Medicine in the Progressive Era: The Move toward Monopoly* (Baltimore: Johns Hopkins University Press, 1977), pp. 15–28. For accounts of the AMA's nineteenth-century activities in therapeutics, see Paul Starr, *The Social Transformation of American Medicine* (New York: Basic Books, 1982), pp. 127–129 and Pernick, *A Calculus of Suffering* (n. 10), pp. 26–29, 41, 69–70. Both scholars agree that the AMA failed to do much about regulating therapeutics before the twentieth century, but Starr places slightly greater emphasis on the AMA's inability to command the necessary political resources to enforce their views on the profession as a whole and society at large, while Pernick emphasizes divisions of opinion within the organization that led to a lack of political will.

19 On Simmons's career and role in the reorganization, see Morris H. Fishbein, "George Henry Simmons, 1852–1937," *Proceedings of the Institute of Medicine of Chicago* 11 (November 15, 1937), 397–401; on the role of previous JAMA editors, see Elizabeth Knoll, "The American Medical Association and Its Journal," in W. F. Bynum, Stephen Lock, and Roy Porter, eds., *Medical Journals and Medical Knowledge: Historical Essays* (New York: Routledge, 1992), esp. pp. 146–159.

suggested that the AMA create a body, subsidized by manufacturers' fees, to analyze the quality and composition of new drugs. As *JAMA*'s editor, Simmons had sought an independent basis for judging the therapeutic claims published by the journal's advertisers. After an initial rejection by the AMA's House of Delegates, the proposal to create a Council on Pharmacy and Chemistry was approved by a vote of the Board of Trustees on February 3, 1905.[20]

As a creation of the Board of Trustees, the newly established council represented the views of the profession's national leadership, heavily weighted toward specialists and medical educators, rather than the local practitioners whose base was in the AMA's newly organized House of Delegates.[21] Composed of individuals selected for their interest and eminence in pharmacological research, the new council placed its greatest emphasis on regulating drugs and drug promotions. Of ten initial members, seven (Arthur Cushny, M.D.; Lewis Diehl, Ph.M.; C. S. N. Hallberg, M.D., Ph.G.; Robert A. Hatcher, M.D., Ph.G.; W. A. Puckner, Ph.G.; J. O. Schlotterbeck, Ph.G., Ph.D.; and Torald Sollman, M.D.) were professors of pharmacology, pharmacy, or chemistry, while two (Lyman F. Kebler, Ph.G, M.S., M.D., and M. I. Wilbert, Ph.M) worked in government laboratories responsible for the evaluation of vaccines and drugs. (Simmons, *JAMA*'s editor, was the tenth.) In a era when influence in the medical community was still measured first by local, and then by national reputation, the council's composition placed it at a disadvantage. Although six of the ten held medical degrees, none was regarded as engaged in the practice of medicine, and only George Simmons was widely known in the profession.[22]

20 On the decision to create the council, see James G. Burrow, "The Prescription-Drug Policies of the American Medical Association in the Progressive Era," in John Blake, ed., *Safeguarding the Public: Historical Aspects of Medicinal Drug Control* (Baltimore: Johns Hopkins University Press, 1970), pp. 112–122. For discussions of a federal role, see F. E. Stewart, "Proposed National Bureau of Materia Medica," *JAMA* 35 (April 21, 1901), 1175–1178; Ellis, "Necessity for a National Bureau" (n. 11), 490–491; Victor C. Vaughan, "Discussion," and T. D. Davis, "Discussion," both in *Bulletin of the American Academy of Medicine* 6 (December 1903), 495 and 495–496. For Simmons's views on the government's responsibilities, see George H. Simmons to Surgeon General Walter H. Wyman, January 20, 1906, Public Health Service, General Files 1900–1923, Record Group 90, Box 456, NA. It appears as if Simmons sought over a number of years to enlist manufacturing support for this enterprise, independently of any efforts to "secure federal support": see Prof. Simmons to Prof. Remington, December 8, 1904, Box 51, John Jacob Abel papers, Chesney Archives. See also "Report of the Council on Pharmacy and Chemistry," *JAMA* 46 (March 24, 1906), 896–897.
21 On the structure and leadership of the AMA, see Starr, *Social Transformation* (n. 18), pp. 109–110; William H. Rothstein, *American Medical Schools and the Practice of Medicine: A History* (New York: Oxford University Press, 1987), pp. 107–108. Burrow, "The Prescription-Drug Policies of the AMA" (n. 20), is far and away the best treatment of the early council. For additional information, see J. H. Long, "On the Work of the Council on Pharmacy and Chemistry of the American Medical Association," *Science* 32 (December 23, 1910), 889–901; Austin Smith, "The Council on Pharmacy and Chemistry and the Chemical Laboratory," in Morris Fishbein, ed., *A History of the American Medical Association, 1847 to 1947* (Philadelphia: W. B. Saunders, 1947), pp. 865–886, and Harry Dowling, *Medicines for Man: The Development, Regulation and Use of Prescription Drugs* (New York: Alfred A. Knopf, 1970), pp. 155–185.
22 Kebler and Wilbert worked for the Department of Agriculture and the U.S. Hygienic Laboratory, respectively. These men were soon joined by Samuel Sadtler (Ph.D), J. H. Long (M.S., Sc.D.),

To compensate for its lack of reputation, Simmons provided the council with access to the pages of *JAMA*. There a regular column, aptly named "The Propaganda for Reform," provided "intelligent physicians" with an "unprejudiced examination" of information concerning items "worthy of [their] patronage." Any manufacturer seeking recognition of his product by the council, and thereby the profession, was required to make its composition known, to justify the therapeutic claims made on its behalf, and to avoid exaggerated or misleading advertising. Justly deserving products were accorded recognition in an annual compilation issued by the council, *New and Nonofficial Remedies*.[23]

Like many other Progressive-era reforms, the council's program was an attempt to moderate the excesses of capitalism: "Honest advertising is a necessary feature of civilization – at least it is not an unmitigated evil. Fraudulent advertisements are one of the curses of civilization."[24] Understandably, in the views of council members, drug manufacturers sought to make money. But however appropriate in other walks of life, in therapeutics the profit motive exercised a baneful influence:

> There is a good deal of difference between the introduction of new products to science and new brands of manufacture to commerce. The former belongs the sphere of science and the latter to the sphere of commerce. . . . The exploitation of new products by exaggerating their merits and repressing knowledge of failures is one of the most dangerous forms of quackery.[25]

Unchecked, commercialism threatened to undermine the scientific basis for a "rational therapeutics," "debauching our medical journals" and "tainting our textbooks."[26] The council's efforts were a means for science to fight back.

Although Simmons took the lead in organizing the council, its acknowledged leader over the next four decades was Torald Sollman, professor of pharmacology at Western Reserve University, and author of the first American textbook on the

Julius Stieglitz (Ph.D), F. G. Novy (M.D., Sc.D.), and Harvey W. Wiley (M.D., Ph.D.). Sadtler, Long, and Stieglitz were professors of chemistry; Novy was professor of bacteriology; and Wiley, physician and chemist, was head of the Bureau of Chemistry in the U.S. Department of Agriculture, responsible for administering the 1906 Pure Food and Drug Act. Within the academic community, Novy, Sollman, and Stieglitz were almost certainly well known, and Cushny's reputation was international. What any of these names might mean to the practitioner in Louisville, Kentucky, is, however, another matter. For a partial list of early membership, see Smith, "The Council" (n. 22), pp. 866–869, from which the preceding biographical information is taken.

23 For a list of the council's initial criteria, see Council on Pharmacy and Chemistry, "Preliminary Announcement," *JAMA* 44 (March 4, 1905), 720–721. The first edition of *New and Nonofficial Remedies* was in 1907.

24 Torald Sollman, *The Broader Aims of the Council on Pharmacy of the American Medical Association* (Chicago: AMA, 1908), p. 21.

25 F. E. Stewart, "Proposed National Bureau of Materia Medica," *JAMA* (April 27, 1901), 1177. See also Brace W. Loomis, "Therapeutics and the Drug Manufacturer," *BMSJ* 146 (May 8, 1902), 486–487; Simmons, "Proprietary Medicines" (n. 11).

26 George H. Simmons, "The Commercial Domination of Therapeutics and the Movement for Reform," *JAMA* 48 (May 18, 1907), 1645. Wood, "Proprietary Therapeutics" (n. 11), 333–334, and Blumer, "The Need of Reorganization" (n. 9), 262–264, express similar concerns about the effects of commercialism on the medical literature.

new, laboratory-based, pharmacology.[27] Led by Sollman, the pharmacologists on the council took as their initial targets the manufacturers of "secret" remedies: variations on standard compounds whose uselessness (or potential toxicity) was concealed behind names invoking occult powers (Bioplasm) or suggesting safe narcotics (Sal-codeia).[28] Forcing manufacturers to reveal the contents of these drugs would enable physicians to discard redundant or impotent drugs. But the truth-telling principle applied equally to medicines "that have merit and that would be used even if the simple unvarnished truth were told about them." For Sollman and the other council members, the campaign against secret remedies was merely "preliminary to a larger and broader aim, the general reformation of what is debased and debasing in the present status of therapy."[29]

For the products with which the AMA council was concerned, the physician was the ultimate consumer. A rational therapeutics required not only a scientific assessment of the accomplishments and limitations of specific drugs, but practitioners capable of recognizing and acknowledging those limitations in their practice. Even the carefully screened compounds appearing in the official pharmacopeias did not "constitute an advance" when "used as uncritically, with the same exaggerated expectations, as are the proprietary articles."[30]

The council benefited from the support of "the better element of the medical profession," which endorsed its program. But the council's authority with manufacturers rested with its ability to reshape the attitudes of the profession at large. The reformers' program of publicity made sense only if the medical public acted on the information provided:

In whatever way we look at it, the responsibility always returns to the individual physician – he is the man who carries the arms. It comes to him not so much on the day when he votes for a resolution, but every day, every time when he writes a prescription. Whenever he picks up a prescription blank, he is not only directing the treatment of his patient; he is also directing the proprietary business, in all its ramifications; and beyond this, he is directing the future of therapeutics. With each prescription, he renders a decision whether truth or falsehood shall prevail; whether therapeutics shall be scientific or unscientific; whether the abuse of indiscriminate self-medication shall continue or not.[31]

---

27 On Sollman's career, see Torald Sollman, "Why An Annual Review of Pharmacology?," *Annual Review of Pharmacology* 1 (1961), 3–6. I owe this reference to John Parascandola. Sollman was not formally chairman of the council until 1936, however. "Torald Sollman, MD, Dies," *JAMA* 191 (March 1, 1965), 38.

28 "The Secret Nostrum vs. the Ethical Proprietary," *JAMA* 44 (March 4, 1904), 718–721. On the ingenuity of cure peddlers in naming their products, see Young, *Medical Messiahs* (n. 6).

29 Sollman, *Broader Aims of the Council* (n. 24), p. 3. See also the discussion by Julius Stieglitz of chemical compounds that were potentially worthwhile, but for which exaggerated therapeutic claims were made and whose quality varied from lot to lot and manufacturer to manufacturer. "The Problem of the Synthetic Chemical Compound," *JAMA* 46 (May 5, 1906), 1341–1342.

30 Sollman, *Broader Aims of the Council* (n. 24), p. 33.

31 Ibid., p. 46. See also David L. Edsall, "The Work of the Council on Pharmacy and Chemistry," *JAMA* 55 (November 12, 1910), 701; Augustus A. Eschner, "The Objection to Prescribing Medicines of Unknown Composition," *JAMA* 40 (May 2, 1903), 1189; Charles Wallis Edmunds, "Therapeutic Progress," *JAMA* 52 (February 13, 1909), 523.

As with other AMA-sponsored reforms, in physician licensure and medical education, new legislation abetted the movement for a rational therapeutics. Harvey Wiley, the crusading chief of the federal Bureau of Chemistry, responsible for administering the Pure Food and Drug Act of 1906, and John Anderson and George McCoy, responsible for testing vaccines and serums under the federal Biologics Control Act of 1902, held seats on the council and worked closely with it.[32] Likewise, the council accepted the support of the consumer movement in its efforts to chasten industry, and welcomed the cooperation of progressive drug firms.[33] But the council's program depended less on legislative and institutional remedies than on the moral conversion of the individual physician.[34] As council members put it, the physician who benefited from the enhanced status of medicine had an obligation to exercise his new powers responsibly and intelligently.[35]

Ultimately, it was the medical profession and not the pharmaceutical trade that the reformers found lacking: "We cannot blame manufacturing chemists for finding new things or advertising them as cleverly as possible. That they and the nostrum vendor are surprisingly successful in selling their wares is largely our fault."[36] If physicians were equipped to make competent judgments on the merits of new drugs, the desire of each manufacturer to produce and sell its own unique compounds would present few problems: "Unfortunately, however, the physician's training is likely to be such that he can not distinguish the rank fraud from the efficacious remedy, honestly made and sold."[37]

At the time the council was formed, the teaching of therapeutics was nearly as dismal as its practice. Only a handful of schools provided instruction beyond *materia medica*, the learning by rote of a repertoire of medications and their uses.

32 See Smith, "The Council" (n. 21), pp. 868–869. On the Bureau of Biologics, see Ramunas Kondratas, "The Biologics Control Act of 1902," in James Harvey Young, ed., *The Early Years of Federal Food and Drug Control* (Madison, WI: American Institute of the History of Pharmacy, 1982), pp. 8–27. On Wiley and his successors at the early Food and Drug Administration, see Young, *Medical Messiahs* (n. 6), pp. 41–65. On the connections between university and government pharmacology more generally, see John Parascandola, *The Development of American Pharmacology: John J. Abel and the Shaping of a Discipline* (Baltimore: Johns Hopkins University Press, 1992), pp. 91–100. For further discussion of the links between therapeutic reformers and federal officials, see Chapter 3.

33 For the response of various firms to the council's initial announcement, see "Expressions on the Announcement," *JAMA* 44 (March 25, 1905), 971. On the support of consumer advocates for the campaign against quackery, see Young, *Medical Messiahs* (n. 6), pp. 29–32. Paul Starr reports that the AMA distributed over 150,000 copies of "The Great American [drug] Fraud," a muckraking account of the drug industry published by *Collier's Weekly* in 1905. See his *Social Transformation* (n. 18), p. 131.

34 On the council's reservations about the 1906 drug law and its recognition of the need to go beyond either federal or state legislation to accomplish its aims, see especially Burrow, "Prescription Drug Policies" (n. 20), pp. 115–117.

35 Hatcher, "The Duty of the Medical Profession" (n. 16), 1339, 1341; Edsall, "The Work of the Council" (n. 31), 1703–1704.

36 Davis, "Effect of Proprietary Literature on Medical Men" (n. 9), 1339. See also Simmons, "The Commercial Domination of Therapeutics" (n. 26), 1646.

37 W. A. Puckner, "The Nostrum from the Point of View of the Pharmacist," *JAMA* 46 (May 5, 1906), 1340.

The new therapeutics altered somewhat the drugs covered, but the atheoretical, didactic character of the instruction remained unchanged. As might be expected, several of the council's founding members were extensively involved in efforts at educational reform.[38] But educating the medical public was more than a matter of changing classroom instruction. Members of the council expected no less than an intellectual transformation in the profession: cultivation of an experimental orientation toward therapeutic practice.

THE IDEA OF AN EXPERIMENT

> Considered in itself, the experimental method is nothing but reasoning by whose help we methodically submit our ideas to experience – the experience of facts.[39]

In the last quarter of the nineteenth century, medicine experienced a scientific revolution. The revolution occurred not in the practice of medicine but in what came to be known as the medical sciences: bacteriology, physiology, physiological chemistry, and pharmacology, each of which in turn acquired the means to produce and manipulate in the laboratory the phenomena of disease.[40] To a small community of elite physicians, European trained and inspired, the future of medicine would be shaped in the laboratory. Like others of their generation, council members were converts to the gospel of experimental truth: "Experiment is the only certain way of progress."[41]

38 On the teaching of pharmacology, see David L. Cowen, "Materia Medica and Pharmacology," in Ronald L. Numbers, ed., *The Education of American Physicians: Historical Essays* (Berkeley: University of California Press, 1980), pp. 105–110. Cowen's discussion of the period from 1900–1930 is extremely cursory. Three of the nine scientists Cowen singles out for mention were founding members of the council (Sollman, Hatcher, and Cushny) while several others (S. J. Meltzer, A. N. Richards, John J. Abel) were prominent in efforts to establish the practice of therapeutics on a rational basis (ibid., 112).

39 Claude Bernard [1865], *An Introduction to the Study of Experimental Medicine* (New York: Dover Publications, 1957), p. 2.

40 From the large and growing literature on the history of laboratory sciences and medicine, see especially John Harley Warner, "Ideals of Science" (n. 13), and Bruno Latour, "Give Me a Laboratory and I Will Raise the World," in Karin D. Knorr-Cetina and Michael Mulkay, eds., *Science Observed: Perspectives on the Social Study of Science* (London: Sage Publications, 1983), pp. 141–170. On the specific disciplines mentioned, see Patricia Peck Gossel, *The Emergence of American Bacteriology, 1875–1900* (Ph.D. thesis, Johns Hopkins University, 1989); Gerald L. Geison, ed., *Physiology in the American Context, 1850–1940* (Bethesda, MD: American Physiological Society, 1987); Robert E. Kohler, *From Medical Chemistry to Biochemistry: The Making of a Biomedical Discipline* (Cambridge: Cambridge University Press, 1992); Parascandola, *The Development of American Pharmacology* (n. 32). For a further discussion of laboratories and therapeutic research, see Chapter 2.

41 Sollman, *Broader Aims of the Council* (n. 24), p. 47; John Harley Warner, "The Fall and Rise of Professional Mystery: Epistemology, Authority and the Emergence of Laboratory Medicine in Nineteenth-Century America," in Andrew Cunningham and Perry Williams, eds., *The Laboratory Revolution in Medicine* (Cambridge: Cambridge University Press, 1992), pp. 110–141. On the European influence in American medicine, see Thomas Neville Bonner, *American Doctors and German Universities: A Chapter in International Intellectual Relations, 1870–1914* (Lincoln: University of

In its work, the council neglected none of the available tools for reform – legislation, publicity, education – but it relied most on the expectation that physicians would emulate medicine's scientific elite. First and foremost, council reformers sought to change the way physicians *thought* about therapeutics. In particular, reformers hoped that physicians would adopt their own, experimental, attitude toward therapeutic claims. Their chosen instrument for reformation, accordingly, was the idea of an experiment. Among active researchers, appeals to experimentation were clear enough. Experimental studies were the ideal means for producing and evaluating beliefs about the causes and treatment of disease. Most physicians, however, were not engaged in research. Reformers nonetheless expected that practicing physicians would adopt the experimenter's critical and provisional approach toward therapeutic knowledge.

First and foremost, the belief in experimental method denoted confidence in the virtues of a specific cast of mind, an intelligence capable of clear reasoning and unprejudiced judgment. The application of experimental reasoning to the facts of the clinic was no less a scientific accomplishment than a laboratory experiment:

The patient's history, conditions, symptoms, form [the physician's] data. Thereupon he, too, frames his working hypothesis, now called a diagnosis. It suggests a line of action. Is he right or wrong? Has he actually amassed all the significant facts? Does his working hypothesis properly put them together? The sick man's progress is nature's comment and criticism. . . . The progress of science and the scientific or intelligent practice of medicine employ, therefore, exactly the same technique.[42]

Experimental knowledge, in this sense, was within the reach of all physicians: "The essential conditions are . . . in the mental equipment of the investigator. What is needed is, first of all, a frank dislike for cant."[43] Sound research was as much a matter of "attitude" as of "technic": the novice investigator must learn to accept agnosticism "in regard to what is not proved."[44] The hastiness with which some researchers endorsed new treatments stemmed from a failure of intellect and character: "The man who makes an empirical discovery, who believes it to be a fact, has the moral obligation to establish by exact observation that it is a fact and not just a figment of his imagination."[45] The same standards applied to the

Nebraska Press, 1987); Robert G. Frank, "American Physiologists in German Laboratories, 1865–1914," in Geison, *Physiology in the American Context* (n. 40), pp. 11–46.

42 Abraham Flexner, *Medical Education in the United States and Canada: A Report to the Carnegie Foundation for the Advancement of Teaching* (New York: Carnegie Foundation for the Advancement of Teaching, 1910), p. 55. See also Solis-Cohen, "Progress in Therapeutics" (n. 15), 121; Louis Fugueres Bishop, "A Plea for Greater Simplicity in Therapeutics," *JAMA* 35 (November 24, 1900), 1333; Lewellys F. Barker, "Medical Laboratories: Their Relation to Medical Practice and Medical Discovery," *Science* 27 (April 17, 1908), 607; Richard F. Pearce, "The Experimental Method: Its Influence on the Teaching of Medicine" [1910], in *Medical Research and Education* (New York: Science Press, 1913), p. 110.

43 Torald Sollman, "Experimental Therapeutics," *JAMA* 58 (January 27, 1912), 244.

44 Torald Sollman, "The Evaluation of Therapeutic Remedies in the Hospital," *JAMA* 94 (April 26, 1930), 1279–1280.

45 Sollman, "Experimental Therapeutics" (n. 43), 242.

practicing physician: only "laziness" prevented physicians from "using their own brains" to determine what drugs to use and whether they were working.[46]

Considered as an attitude, experimentalism was potentially accessible to all. Considered as a technology, however, experiments were the domain of the few – experts with the training, intelligence, and resources to produce and interpret their findings.[47] The dual character of experimental knowledge was most acutely felt in areas closest to the actual conduct of medical practice, such as therapeutics. By its very nature, therapeutic experimentation was an esoteric subject. Experience alone provided knowledge about the vagaries of specific diseases necessary to complement more general training in research techniques. The expertise required to design an experiment on treating heart failure was not the same as that needed to judge the worth of a new bactericidal compound.[48]

The value of an experiment depended on the degree to which an experimenter anticipated potential sources of error: "It is the purpose of an experimental science to replace accident by design."[49] Therapeutic reformers took their counsel from Francis Bacon, who advised men of science to be ever on the alert for self-deception. The laboratory sciences provided the model for their work: "the laboratory worker plans a series of experiments, and he endeavors to eliminate errors by repetition, and by controlling the various factors which might influence his results."[50] Experimentation was an aid to methodical self-doubt.

Clinical evaluation, no less than preclinical testing, needed to be conducted according "to the canons of other scientific experimentation. Otherwise, its scientific usefulness is nil, and even its practical usefulness is, at best, doubtful."[51] Placing therapeutics on an experimental basis meant more than subjecting a series of patients to treatment: "Experiments may be framed so loosely, the observations may be so superficial, the analysis of results so careless, the deductions so illogical, that the experiment has no permanent value – it is not an experiment in the precise sense of the word."[52] Like the laboratory study, the clinical investigation

46 Solis-Cohen, "Progress in Therapeutics" (n. 15), 124; Blumer, "The Need of Reorganization" (n. 9), 261.

47 John Jacob Abel, "On the Teaching of Pharmacology, Materia Medica and Therapeutics in Our Medical Schools," *Philadelphia Medical Journal* 6 (September 1, 1903), 385; Frederick P. Gay, "Specialization and Research in the Medical Sciences," *Science* 45 (January 12, 1917), 25–33. The ambiguous nature of the appeal to experiment may have been part of its appeal. See Daniel M. Rodgers, "In Search of Progressivism," *Reviews in American History* 10 (1982), 122–127. For a different reading of the laboratory, emphasizing its elitist and exclusionist tendencies, see Warner, "The Fall and Rise of Professional Mystery" (n. 41).

48 Gold, "Recent Advances in Drug Therapy" (n. 16), 97–102; Walter Houston, "Standards in Therapeutics," *International Clinics* (June 1933), 191; Harry M. Marks, *Local Knowledge: Experimental Communities and Experimental Practices, 1918–1950*, a paper presented at the conference on Twentieth Century Health Sciences: Problems and Interpretations, University of California, San Francisco, May 1988.

49 Frederick P. Gay, "Immunology: A Medical Science Developed through Animal Experimentation," *JAMA* 56 (February 25, 1911), 579.

50 Albion Walter Hewlett, "The Cooperation between Pharmacology and Therapeutics," *JAMA* 59 (October 6, 1917), 1123.

51 Sollman, "Experimental Therapeutics" (n. 43), 244.

52 Ibid., 242.

must be planned and regulated: "The results in ten well controlled cases are of more value than the haphazard impressions from a thousand cases."[53]

A "well controlled" experiment was not necessarily one with an untreated series of patients, but one in which a knowledgeable and experienced investigator had anticipated the "multitude of factors" that might affect the outcome: patient selection, dosage, laboratory technique, and the natural history of the disease. Most references to "controlled" studies refer to more than the use of an untreated control series, even where that practice is advocated. Employing a series of untreated cases was one aid to interpreting experimental results, but not necessarily the only means, or the best. Where the use of untreated controls led investigators to neglect "the individuality of cases," they were of "limited or doubtful" value.[54]

Replicating the mastery of a laboratory experiment was difficult to accomplish in the physician's office.[55] The hospital accordingly formed an essential adjunct to the conduct of "well-controlled" experiments:

In a case of hypertension it is not usually feasible – though it is quite justifiable – to have a patient make ten or more office visits without any treatment in order to ascertain the spontaneous variations in that patient's blood-pressure, yet unless that is done one can rarely draw any conclusions about the action of a drug upon the blood-pressure with any assurance that the change was not entirely independent of the drug.[56]

Hospitals afforded the opportunity not only to record observations but, if needed, to regulate the behavior of experimental subjects. Where the activity of patients constituted an aspect of the experimental conditions, this too could be "controlled" best in the hospital.[57]

The special requirements of facilities, equipment, and expertise placed therapeutic investigation beyond the means of most physicians. Controlled experiments nonetheless remained a standard by which other evidence was found wanting. Advocates of an experimental philosophy saw no contradiction in believing that experimental knowledge was within the reach of all physicians while maintaining that proper therapeutic experimentation demanded special talents and resources. If the average physician was no longer able to participate in the production of experimental truth, in reformers' eyes he still belonged to a community bound to

53 Rowntree, "The Role and Development of Drug Therapy" (n. 16), 1064. See also Torald Sollman's remarks in "Therapeutic Research," *JAMA* 58 (May 4, 1912), 1390; Blumer, "The Need of Reorganization" (n. 9), 262–263.

54 For advocacy of using untreated cases, see Joseph L. Miller, "How May the Science of Therapeutics Be Advanced?," *JAMA* 59 (September 21, 1912), 915. For some objections to untreated controls, see Torald Sollman, "The Crucial Test of Therapeutic Evidence," *JAMA* 69 (July 21, 1917), 199.

55 Sollman, "Evaluation of Therapeutic Remedies in the Hospital" (n. 44), 1278. Contrast Sollman's remark in "Experimental Therapeutics" (n. 43), 243.

56 Gold, "Recent Advances in Drug Therapy" (n. 16), 96. See also Torald Sollman, "Research Problems of Pharmacology," *JAMA* 41 (November 28, 1903), 1330; George Blumer, "The Need of Reorganization" (n. 9), 265; John F. Anderson, "Some Unhealthy Tendencies in Therapeutics," *JAMA* 63 (July 14, 1914), 2; W. I. Wilbert, "Materia Medica and Pharmacy in Hospital Practice," *JAMA* 49 (November 16, 1920), 1661.

57 Sollman, "Evaluation of Therapeutic Remedies in the Hospital" (n. 44), 1279.

be guided by that truth in its actions. Even the physician who could not produce new therapeutic knowledge was obligated to accept the authority of those who did.

THE WORK OF THE COUNCIL: KNOWLEDGE AND VIRTUE

Nearly all abuses arise because someone profits thereby.[58]

In theory, establishing a rational therapeutics meant providing an experimentally based chain of evidence linking laboratory and bedside. In the practical work of the council, many of the necessary links were missing and others were weaker than desired. As a consequence, the council's deliberations reflect a curious mixture of judgments about the quality of evidence and opinions about the motives of the men who provided it. Where evidence of therapeutic value was equivocal, evidence of character aided the decision. The products of firms that had proved reliable in the past were scrutinized less carefully than those of habitual offenders.[59] The most trustworthy data were offered by those who lacked economic motives entirely: the "high-minded men" and "institutions" of clinical science.[60]

Where secure evidence from the laboratory existed, the council had few difficulties in arriving at a decision. Following a well-established pharmacological tradition, council members began by analyzing the chemical identity of commercial products.[61] For many of their assessments, the chemistry laboratory proved adequate. Drugs whose principal ingredients were found to be inert or whose active ingredients varied wildly from lot to lot could be readily dismissed.[62] So-

---

58 Robert Hatcher to Torald Sollman, November 25, 1936, Torald Sollman papers, Archives, Cleveland Health Sciences Library, Cleveland, Ohio [hereafter Sollman papers].

59 Distinguishing between the trustworthy and the untrustworthy firm was no simple matter, as Harvard Medical School's David Edsall noted shortly after his appointment to the council. And nothing, he warned, keeps a "reputable" firm from hiring disreputable individuals or itself taking advantage of the council's lack of scrutiny. See Council on Pharmacy and Chemistry, *Bulletin* 7 (April 2, 1908), 152–153, American Medical Association Archives, Chicago. I am extremely grateful to the American Medical Association for permitting me to consult its collection of the *Bulletin,* which records the minutes of the council's weekly meetings, and to Ms. Terry Austin and Ms. Marguerite Falucco for assisting me with the collection.

60 The term is Torald Sollman's, from "Evaluation of Therapeutic Remedies in the Hospital" (n. 44), 1279. See also Lewellys Barker, "Organization of the Laboratories in the Medical Clinic of the Johns Hopkins Hospital," *Bulletin of the Johns Hopkins Hospital* 18 (1907), 195. On the historical sources of the emphasis on character in science, see Steven Shapin, *A Social History of Truth: Civility and Science in Seventeenth-Century England* (Chicago: University of Chicago Press, 1994).

61 On the tradition of identifying (and revealing) the components of proprietary remedies through chemical analysis, see Bouvet, "Sur l'essai des médicaments" (n. 10), and Matthew Ramsey, "Property Rights and the Right to Health: The Regulation of Secret Remedies in France, 1789–1815," in W. F. Bynum and Roy Porter, eds., *Medical Fringe and Medical Orthodoxy, 1750–1850* (London: Croom Helm, 1987), pp. 79–105.

62 Torald Sollman, "Yesterday, Today and Tomorrow: The Activities of the Council on Pharmacy and Chemistry," *JAMA* 61 (July 12, 1912), 5–6; Paul Nicholas Leech, "Chemistry in the Service of Pharmaceutical Medicine," *JAMA* 85 (July 11, 1925), 139–140.

called irrational mixtures, proprietary combinations that contained either too little of one drug or too much of another to obtain the desired effects, were similarly disdained.[63] The intrepid chemist could even discover honesty, or at least, its absence: "misstatements as to therapeutic efficiency . . . may be due to ignorance or excusable prejudice; but misstatements as to composition cannot be due to these causes, but only to downright dishonesty and intentional fraud."[64]

If it had been possible to resolve all therapeutic questions in the chemical laboratory, council members might have been content. But manufacturers continued to pose claims which that laboratory could not address. Take the case of glandular extracts, a hotbed of innovative activity in the early 1900s. A package might well consist of what the manufacturer said it did: red bone marrow extract. That claim could be tested in the chemistry laboratory. But did red bone marrow do what physicians thought it might? And if the council approved red bone marrow extract, what about ovarian extract, parotid gland extract, and a platoon of other products waiting in the wings?[65] For these questions, the chemical laboratory would not suffice.

Animal experimentation provided the next step in judging a drug's merit. By 1900, the practice of evaluating vaccines and antiinfective agents on experimentally infected animals was already well established.[66] The practice readily generalized to other kinds of drugs. The animal study was the exemplar of the well-controlled experiment. For animals, unlike sick patients, conditions could be varied at will: the selection of subjects, the range of doses, and even the intensity of pathology were manipulable at the experimenter's wish. Research on animals provided rapid and extensive information about a drug's safety, or lack thereof. For compounds that eventually proved useful, such studies would aid in determining the range of effective dosages and circumstances under which the drug might be used.[67] Their

63 On the whole, the members of the council favored the view of pharmacologists that when multiple drugs were to be used, the physician ought to prescribe them individually, but the council nonetheless had difficulties in setting a blanket policy on such mixtures. For discussion, see *Bulletin* 1 (March 9, 1905), 15; *Bulletin* 1 (March 16, 1905), 24, 26; *Bulletin* 1 (March 23, 1905), 31–33. Although a ban was ultimately adopted, the issue continued to be debated through the 1920s. See *Bulletin* 26 (April 4, 1918), 167; *Bulletin* 43 (1926), 67, 84, 100; *Bulletin* 47 (March 28, 1928), 232– 233.

64 *Bulletin* 3 (March 20, 1906), 99. On the distinction between the motives of industrial researchers and the honest, but sometimes mistaken, professional, see also Rowntree, "The Role and Development of Drug Therapy" (n. 16), 1064. On the notion of "chemical honesty" and truth in labeling, see Robert M. Crunden, *Ministers of Reform: The Progressives' Achievement in American Civilization 1889–1920* (New York: Basic Books, 1983), p. 186.

65 In the case of red bone marrow, the council recommended its approval on the grounds that it was "honestly exploited." *Bulletin* 4 (August 9, 1906), 97; *Bulletin* 4 (August 23, 1906), 127. Questions about the adequacy of the chemistry laboratory to resolve therapeutic issues continued to recur: see *Bulletin* 27 (January 10, 1918), 27.

66 Barker, "On the Present Status of Therapy" (n. 12), 154; Paul Ehrlich, "Address Delivered at the Dedication of the Georg-Speyer-Haus" [1906], in *The Collected Papers of Paul Ehrlich,* ed. F. Himmelwiet (London: Pergamon Press, 1960), vol. III, pp. 59, 61–62; Horatio C. Wood Jr., "The Limits and Purpose of Bio-Assay," *JAMA* 59 (October 19, 1912), 1433–1434.

67 On the advantages of animal studies, see Hewlett, "Cooperation between Pharmacology and Therapeutics" (n. 50), 1123.

essential virtue, however, was in providing experimenters with the means to guard against the pitfalls of clinical experimentation: mice were far less likely than humans to recover solely on the basis of their keepers' kind attentions and encouraging wishes.[68]

However essential a tool, animal experimentation, too, had its limitations. Some drugs presented to the council could not be reliably tested on animals.[69] A growing awareness of the differences between laboratory animals and humans made it increasingly necessary to interpret data from such studies with caution.[70] For clinicians, as well as for an older generation of pharmacologists, the testing of drugs on humans remained the ultimate court.[71] Clinical skepticism regarding the laboratory made it difficult for the council to dismiss a compound out of hand on the basis of animal studies.[72]

Clinical investigations constituted the "weakest link" in therapeutic research.[73] Strengthening the link meant keeping clinical evaluation out of the "average" practitioner's hands: "the approximate value of a new drug should be determined exhaustively, on patients as well as animals, before it is advertised to the profession."[74] In the hopes of obtaining evaluation by experienced clinical investigators, promising drugs that passed the council's initial laboratory screening were deemed

---

68 "Report of the Council on Pharmacy and Chemistry: Cactus Grandiflorus," *JAMA* 54 (March 12, 1910), 889.

69 See, for example, the discussion of the antipyretic agent A-S-Phen and Sollman's opinion that "animal experimentation is not very satisfactory for determining antipyretic action," *Bulletin* 7 (February 20, 1908), 86.

70 George B. Wallace, "The Influence of Pathologic Conditions on the Actions of Drugs," *JAMA* 59 (September 9, 1912), 839–841; John A. Kolmer, "The Chemotherapy of Experimental Bacterial Infections," *Annals of Surgery* 65 (1917), 142–146.

71 Horatio C. Wood Jr., "Pharmacological Superstitions," *JAMA* 66 (April 6, 1916), 1068. For the continuing skepticism of clinicians regarding the superiority of laboratory studies over clinical evidence in questions of therapeutics, see "Discussion on the Papers of Drs. Cushny, Tyrode and Sollman," *JAMA* 41 (November 28, 1903), 1333–1334; A. Jacobi, "Phases in the Development of Therapy," *Yale Medical Journal* 41 (1905-1906), 493–494; Warren Coleman, "The Present Status of Drug Therapy," *New York State Journal of Medicine* 17 (August 1917), 362; Charles L. Minor, "On the Present Tendency to Nihilism in Drug Therapeutics," *Therapeutic Gazette* 42 (1918), 312–317; Lewellys F. Barker, "The Value of Drugs in Internal Medicine," *JAMA* 77 (October 8, 1921), 1154.

72 On the necessity of conducting animal studies, despite the difficulties of extrapolating between species, see Sollman, "Experimental Therapeutics" (n. 43), 243–244; Hewlett, "Cooperation between Pharmacology and Therapeutics" (n. 50), 1123–1124. Council member Robert Hatcher was responsible for demonstrating the variability of absorption and excretion of different drugs in different species. Rather than making Hatcher a skeptic about the role of animal studies, it made him insist on studying drug effects on an even wider range of species. See Robert A. Hatcher and Cary Eggleston, "Studies on the Absorption of Drugs," *JAMA* 63 (August 8, 1914), 469–473.

73 Arthur Cushny to Torald Sollman, July 9, 1909, Sollman papers. Cushny's remark was meant as a description of the state of affairs which council members hoped to improve. To some degree, however, it reflects the beliefs of pharmacologists on the council in a hierarchy of evidence, with laboratory studies being the most secure and clinical investigations the least reliable. For an explicit discussion of this hierarchy of evidence, and the problem of inconsistencies in the criterion used to judge therapeutic claims, see *Bulletin* 49 (March 20, 1929), 237.

74 Sollman, "Yesterday, Today and Tomorrow" (n. 62), 6. On the importance of qualified observers, see also *Bulletin* 11 (March 24, 1910), 156; *Bulletin* 40 (July 2, 1924), 2–3; *Bulletin* 48 (November 7, 1928), 347–348.

"experimental." Once the drugs were granted "provisional" approval, however, physicians no longer regarded them as experimental. They were used by "incompetent observers" with little interest in producing evidence the council might find acceptable.[75] Controlling the quality of experimental studies proved as difficult as controlling the quality of therapeutic practice more generally.

Lacking access to patients, and already overburdened by their laboratory work, the pharmacologists on the council were in no position to produce their own clinical data. From the outset, they acknowledged the need for a pool of capable clinical observers who would "be in a position" to help them in assessing therapeutic claims.[76] The difficulty was in finding "suitable" individuals. Initially, the laboratory researchers on the council doubted the possibility of finding intellectually qualified and politically sympathetic clinicians.[77] Early in 1908, however, a staff of clinical consultants to advise the council was selected and, at the suggestion of the AMA's Board of Trustees, two university clinicians, David Edsall and Joseph Capps, were appointed to the council.[78]

The council's consultants were generally medical school faculty, expert on either the disease or type of drug in question. Knowledgeable though they might be, these consultants rarely had their own data to guide them. Their first line of offense, accordingly, was to scrutinize the manufacturer's behavior: how "aggressively" was the product being promoted and how "excessive" did the therapeutic claims seem?[79] In scrutinizing manufacturers' promotions, referees sought refuge where possible in laboratory knowledge of a drug's action.[80] But the council's minutes are replete with reports from referees who doubt the value of a compound but lack the evidence to prove it worthless. Where "honest differences" of opinion existed among responsible observers, the council was powerless to act, even when several members had strong reservations about a compound.[81] At best, they could negotiate with the manufacturer to tone down the therapeutic claims somewhat.

The case of Ceanothyn, a new anticoagulant first reviewed in 1926, illustrates the council's difficulties. The council's referee recommended publication of a

---

75 *Bulletin* 21 (June 17, 1915), 354; *Bulletin* 22 (July 29, 1915), 68. The problem of when to grant experimental approval continued to recur through the end of the decade: *Bulletin* 32 (February 23, 1920), 104; *Bulletin* 32 (March 16, 1920), 142.

76 *Bulletin* 1 (June 15, 1905), 147. On Sollman's interest in promoting a role for clinicians in pharmacology, see Parascandola, *Development of American Pharmacology* (n. 32), p. 131.

77 See the discussions in *Bulletin* 6 (October 24, 1907), 184; *Bulletin* 6 (October 31, 1907), 194; *Bulletin* 6 (November 7, 1907), 202; *Bulletin* 6 (November 14, 1907), 214–215.

78 *Bulletin* 7 (January 23, 1908), 46, 49–50; and *Bulletin* 7 (February 7, 1908).

79 *Bulletin* 21 (May 20, 1915), 298; *Bulletin* 32 (September 8, 1920), 80; *Bulletin* 34 (September 21, 1921), 194–195; *Bulletin* 39 (January 30, 1924), 91; *Bulletin* 40 (July 30, 1924), 73–73.

80 *Bulletin* 7 (May 28, 1908), 329–330; *Bulletin* 15 (February 8, 1912), 79; *Bulletin* 29 (May 1, 1919), 168; *Bulletin* 40 (November 12, 1924), 458–461; *Bulletin* 43 (August 11, 1926), 67; *Bulletin* 49 (April 17, 1929), 312.

81 *Bulletin* 21 (May 5, 1915), 298; *Bulletin* 22 (July 29, 1915), 431; *Bulletin* 23 (March 16, 1916), 108–112; *Bulletin* 23 (April 6, 1916), 149; *Bulletin* 31 (March 31, 1920), 141; *Bulletin* 32 (October 20, 1920), 159; *Bulletin* 45 (March 30, 1927), 247–255; *Bulletin* 47 (March 14, 1928), 195; *Bulletin* 47 (March 28, 1928), 237, 248; *Bulletin* 48 (October 17, 1928), 250.

favorable report, based on laboratory evidence that the compound increased clotting times. Two pharmacologists on the council questioned the referee's report on prima facie grounds, arguing that the small amounts of active agent present in the compound could not possibly have such an effect. The pharmacologists – Torald Sollman and Robert Hatcher – joined Columbia clinician Walter Palmer in arguing that only evidence from clinical studies could resolve the question.[82] The referee countered that "if the question of approved therapeutic value is in every case the acid test of acceptance by the Council, this will in most cases result in many years delay of definite action by the Council."[83] When subsequent clinical tests proved negative, the council's Anton Carlson, who favored the drug, questioned the new researchers' qualifications. Even after a "blinded" clinical test, in which the researchers did not know when the active agent was administered, the council continued to debate how critical of the drug its report should be. Only in 1930, after nearly five years of discussion, did the council publish a final report rejecting the drug.[84]

Ideally, the council would have routinely commissioned its own clinical studies, independently assessing manufacturers' therapeutic claims just as the AMA Chemical Laboratory tested commercial statements about the composition and purity of drugs. The council's founders had envisioned such organized therapeutic investigations as part of their reform program.[85] In 1911, the AMA authorized a research grants program to be administered by the council, but the limited funding went largely to relatively small-scale pharmacologic studies.[86] Occasionally, successful clinical studies were mounted by council referees. But overworked council members rebuffed or ignored the occasional suggestions of referees that the council itself coordinate clinical studies to resolve disputed questions.[87]

82 *Bulletin* 48 (October 38, 1928), 304–309; *Bulletin* 48 (November 7, 1928), 326–327; *Bulletin* 48 (November 28, 1928), 419; *Bulletin* 48 (December 5, 1928), 439–440.

83 *Bulletin* 48 (October 31, 1928), 306.

84 *Bulletin* 50 (September 25, 1929), 245–248; *Bulletin* 50 (October 23, 1929), 306–307; *Bulletin* 50 (October 30, 1929), 325; *Bulletin* 50 (November 13, 1929), 24, *Bulletin* 50 (December 31, 1929), 585–586; *Bulletin* 51 (January 8, 1930), 12; *Bulletin* 51 (January 15, 1930), 38; Council on Pharmacy and Chemistry, "Ceanothyn Not Acceptable for N.N.R. II," *JAMA* 94 (February 8, 1930), 419.

85 See Torald Sollman, "Research Problems of Pharmacology" (n. 56), 1330–1333, which variously suggests that scientific societies, medical schools, and the AMA Section on Pharmacology and Therapeutics coordinate such clinical investigations; F. E. Stewart, "Proposed National Bureau of Materia Medica" (n. 20), 1175–1177. For further discussions of the need for the council to organize research, see *Bulletin* 6 (November 7 1907), 202; *Bulletin* 10 (October 21, 1909), 223; J. H. Long, "On the Work of the Council" (n. 21), 899.

86 *Bulletin* 13 (1911), 83, 105–106, 114, 311–313. On the subsequent work of the committee, see *Bulletin* 24 (February 15, 1917), 91–92. See also the detailed published reports of the committee, American Medical Association, Council on Pharmacy and Chemistry, Committee on Therapeutics, *Annual Report* (1912–1931), on which this judgment is based.

87 For examples of successful studies, see *Bulletin* 39 (April 23, 1924), 274–275; A. W. Hewlett, "Clinical Effects of 'Natural' and 'Synthetic' Sodium Salicylate," *JAMA* 61 (August 2, 1913), 319–320 (a "double blinded" comparison of natural and sodium salicylate). As late as 1916 Torald Sollman was still citing this innovative study as the principal example of the council's work in clinical investigation: "The Therapeutic Research Committee of the Council on Pharmacy and Chemistry of the American Medical Association," *JAMA* 67 (November 11, 1916), 1440.

Publicly, council members continued to propagandize for more careful clinical experimentation. Privately, they relied on the opinions and recommendations of trusted colleagues in cases where evidence from the laboratory would not suffice.[88] In the absence of reliable evidence, the council turned to reliable men. The opinions of experts were an imperfect substitute for facts, but their allegiance to science meant that they would only err. They would not deceive:

In their entrance through scientific channels exaggerated therapeutic claims are made at times, as the result of a lack of critical judgment and adequate controls. But in their introduction through commercial channels, financial consideration and lack of true appreciation of the fundamental problems preclude unbiased observations.[89]

Belief in the integrity of scientists formed no part of the council's official pronouncements on experimental method, but where a particular truth could not be established, a proven dedication to truth might suffice. The assurance of reformers in the contribution of experimental method to medicine was premised on a relentless confidence in the future: truth will out.

THE LEGACY OF THE COUNCIL, 1900–1930

It may seem strange that I should put forward three sentiments, namely, interest in an indefinite community, recognition of the possibility of this interest being made supreme, and hope in the unlimited continuance of intellectual activity, as indispensable requirements of logic.[90]

Historians have puzzled over the seemingly deluded faith in experts that characterized early twentieth-century reform movements. The aspirations of science so far exceeded its visible accomplishments that any confidence in the authority of science seems misplaced, a product either of conspiracy or false consciousness.[91]

Proposals for council-organized clinical research are discussed in *Bulletin* 19 (February 12, 1914), 105; *Bulletin* 23 (March 30, 1916), 130; *Bulletin* 43 (March 31, 1926), 206–207, 215–217, 229; *Bulletin* 43 (July 28, August 11, August 25, 1926), 46, 58, 81; *Bulletin* 45 (March 30, 1927), 237–238; *Bulletin* 45 (April 6, 1927), 267; *Bulletin* 57 (March 22, 1933), 470b; Eugene DuBois to Linsley R. Williams, April 13, 1933, and Morris Fishbein to DuBois, April 27, 1933, Box 2, Morris Fishbein papers, University of Chicago [hereafter Fishbein papers].

88 For reliance on testimony, see *Bulletin* 15 (February 8, 1912), 81; *Bulletin* 32 (October 13, 1920), 142; *Bulletin* 48 (October 17, 1928), 250, 263–264; *Bulletin* 48 (October 24, 1928), 293–294 and, for a critical discussion of testimonials, see *Bulletin* 39 (February 23, 1924), 120.

89 Rowntree, "The Role and Development of Drug Therapy" (n. 16), 1064. See also Wilbert, "Materia Medica and Pharmacy" (n. 56), 1661; *Bulletin* 46 (September 28, 1927), 222; *Bulletin* 50 (October 29, 1929), 325; *Bulletin* 50 (November 13, 1929), 414.

90 C. S. Peirce, "On the Doctrine of Chances, with Later Reflections," in Justus Butler, ed., *Philosophical Writings of Peirce* (New York: Dover Publications, 1955), p. 163.

91 See, for example, E. Richard Brown, *Rockefeller Medicine Men: Medicine and Capitalism in America* (Berkeley: University of California Press, 1979). Paul Starr's account of the "cultural authority" of the physician, while warily avoiding either extreme of interpretation, likewise steers clear of examining the profession's scientific claims and conduct in any detail, while remaining doubtful that such an examination could yield much of use. See *Social Transformation* (n. 18), esp. pp. 134–140.

Certainly the fruits of the council's labors through the 1920s seem meager, with the majority of physicians continuing to rely on their own limited clinical impressions or the uncontrolled testimonials of others.[92] Yet for reformers, the shortcomings of actual therapeutic experimentation and its failure to guide the conduct of practicing physicians were a cause for disappointment but not doubt.

Their unquenched optimism rested on the equation, curious to us but recognizable to their contemporaries, between science and morality.[93] The conduct of therapeutic experimentation was meant as an exercise in morality as much as intelligence. The reliance on certain experimental procedures – adequate controls and "blind" testing – were but the visible signs of an inner conviction, a commitment to the "merciless search for errors."[94] So long as a small community of likeminded individuals endorsed the experimental standards of the council, reformers remained confident of eventual success. If some physicians were motivated by an interest in knowledge, then so all might be someday.

Along with a belief in science's morality went suspicions of the immorality of commerce. A loyalty to theories was regrettable but excusable; a loyalty to products and firms was more damning. Corporate interests and the interests of science were seen as antagonistic: "proprietary-ship [*sic*] in pharmaceuticals, in medicine, is unscientific."[95] In the council's view, the advertising department "held sway" at the "reputable" drug manufacturer no less than at the patent medicine vendor.[96]

---

92 Joseph E. Capps, "Irrational Tendencies in Modern Therapy," *JAMA* 83 (July 5, 1924), 2; Hatcher, "The Duty of the Medical Profession" (n. 16), 1339–1342; Chauncey D. Leake, "The Pharmacologic Evaluation of New Drugs," *JAMA* 93 (November 23, 1929), 1632; *Bulletin* 50 (November 13, 1929), 508; "Verbatim Report, Special Fall Meeting, Council on Pharmacy and Chemistry with the Board of Trustees, November 15, 1934," *Bulletin* 62 (December 6, 1934), a12–a18; Albert E. Bulson to Morris Fishbein, October 3, 1927, Box 1, Fishbein papers.

93 Christian A. Herter, "Imagination and Idealism in the Medical Sciences," *JAMA* 54 (February 5, 1910), 423–430. On the late nineteenth-century background to such views, see the introduction to Charles E. Rosenberg's *No Other Gods: On Science and American Social Thought* (Baltimore: Johns Hopkins University Press, 1978), pp. 1–21; the essays by David A. Hollinger, "Inquiry and Uplift: Late NineteenthCentury American Academics and the Moral Efficacy of Scientific Practice," and Thomas L. Haskell, "Professionalism *versus* Capitalism: R. H. Tawney, Emile Durkheim and C. S. Peirce on the Disinterestedness of Professional Communities," both in Thomas L. Haskell, ed., *The Authority of Experts: Studies in History and Theory* (Bloomington: Indiana University Press, 1984), pp. 142–156, 180–225; and Owen Hannaway, "The German Model of Chemical Education in America: Ira Remsen at Johns Hopkins (1876–1913)," *Ambix* 23 (November, 1976), esp. 153–154. On the moral and religious impetus to Progressive-era reforms in general, see Crunden, *Ministers of Reform* (n. 64).

94 The phrase is Torald Sollman's, from "Evaluation of Therapeutic Remedies in the Hospital" (n. 44), 1280.

95 George H. Simmons to John Jacob Abel, January 18, 1916, John Jacob Abel papers, Box 51, Chesney Archives. As late as 1909, Reid Hunt was proposing that new drug development and evaluation be conducted in the "pharmacologic laboratories of the medical schools, of the Government and of medical associations." Hunt, "What the Individual Physician Can Do" (n. 9), 502. Interestingly, the chemist Ira Remsen, who had aspired to be a physician, was similarly antagonistic to industrial influences on chemistry, although his reasons were somewhat different from those of therapeutic reformers. See Owen Hannaway, "The German Model" (n. 93), 156–157.

96 Leech, "Chemistry in the Service of Pharmaceutical Medicine" (n. 62), 139. See also Simmons, "The Commercial Domination of Therapeutics" (n. 26), 1650; G. W. McCoy, "Official Methods

Even when not actively subverting rational therapeutics, companies put other interests ahead of the truth. Despite occasional doubts about the wisdom of attacking those they sought to reform, council members' suspicions of commercial motives were deeply ingrained.[97]

As historian Richard McCormick has noted, concerns about the "corrupting" influence of business were widespread in the decade when the council began its work.[98] George Simmons's conviction that business and medical science are inherently at odds places therapeutic reformers closer to capitalism's contemporary academic critics, the social scientists Thorstein Veblen and Richard Ely, than to the university chemists and engineers who by the First World War went avidly in search of industrial patronage. Unlike Ely or Veblen, none of the therapeutic reformers could ever be called a socialist. Their critique of business was partial and limited to medicine. They sought not to eliminate business from American society, but to subordinate it to the authorized voices of medical science.[99]

The path charted by therapeutic reformers is distinctive in other respects. Unlike contemporaneous efforts in hospital and educational reform, therapeutic reformers sought few allies outside the profession.[100] The council's energies were directed inward, toward changing the practice of medicine itself.

In changing medical practice, the council had the support, it hoped, of the AMA's Board of Trustees and of like-minded university clinicians and scientists.[101]

of Control of Remedial Agents for Human Use," *JAMA* 74 (June 5, 1920), 1554; *Bulletin* 51 (January 8, 1930), 14.

97 *Bulletin* 31 (March 20, 1920), 91; and *Bulletin* 31 (March 27, 1920), 110.

98 Richard L. McCormick, "The Discovery That Business Corrupts Politics: A Reappraisal of the Origins of Progressivism," *American Historical Review* 86 (April 1981), 247–274. McCormick's account emphasizes the suddenness of the "discovery," which he dates precisely to the years 1905–1908. For accounts that stress the longer-term development of regulatory legislation, see William R. Brock, *Investigation and Responsibility: Public Responsibility in the United States* (Cambridge: Cambridge University Press, 1984), and, in the area of food and drug legislation, James Harvey Young, *Pure Food: Securing the Federal Food and Drugs Act of 1906* (Princeton: Princeton University Press, 1989).

99 On Ely and Veblen, see Dorothy Ross, *The Origins of American Social Science* (Cambridge: Cambridge University Press, 1991), pp. 109–138, 204–216. See, by comparison, the physical scientists discussed in David F. Noble, *America by Design: Science, Technology and the Rise of Corporate Capitalism* (New York: Oxford University Press, 1979), pp. 128–147, 182–195, 234–256; Swann, *Academic Scientists* (n. 4), pp. 59–65; John W. Servos, "The Industrial Relations of Science: Chemical Engineering at M.I.T., 1900–1939," *Isis* 71 (1980), 531–549.

100 Philanthropic foundations, for example, played a key role in the movement for hospital and medical education reform between 1910 and 1930. On hospital reform, see Rosemary Stevens, *In Sickness and in Wealth: American Hospitals in the Twentieth Century* (New York: Basic Books, 1989), pp. 114–118, 129–130, and Peter Buck, "Why Not the Best? Some Reasons and Examples from Child Health and Rural Hospitals," *Journal of Social History* 18 (1985), 413–431, which also discusses the important role of life insurance companies. For medical education, see Gerald E. Markowitz and David Rosner, "Doctors in Crisis: Medical Education and Medical Reform in the Progressive Era, 1895–1915," in Susan Reverby and David Rosner, eds., *Health Care in America: Essays in Social History* (Philadelphia: Temple University Press, 1979), pp. 185–205.

101 The council nonetheless doubted on occasion the degree to which the AMA Board of Trustees supported it. See *Bulletin* 31 (March 20, 1920), 97–98. For criticisms of the council's policies in specific cases, see Leslie T. Gager, "Abstract of Discussion," *JAMA* 93 (November 23, 1929), 1634;

But successful therapeutic reform depended on changing physicians at the bottom, not the top, of the profession. For these physicians to change, medicine, no less than the market, had to be governed by science. Few physicians shared in the full strength of reformers' convictions that the future of therapeutic progress lay in the laboratory. Appeals to the "art" of medicine evoked the authority of the physician at the bedside.[102] But beyond differences about the ultimate sources of medical knowledge lay a more fundamental divide.

Reformers assumed that practitioners shared a community of interests with men of science. Diagnosis and treatment – the "work" of clinical practice – were understood as exercises in scientific reasoning, akin to the formulation and testing of experimental hypotheses. In an era when diagnostic acumen was the accepted measure of the accomplished practitioner, reformers often presented therapeutic decisions as problems in applied diagnosis: study the patient carefully, reason methodically, arrive at a correct diagnosis, and the therapeutic problem is solved.[103]

For reformers, what distinguished the man of science from other medical practitioners was not that he possessed the truth about diagnosis and treatment, but that he renounced false complacency. Recognizing the limits of one's knowledge was of equal importance with having a supply of it in the first instance. Putatively men of science, practicing physicians were eligible and expected to join its community. But to the practicing physician, concerned with accommodating (and keeping) his patients, arriving at the truth was a problem best left to others. The practice of medicine may have been, in the ideology of the era, more than a mere business but it was a business no less.[104]

Albert E. Bulson to Morris Fishbein, October 3, 1927, Box 1, Fishbein papers. For concerns over lack of support for the council from rank-and-file members of the profession, see Chauncey D. Leake, "The Pharmacologic Evaluation of New Drugs," *JAMA* 93 (November 23, 1929), 1634. See also the debate over whether the council's criticisms about the promotion of Salvarsan would damage its reputation: *Bulletin* 13 (February 2, 1911), 55–57; *Bulletin* 13 (February 9, 1911), 74–76.

102 The issue has been best addressed for the contemporary British medical profession. See Judy Sadler, "Ideologies of 'Art' and 'Science' in Medicine: The Transition from Medical Care to the Application of Technique in the British Medical Profession," in Wolfgang Krohn, Edwin Layton Jr., and Peter Weingart, eds., *The Dynamics of Science and Technology: Sociology of the Sciences Yearbook 1978* (Dordrecht: D. Reidel, 1978), pp. 177–218; Christopher Lawrence, "Incommunicable Knowledge: Science, Technology and the Clinical Art in Britain, 1850–1914," *Journal of Contemporary History* 20 (1985), 503–520.

103 See A. Jacobi, "Phases in the Development" (n. 15), 502; George M. Dock, "The Movement for Exact Treatment" (n. 17), 92–93; Richard F. Pearce, "The Experimental Method" (n. 42), 110; C. M. Jackson, "The Role of Research in Medicine," *Science* 60 (September 12, 1924), 231.
   On diagnostic accomplishment as a standard, see Paul B. Beeson and Russell C. Maulitz "The Inner History of Internal Medicine," in Russell C. Maulitz and Diana E. Long, eds., *Grand Rounds: One Hundred Years of Internal Medicine* (Philadelphia: University of Pennsylvania Press, 1988), pp. 33–35; on the metaphoric uses of medical diagnosis, see JoAnne Brown, *The Definition of a Profession: The Authority of Metaphor in the History of Intelligence Testing, 1890–1930* (Princeton: Princeton University Press, 1992), pp. 90–94.

104 On the discovery that practitioners had economic motives, see Peter Buck, "Why Not the Best?" (n. 100).

Circumstances as well as ideology constrained reformers in their dealings with the medical profession at large. Dependent on practitioners' goodwill for clientele and reputation, academic physicians exercised few powers over their colleagues in the community.[105] To tell physicians what they *must* do, rather than instruct them in what they *should* do, went beyond the limits of the council's authority. With noncompliant physicians, they were armed only with persuasion. Speaking in the name of science, reformers could only hope that they would eventually be heard above the noise of the market.

Long after George Simmons had left his job as editor of *JAMA*, the council he had created sought to ensure that university scientists, not corporate copywriters, had the last word on therapeutics. The standards of evidence articulated by the council were widely endorsed within academic medicine. As discussed in Chapter 3, these standards formed the basis for federal drug regulation in the 1930s and 1940s. For some reformers, however, relying on the isolated, experienced investigator of Simmons's and Sollman's era was not enough. Modern medicine, like modern business, had to be organized. The following chapter considers the development of cooperative clinical research in the decades between the two world wars.

105 On the importance of referrals and the income from them, see A. T. Cabot, "Realism in Medicine," *BMSJ* 142 (June 21, 1900), 650. As late as 1940, part-time clinical faculty at medical schools outnumbered full-time 4.6 to 1. On this, and the dependence of full-time faculty on clinical income, see Rothstein, *American Medical Schools* (n. 21), pp. 165–169.

2

Memories of underdevelopment: Therapeutic research in the United States, 1900–1935

> The more we increase the number of our observations, the more do individual peculiarities, and exceptions to the general rule, disappear; and the more certainly do the averages obtained represent the normal condition of the objects observed.[1]

Over the course of the nineteenth century, researchers working in a variety of fields noticed a common problem: individual observers, putatively studying the same phenomenon with similar techniques, gave divergent accounts of it. Even in a science as exact as astronomy, two observers working in the same observatory, under similar conditions, and with identical equipment reported measurements that did not agree. As with the observations themselves, understanding of the problem varied with the science and the decade. Solutions ranged from the "technical fix" (eliminate, by the use of improved instrumentation, dependence on human observers and their frailties) to institutional reforms (standardize the procedures by which data were collected).[2]

As contemporary observers emphasized, the phenomena of disease were far more variable in appearance and behavior than the objects studied in astronomy.[3]

1 William A. Guy, "On the Value of the Numerical Method As Applied to Science, but Especially to Physiology and Medicine," *Journal of the Royal Statistical Society* 2 (1839), 38.
2 Edwin G. Boring, "The Personal Equation," in idem, *A History of Experimental Psychology* (New York: Appleton Century Crofts, 1957), pp. 134–156; Stephen M. Stigler, *The History of Statistics: The Measurement of Uncertainty before 1900* (Cambridge: Harvard University Press, 1986), pp. 240–242; Simon Schaffer, "Astronomers Mark Time: Discipline and the Personal Equation," *Science in Context* 2 (Spring 1988), 115–145; Anson Rabinbach [on the work of the physiologist Etienne-Jules Marey], *The Human Motor: Energy, Fatigue and the Origins of Modernity* (New York: Basic Books, 1990), pp. 88–119. Ian Hacking presents the interesting case of C. S. Peirce who through repeated training exercises conditioned the response times of a small boy so that the variability of his observations was minimal. See his *The Taming of Chance* (Cambridge: Cambridge University Press, 1990), pp. 202–204.
3 Elisha Bartlett, *An Essay on the Philosophy of Medical Science* (Philadelphia: Lea and Blanchard, 1844), pp. 148–152; Guy, "Value of the Numerical Method" (n. 1), 26–30; Jules Gavarret, *Principes généraux de statistique médicale; ou, Developpement des règles qui doivent présider à son emploi* (Paris: Bechet jeune et Labe, 1840), pp. 114–115. On the uses of statistics in nineteenth-century French and German medicine, see, in addition to the works in note 6, Joseph Schiller, *Claude Bernard et les problèmes*

The problem was compounded by the conditions of observation: a single physician rarely got to observe the great variety of individual responses to a particular disease. To accumulate an accurate picture of disease, either someone must gather observations from a large number of physicians; or a single physician, suitably based in a hospital ward, must gather observations on large numbers of patients with a given disease. The first strategy informed the meteorological and epidemiological observations of the late eighteenth and mid-nineteenth centuries. The second was the modus operandi of the Paris clinical school whose physicians controlled admissions to a few select wards in the city's large hospitals.[4]

Physicians returning to the United States from training in Paris in the 1840s found few opportunities to emulate the close hospital observations of their teachers.[5] In the United States, the independent practitioner remained the repository of knowledge. Physicians accumulated knowledge of disease over the course of a long career, making age synonymous with expertise. Those who aspired to transcend the limitations of individual investigators turned to surveying large numbers of physicians about their experience (and opinions) of therapies.[6] Such "collective investigation," as it came to be known, enjoyed a brief flurry of interest

scientifiques de son temps (Paris: Les Editions du Cèdre, 1967), pp. 154–171; William Coleman, "Experimental Physiology and Statistical Inference: The Therapeutic Trial in Nineteenth-Century Germany," in Lorenz Krüger, Gerd Gigerenzer, and Mary S. Morgan, eds., *The Probabilistic Revolution* (Cambridge: MIT Press, 1987), vol. 2, pp. 201–228; J. Rosser Matthews, *Quantification and the Quest for Medical Certainty* (Princeton: Princeton University Press, 1995), pp. 14–85.

4 On the collection of meteorological and epidemiological data, see Jean Meyer, "Une enquête de l'Académie de médecine sur les épidemies (1774–1794)," *Annales: E. S. C.* (August 1966), 729–749; Jean-Pierre Peter, "Une enquête de la Société Royale de Médecine (1774–1794): Malades et maladies à la fin du XVIIIe siècle," *Annales: E. S. C.* 22 (July–August 1967), 711–751; Caroline G. Hannaway, "The Société Royale de Médecine and Epidemics in the 'ancien regime,'" *BHM* 46 (1972), 257–273. In the United States, the army and local medical societies encouraged the collection of such data. See James H. Cassedy, *Medicine and American Growth, 1800–1860* (Madison: University of Wisconsin Press, 1986), pp. 29–35, 44–50, 129–137; John Harley Warner, *The Therapeutic Perspective: Medical Practice, Knowledge and Identity in America, 1820–1885* (Cambridge: Harvard University Press, 1986), pp. 73–75. On data gathering in the Paris Clinic, see Erwin H. Ackerknecht, *Medicine at the Paris Hospital, 1794–1848* (Baltimore: Johns Hopkins University Press, 1967); L. S. Jacyna, "Au Lit des Malades: A. F. Chomel's Clinic at the Charité, 1828–1829," *Medical History* 33 (1989), 420–449.

5 Bartlett, *Essay* (n. 3), p. 310. The few isolated exceptions to the pattern, most notably, James Jackson's and William Gerhard's investigations into typhoid, do not alter the general picture. See Dale C. Smith, "Gerhard's Distinction between Typhoid and Typhus and Its Reception in America, 1833–1860," *BHM* 54 (1980), esp. 373–376. For a more positive assessment of American capacities, see James H. Cassedy, *American Medicine and Statistical Thinking, 1800–1860* (Cambridge: Harvard University Press, 1984), pp. 68–91.

6 Most such studies concerned the etiology and natural history of the more common diseases. Opportunities for therapeutic investigations were even more limited, but see the discussion of earlier European work in Ian Hacking, *The Taming of Chance* (n. 2), pp. 81–86; George Weisz, "Academic Debate and Therapeutic Reasoning in Mid-19th Century France," in Ilana Löwy, Olga Amsterdamska, John Pickstone, and Patrice Pinell, eds., *Medicine and Change: Historical and Sociological Studies in Medical Innovation* (London: John Libbey Eurotext, 1993), pp. 287–315; George Weisz, *The Medical Mandarins: The French Academy of Medicine in the Nineteenth and Twentieth Centuries* (Oxford: Oxford University Press, 1995), pp. 159–188. Weisz provides a more nuanced and informed account than Matthews, *Quantification and the Quest for Medical Certainty* (n. 3).

in England and the United States between the 1860s and the 1890s.[7] But collective investigation presupposed an equality of observers which physicians in the late nineteenth century increasingly began to question.[8] That some observers were more qualified than others was a contention few therapeutic reformers doubted. Just who those more qualified observers were was a matter for some dispute.

Collective investigations initially sought out the experience and opinions of the general practitioner.[9] Those who criticized collective investigation in the 1890s questioned the value of the observations made by the ordinary practitioner who lacked, according to critics, both the facilities and the skill to make reliable and pertinent observations. But critics equally eschewed therapeutic evaluations conducted under the auspices of hospitals whose "surroundings . . . are so different from those of private practice that the measure of success in hospital cases cannot be taken as an index" of the value of a treatment in routine practice.[10] Specialty societies collected data from their members, who were said to offer a collective experience more relevant than that of the hospital-based practitioner, and more reliable than that of the general practitioner. Yet not all specialists agreed that it was proper to rely on the "observations of people that [one] knows very little about." A contentious debate at the American Pediatric Society about the value of

7 "Collective investigation" appears to have escaped the attention of both historians of statistics and therapeutics; the movement needs more attention and analysis than I can give it here. On the British initiative, see "Report of the Committee on the Action of Medicines," *British Medical Journal* ii (August 16, 1862), 177; "An Investigation into the Effects of Remedies," *British Medical Journal* ii (August 16, 1862), 175–176; "The Work of the Collective Investigation Committee," *British Medical Journal* ii (1882), 1242–1243; *The Collective Investigation Record Containing the Reports of the Collective Investigation Committee of the British Medical Association,* 3 vols. (London: British Medical Association, 1887). For brief historical accounts, see R. M. S. McConaghey, "The B. M. A. and Collective Investigation," *British Medical Journal* i (February 25, 1956), Supplement, 59–61; Ernest Muirhead Little, *History of the British Medical Association, 1832–1932* (London: British Medical Association, 1932), 301–305.

   For American examples, see Ephraim Cutter, Alonzo Chapin, and S. A. Toothaker, "Report of the Committee . . . into the Therapeutical Action of Medicinal Agents," *BMSJ* 68 (1863), 342–347; "Collective Investigation of Diseases," *JAMA* 1 (August 1883), 216–218; Henry B. Baker, "Collective Investigation of Disease," *JAMA* 9 (1887), 486–490.

8 Such objections were already noted by proponents of the method. See Cutter et al., "Report" (n. 7), 344. The fate of "collective investigation" may also have been affected by drug manufacturers' appropriation of the term to obtain case reports on new drugs, which were then incorporated into drug promotions. See *The Ethical Relations Existing between Medicine and Pharmacy: With Illustrations of an Improved Method for the Collective and Scientific Investigation of New Drugs* (Detroit: Scientific Department of Parke, Davis & Company, 1887).

9 See especially William W. Gull, "An Address on the International Collective Investigation of Disease," *British Medical Journal* ii (August 16, 1884), 306; Cutter et al., "Report" (n. 7), 344.

10 "Report of the American Pediatric Society's Collective Investigation into the Use of Antitoxin in the Treatment of Diphtheria in Private Practice," *JAMA* 27 (July 4, 1896), 27–35; John W. Kyger, "A Protest against Accepting the Conclusions of Hospital Physicians As to the Value of Antitoxine in Diphtheria," *New York Medical Journal* 63 (1895), 151; D. J. Leech and William Hunter, "An Inquiry Regarding the Importance of Ill-Effects following the Use of Antipyrin, Antifebrin and Phenacetin Conducted by the Therapeutic Committee of the British Medical Association," *British Medical Journal* i (1894), esp. 85. The British objections to hospital-based surveys directly informed at least one analysis in the United States. See L. F. Kebler, F. P. Morgan, and Philip Rupp, *The Harmful Effects of Acetanilid, Antipyrin and Phenacetin,* U.S. Department of Agriculture, Bureau of Chemistry, Bulletin No. 126 (Washington, DC: Government Printing Office, 1909), pp. 10, 12.

collective investigation apparently put an end to that society's efforts at organized inquiry.[11]

Similar difficulties beset the newly emerging laboratory sciences. Historians of medicine and science have emphasized the institutional growth of the laboratory sciences in the last third of the nineteenth century.[12] After the successful introduction of diphtheria antitoxin in 1894, few physicians doubted that laboratory scientists could produce potent and effective therapeutic agents. The production of reliable therapeutic *knowledge* was another matter. Laboratory scientists challenged the physician's traditional reliance on clinical experience. It took correspondingly little time for clinicians to question the relevance of laboratory studies to human disease.[13]

In describing medicine's intellectual and social landscape at the turn of the century, historians have emphasized conflicts between laboratory-based scientists and clinicians.[14] In therapeutics, however, the potential sources of authority were plural, not dual, and the potential for conflict was not confined to individuals with different scientific orientations or professional training. Institutional settings, no less than disciplinary traditions and specialty orientations, influenced the kinds of research attempted and achieved.[15]

11 Collective investigations organized by specialty societies are "Report of the Committee on Collective Investigation concerning the Ocular Muscles," *JAMA* 53 (September 4, 1900), 794–796; "The Report of the American Pediatric Society's Collective Investigation into the Use of Antitoxin in the Treatment of Diphtheria in Private Practice," *Transactions of the American Pediatric Society* 8 (1896), 21–45 [this is the full report of the study reported in n. 10]; "The American Pediatric Society's Report on the Collective Investigation of the Antitoxin Treatment of Laryngeal Diphtheria in Private Practice, 1896–1897," *Transactions of the American Pediatric Society* 9 (1897), 32–38; "The American Pediatric Society's Collective Investigation on Infantile Scurvy in North America," *Transactions of the American Pediatric Society* 10 (1898), 5–33. This last is a pathological and epidemiologic study, as was the ophthalmological inquiry.

12 See, most recently, the introduction and studies gathered in Andrew Cunningham and Perry Williams, eds., *The Laboratory Revolution in Medicine* (Cambridge: Cambridge University Press, 1992), and especially the article by John Harley Warner, "The Rise and Fall of Professional Mystery: Epistemology, Authority and the Emergence of Laboratory Medicine in Nineteenth-Century America," pp. 110–141.

13 See Warner, "The Rise and Fall of Professional Mystery" (n. 12); idem, "Ideals of Science and Their Discontents in Late Nineteenth-Century American Medicine," *Isis* 82 (September 1991), 454–478.

14 On conflicts between clinicians and laboratory scientists, see Russell C. Maulitz, " 'Physician versus Bacteriologist': The Ideology of Science in Clinical Medicine," and Gerald L. Geison, "Divided We Stand: Physiologists and Clinicians in the American Context," both in Morris J. Vogel and Charles E. Rosenberg, eds., *The Therapeutic Revolution: Essays in the Social History of American Medicine* (Philadelphia: University of Pennsylvania Press, 1979), pp. 91–109 and 67–90; Steve Sturdy, "From the Trenches to the Hospitals at Home: Physiologists, Clinicians, and Oxygen Therapy, 1914–1930," and Michael Worboys, "Vaccine Therapy and Laboratory Medicine in Edwardian Britain," both in John V. Pickstone, ed., *Medical Innovations in Historical Perspective* (New York: St. Martin's Press, 1992), pp. 104–123 and 84–103; and Christopher Lawrence, "Experiment and Experience in Anaesthesia: Alfred Goodman Levy and Chloroform Death, 1910–1960," in Christopher Lawrence, ed., *Medical Theory, Surgical Practice* (London: Routledge, 1992), pp. 263–294.

15 See John Higham, "The Matrix of Specialization," in Alexandra Oleson and John Voss, eds., *The Organization of Knowledge in Modern America, 1860–1920* (Baltimore: Johns Hopkins University Press, 1979), pp. 3–18. Though not speaking of medicine per se, Higham, unlike recent historians of medicine, stresses both the elitist ethos and the countervailing pluralism engendered by the proliferation of new scientific specialties and institutions.

Between 1880 and 1930, physicians sought reliable therapeutic evidence in the laboratory, at the hospital, from medical school faculty, and in the offices of specialists and general practitioners.[16] While some physicians interested in therapeutic reform struggled with the difficulties of translating the methods and culture of the laboratory researcher to the clinic, others, entirely based in the clinic, devised new organizational forms for combining and comparing the experiences of individual physicians.[17]

Regardless of whether they worked in the laboratory or the clinic, therapeutic researchers sought to overcome the limitations – inherent, they alleged – in knowledge based on the clinical experiences of individual practitioners. Yet as physicians trained in a professional culture that placed its greatest emphasis on the individual's accumulated experience, researchers encountered great difficulties in escaping that tradition. Even those investigators who most emphasized the limitations of individual experience as a source of therapeutic knowledge found it difficult to surrender their intellectual autonomy to an organized program of therapeutic research.

The culture of individualism – no less influential in medical science than in medical practice – posed one barrier to reformers' efforts to produce reliable, clinically relevant therapeutic knowledge. The widening gap between medicine as practiced in elite university clinics and hospitals and that encountered in general practice proved an even greater obstacle. Physicians who employed innovations such as oxygen therapy, intravenous fluids, or serum treatment for pneumonia depended on facilities and personnel that were simply unavailable to the vast majority of private practitioners.[18] Consequently, even those researchers who overcame the limitations imposed by a culture of individualism found themselves ignored by practitioners who lacked the means and motives to make use of the era's "high-technology" therapeutics.

In the following section, I examine the diversity of settings – from the laboratory to the practitioner's office – in which early twentieth-century medical researchers worked. I then review in detail the history of two efforts devised specifically to overcome the difficulties associated with traditional therapeutic research: the Cooperative Clinical Group study of syphilis treatments and the Commonwealth Fund's experiments with serum treatment of pneumonia.

16 In addition to the sources cited in nn. 7–11, see Victor Robinson, "A Symposium on Drugs," *Review of Reviews* 22 (1916), 15–26; Henry P. Loomis, "A Comparative Study of the Routine Treatment of Certain Diseases in Four of the Largest New York Hospitals," *Medical Record* 63 (January 10, 1903), 41–46.

17 On organizational reforms in early twentieth-century medicine, see Roger Cooter and Steve Sturdy, "Science, Scientific Management and the Medical Revolution in Britain c. 1870–1948," unpublished manuscript. I am grateful to the authors for making this available to me.

18 On the uneven distribution of innovative medical therapies, see Harry M. Marks, "Medical Technology: Social Contexts and Consequences," in W. F. Bynum and Roy Porter, eds., *Companion Encyclopedia of the History of Medicine* (London: Routledge, 1993), vol. 2, pp. 1601–1603; Steve Sturdy, "From the Trenches to the Hospitals" (n. 14), pp. 120–123; Naomi Rogers, *Dirt and Disease: Polio before FDR* (New Brunswick, NJ: Rutgers University Press, 1992), p. 74.

A PLACE FOR CLINICAL INVESTIGATION

From the vantage point of the late twentieth century, we are accustomed to thinking of university-based medical schools as the "natural" location in which to conduct medical research. Yet during the first two decades of the century, medical research flourished in a variety of institutions: research institutes vied with government laboratories, specialty clinics, and universities to provide settings suited to the development of medical knowledge.[19] This organizational diversity permitted researchers to "experiment" with various strategies for linking the scientific work of the laboratory with the problems seen in the clinic.[20] While each site provided certain specific advantages, researchers at each kind of institution experienced characteristic problems in linking the laboratory and the clinic.

The European-trained physicians who organized public health laboratories were the first to introduce German innovations in serum therapy to the United States, beginning in 1894. Researchers in the New York City Health Department made use of the city hospital in evaluating the worth of diphtheria antitoxin.[21] But the public laboratories' subsequent role in developing and distributing serums and vaccines was considerably circumscribed by physicians and vaccine manufacturers who objected to the competition from public enterprises. Although some research on vaccines and serums continued in the health departments of New York City, New York State, Philadelphia, and Massachusetts, bench studies in diagnostic methods and disease etiology predominated in these and other public health department laboratories.[22]

19 The situation in medicine was simply an important subset of the general situation of scientific research. See Charles E. Rosenberg, "Towards an Ecology of Knowledge: On Discipline, Context and History," in Oleson and Voss, *The Organization of Knowledge* (n. 15), pp. 440–455; Robert E. Kohler, "Science, Foundations, and American Universities in the 1920s," *Osiris,* 2nd ser., 3 (1987), 135–138; and Nathan Reingold, "The Case of the Disappearing Laboratory," reprinted in *Science, American Style* (New Brunswick, NJ: Rutgers University Press, 1991), pp. 224–246. The growing importance of universities as a base for research in one medical science – biochemistry – is nicely documented in Robert E. Kohler, "Medical Reform and Biomedical Science: Biochemistry – A Case Study," in Vogel and Rosenberg, *The Therapeutic Revolution* (n. 14), pp. 27–66.
20 In the idiom of the day, Simon Flexner described both the Rockefeller Institute for Medical Research and the innovations in "full-time" salaried clinical faculty as experiments. See Flexner to Lusk, December 15, 1920, and Lusk's reply (December 16, 1920) that, having "lived in a medical school," he "possibly" saw "the realities [of full-time] from a little different viewpoint than" Flexner was "able to do." B/F365, Simon Flexner papers, APS.
21 William Hallock Park, "Clinical Use of Diphtheria Antitoxin," *Medical Communications of the Massachusetts Medical Society* 16 (1894), 749–776. For skepticism regarding the representativeness of cases treated in hospital, see Kyger, "A Protest against Accepting the Conclusions of Hospital Physicians" (n. 10), 151; "Report of the American Pediatric Society's Collective Investigation" (n. 10), 27. The most comprehensive account of the New York City evaluations of diphtheria antitoxin is provided by Evelynn Maxine Hammonds, *The Search for Perfect Control: A Social History of Diphtheria, 1880–1930* (Ph.D. thesis, Harvard University, 1993), pp. 181–200.
22 David Anthony Blancher, *Workshops of the Bacteriological Revolution: A History of the Laboratories of the New York City Department of Health, 1892–1912* (Ph.D. thesis, City University of New York, 1979); Anna M. Sexton, *A Chronicle of the Division of Laboratories and Research, New York State Department of Health, the First Fifty Years: 1914–1964* (Lunenburg, VT: Stinehour Press, 1967); Edward T.

The federal government's Hygienic Laboratory, first established in 1887, had a broader research program than municipal and state laboratories. By 1920, the Hygienic Laboratory's Carl Voegtlin was conducting research not only on serums and vaccines but on chemical compounds used in treating disease.[23] But the Hygienic Laboratory had even less access to patients than local health departments, and its therapeutic investigations were, for all practical purposes, limited to laboratory studies. Questions that could only be resolved in the clinic were not addressed.[24] Research activities at the Hygienic Laboratory were further circumscribed by its regulatory responsibilities: to test the serums, vaccines, and arsenical compounds produced by commercial firms and other laboratories.[25]

Independent research institutes, underwritten by private philanthropy, offered scientists an opportunity to work unencumbered by the teaching responsibilities of the university or the service demands placed on government researchers.[26] Among the wealthiest and most prominent of these was the Rockefeller Institute for Medical Research, established in 1901.[27] A literal embodiment of contempo-

Morman, *Scientific Medicine Comes to Philadelphia: Public Health Transformed, 1854–1899* (Ph.D. thesis, University of Pennsylvania, 1986); Barbara Gutmann Rosenkrantz, *Public Health and the State: Changing Views in Massachusetts, 1842–1936* (Cambridge: Harvard University Press, 1972), pp. 112–127.

23 On Voegtlin's work, see John Parascandola, "Carl Voegtlin and the 'Arsenic Receptor' in Chemotherapy," *JHM* 32 (April 1977), 151–171. Voegtlin's predecessor, Reid Hunt, "did not work actively" on problems of chemotherapy, despite substantial familiarity with and enthusiasm for Ehrlich's program of chemotherapy. E. K. Marshall Jr., "Reid Hunt (1870–1948)," *Biographical Memoirs of the National Academy of Sciences* 26 (1949), 28.

24 On the early research work of the Hygienic Laboratory, see Victoria A. Harden, *Inventing the NIH: Federal Biomedical Research Policy, 1887–1937* (Baltimore: Johns Hopkins University Press, 1986), pp. 18–26, 54–56. See G. W. McCoy, *Memorandum on "Desitin,"* January 5, 1926, on the lack of facilities for clinical research. U.S. Public Health Service (PHS), General Files, 1924–1935, Record Group (RG) 90, Box 66, NA. Where clinical facilities were needed, clinical investigators outside Washington were put on the PHS payroll. See George McCoy to Surgeon General [Cumming], August 4, 1928, and Russell L. Cecil to H. S. Cumming, September 26, 1928, PHS General Files, 1924–1935, RG 90, Box 60, NA.

25 On the regulatory responsibilities of the Hygienic Laboratory, see Laurence F. Schmeckbier, *The Public Health Service: Its History, Activities and Organization* (Baltimore: Johns Hopkins University Press, 1923), pp. 27, 129–133; Ramunas Kondratas, "The Biologics Control Act of 1902," in James Harvey Young, ed., *The Early Years of Federal Food and Drug Control* (Madison, WI: American Institute of the History of Pharmacy, 1982), pp. 8–27. On the burdens such responsibilities imposed on staff time and energy, see G. W. McCoy, *Memorandum for the Surgeon General, Attention Assistant Surgeon General A. M. Stimson,* May 24, 1927, PHS General Files, 1924–1935, RG 90, Box 70, NA; J. W. Schereschewsky to Director, Hygienic Laboratory, August 23, 1919, Public Health Service Central Files, 1897–1923, RG 90, Box 204, NA.

26 On the advantages of research institutes over universities as a site for medical research, see Henry H. Donaldson, "Research Foundations in Their Relation to Medicine," in *Medical Research and Education* (New York: Science Press, 1913), pp. 474–486. On the range and rationale of such institutes more generally, see Kohler, "Science, Foundations and Universities" (n. 19), 135–140; idem, *Partners in Science: Foundations and Natural Scientists, 1900–1945* (Chicago: University of Chicago Press, 1991), pp. 15–53.

27 Although formally established in 1901, the first director, Simon Flexner, was not appointed until June 1902 and research work at the laboratories did not begin until the fall of 1904. See George Washington Corner, *A History of the Rockefeller Institute, 1901–1953: Origins and Growth* (New York: Rockefeller University, 1965), pp. 38, 53, 56–57.

rary ideals of pure science, the institute's formula was to select a handful of individuals, "possessed with the spirit of inquiry and with the ability and training and brains to successfully explore their problems . . . and cherish these men and give them the resources and opportunity they need."[28] Like scientists at the Hygienic Laboratory, the Rockefeller Institute's members conducted most of their research at the bench rather than the bedside. With investigators granted considerable autonomy in the selection of research problems, little of the work done at the Rockefeller Institute had immediate clinical applications. Only Rufus Cole, at the Rockefeller Institute's hospital, and researchers in Simon Flexner's laboratory worked consistently and directly on problems of disease treatment and prevention.[29]

Between 1908 and 1918, Cole, Flexner, and their associates developed treatments or prophylactic vaccines for syphilis, cerebrospinal meningitis, pneumonia, and dysentery. But for Rockefeller researchers, scientific therapeutic research meant more than using the laboratory to produce new treatments: "the scientific element of the profession is looking to us for something more than the usual perfunctory reports of the few drugs which have given some promise of therapeutic activity."[30] Their self-appointed task was to show, not only how new treatments could be developed, but how they should be assessed.

The ideals of Rockefeller researchers were in keeping with the policies of therapeutic reformers. Flexner and his associates would only supply experimental treatments to those physicians able to perform a "scientific trial," so that the "value" of each treatment could be established before it was released to the general medical public.[31] Ability referred both to the investigator's acumen as an observer of disease and to the clinical and technological resources available to him. In doing a proper study, the selection of patients must be verified, by the laboratory and the clinician; the administration of treatment and the patient's response must be carefully monitored, in the laboratory and the clinic; and substantial numbers of

28 The phrases are those of Rufus Cole's, describing the Rockefeller Institute philosophy in a letter to Jerome Greene on plans to develop an institute for research in the social sciences, December 8, 1930, Rufus Cole papers, APS. See also Cole to Francis Blake, May 19, 1919, Cole papers; Corner, *History of the Rockefeller Institute* (n. 27), pp. 58, 152–153, 157–158.

29 See Corner, *History of the Rockefeller Institute* (n. 27), pp. 83–283, for a detailed description of the research programs in the various divisions. On Flexner's laboratory specifically, see ibid., pp. 81–83, 108–114, 144–149, 187–201, 237–244; on the hospital, see pp. 88–107, 249–283. See also Abner McGehee Harvey, "Rufus Cole and the Hospital of the Rockefeller Institute," and Saul Benison, "The Development of Clinical Research at the Rockefeller Institute before 1939," both in *Trends in Biomedical Research, 1901–1976* (North Tarrytown, NY: Rockefeller Archive Center, 1977), pp. 13–26 and 35–36.

30 Wade H. Brown to Simon Flexner, November 25, 1920, Flexner papers, APS; see also Rufus Cole to Francis Neufeld, April 26, 1922, Cole papers, APS.

31 On restrictions to access, see Simon Flexner to John Fordyce, June 15, 1923, and Simon Flexner to Arthur S. Loevenhart, June 19, 1923 (for tryparsamide); Simon Flexner to Dr. McClintock, June 5, 1923 (antimeningitis serum); Simon Flexner to Charles Craig, June 20, 1922, and Craig to Flexner, July 17, 1922 (for pneumonia vaccine). All in Flexner papers, APS. (The phrase "scientific trial" is Charles Craig's.) On pneumonia serum, see Rufus Cole to James W. Jobling, March 12, 1915, Cole papers, APS.

patients should be followed under comparable, "carefully controlled" conditions.[32] At a time when most hospitals were still in the process of acquiring basic laboratory facilities, Flexner's view that the "hospital was, after all, a laboratory" seemed utopian.[33]

Making the hospital into a laboratory for the study of human disease required, in the first instance, that clinical investigators command their own research laboratories, staffed and operated independently of both hospital service laboratories, intended primarily for the care of sick patients, and those research laboratories operated by physiologists, chemists, and other "basic" scientists pursuing their own research programs. Second, clinical investigators required control over the admission and management of patients whose problems they wished to study.[34] Even at the well-endowed Rockefeller Institute, it proved difficult to allow each investigator control over the resources desired for coordinated laboratory and clinical studies of new treatments.[35] Clinical investigators at other institutions found it even more difficult to accomplish their scientific aims, because they lacked the means to compel the cooperation of others. Researchers at the Russell Sage Institute of Pathology, for example, which aspired to do in studying metabolic disorders what the Rockefeller Institute had accomplished in researching infectious disease, were severely handicapped by shortages of funds and a lack of control over "clinical material."[36]

The growing importance of university medical schools as a locus for medical research after 1920 did little to solve the difficulties of clinical researchers.[37] Clinical investigators working in medical schools had to meet the demands of department chairmen to place service obligations before their research. As physi-

32 Simon Flexner to Charles F. Craig, June 20, 1922; Craig to Flexner, July 17, 1922, Flexner papers, APS; Simon Flexner to John A. Fordyce, June 15, 1923, and Fordyce to Flexner, June 18, 1923, Flexner papers; Rufus Cole to Albion Walter Hewett, January 18, 1912, Cole papers, APS.

33 Simon Flexner to Lewellys Barker, March 24, 1905, Lewellys Barker papers, Chesney Archives.

34 Corner, *History of the Rockefeller Institute* (n. 27), pp. 93–94, 106–107; Lewellys Barker, "On the Organization of the Laboratories in the Medical Clinic of the Johns Hopkins Hospital," *Bulletin of the Johns Hopkins Hospital* 18 (June–July 1907), 193–198; Francis Peabody, "Thorndike Memorial Laboratory," in *Methods and Problems of Medical Education: Series 1* (New York: Rockefeller Foundation, 1924), pp. 113–122. See also Rufus Cole to E. P. Lyon, July 29, 1915; Rufus Cole to Warfield T. Longcope, January 21, 1918, Cole papers, APS.

35 This was the case for Wade Brown's planned program for the laboratory and clinical investigation of tryparsamide (and related antisyphilis compounds). See Wade Brown to Simon Flexner, May 31, 1917; *Report of the Biological Work in Chemotherapy to the Board of Scientific Directors: The Rockefeller Institute for Medical Research* [1918]; Wade Brown, "Analysis of the Status of Clinical Work with A 189," [1918]; Brown to Flexner, March 3, 1919; Brown to Flexner, November 25, 1920. All Simon Flexner papers, APS.

36 Graham Lusk to Simon Flexner, February 17, 1920 and May 28, 1920, Flexner papers, APS.

37 Hugh Hawkins, "University Identity: The Teaching and Research Functions," in *The Organization of Modern Knowledge* (n. 15), pp. 285–312. On the development of clinical research in the university-based medical school, see A. McGehee Harvey, "Creators of Clinical Medicine's Scientific Base: Franklin Paine Mall, Lewellys Franklin Barker and Rufus Cole," in idem, *Adventures in Medical Research: A Century of Discovery at Johns Hopkins* (Baltimore: Johns Hopkins University Press, 1976), pp. 124–138.

cians, they faced competition from their medical colleagues for income, for patients to study, and for the allegiance of their students. As scientists, they faced intellectual competition from laboratory-based specialists whose mastery of the relevant intellectual concepts and methodological tools seemed to exceed their own.[38]

Whether clinical investigators were as disadvantaged as they thought with respect to their laboratory colleagues is not clear. Preclinical and clinical scientists were each inclined to emphasize their own group's special problems, and to complain that they were unable to keep pace with the economic and intellectual advances of the other.[39] What is clear is that outside of a few isolated research centers, few clinical specialists controlled the resources called for by their research programs.[40]

The difficulties faced by clinical investigators were as much cultural as material. Following on the traditions of laboratory research, clinical investigators thought in terms of the individual scientist, using his intellect to observe and master the phenomena of nature.[41] American researchers held up the example of Paul Ehrlich who, after laboriously screening hundreds of chemical compounds in the labora-

---

38 On the problems of clinical research, see the contemporary perspectives of Samuel J. Meltzer, "The Science of Clinical Medicine: What It Ought To Be and the Men to Uphold It," *JAMA* 53 (1909), 508–512; and Alfred E. Cohn, "Purposes in Medical Research: An Introduction to the Journal of Clinical Investigation," *Journal of Clinical Investigation* 1 (October, 1924), 1–11; Paul D. White and Catherine Thatcher, "Massachusetts General Hospital Cardiac Department," in *Methods and Problems of Medical Education: Series 8* (New York: Rockefeller Foundation, 1927), esp. pp. 220–221. For a historical perspective on these developments, see Maulitz, " 'Physician versus Bacteriologist' " (n. 14), pp. 91–109; see also R. S. Cunningham, "The Organization of Research in Clinical and Preclinical Departments," *Southern Medical Journal* 26 (July 1933), 615–620, who makes it clear that clinical researchers's problems with the social organization of medical schools were not unique. For the difficulties of recruiting students to research careers, see W. B. Cannon, "The Career of the Investigator," in *Medical Research and Education* (New York: Science Press, 1913), pp. 295–296. Peter English provides an example of the disdain of some physiologists for the work of their physician colleagues in his *Shock, Physiological Surgery and George Washington Crile: Medical Innovation in the Progressive Era* (Westport, CT: Greenwood Press, 1980), pp. 121–154.

39 Yandell Henderson, "Teachers in the Preclinical Sciences," *JAMA* 74 (May 15, 1920), 1416–1417; Joseph Erlanger, C. M. Jackson, Graham Lusk, et al., "An Investigation of Conditions in the Departments of the Preclinical Sciences: Report of a Committee of the Division of Medical Sciences of the National Research Council," *JAMA* 74 (April 17, 1920), 1117–1122. The relative disadvantages of each group apparently varied decade by decade and by locale. Historians have not yet begun to collect the kind of quantitative data on careers in various disciplines that would permit us to adjudicate these claims.

40 For an overview of activities in medical research at specific centers around the country, see A. McGehee Harvey's invaluable *Science at Bedside: Clinical Research in America, 1905–1945* (Baltimore: Johns Hopkins University Press, 1981).

41 The importance of having the individual investigator's mind and hands on the experiment may be seen in William S. McCann, "The Influence of Graham Lusk upon His Students," in *Addresses Given at a Memorial Meeting for Graham Lusk at the New York Academy of Medicine on December 10, 1932* (Baltimore, 1933), 13; Rufus Cole to Henry A. Christian, December 1, 1916, Cole papers, APS; Harry M. Marks, *Local Knowledge: Experimental Communities and Experimental Practices, 1918–1950*, a paper presented at the conference on Twentieth Century Health Sciences: Problems and Interpretations, University of California, San Francisco, May 1988.

tory for antisyphilitic activity, no less carefully screened the clinical investigators who would test the most promising laboratory drug, "606," at the bedside.[42] The Canadian researchers who discovered insulin and the American researchers at Harvard who developed liver extracts for the treatment for pernicious anemia were similarly selective in choosing clinicians to evaluate these therapies. Like Ehrlich, however, the drugs' developers soon found that they could not control research supplies of the drugs.[43]

To reformers interested in improving therapeutic standards, cooperative studies employing the talents of researchers at several institutions seemed a unique device for overcoming the limited vision and opportunities of individual investigators. During the Great War, politicians of science had extended existing opportunities for collaboration among researchers from government, academia, and industry.[44] After the war, such self-appointed spokesmen as the National Research Council's George Ellery Hale and the Carnegie Institution's John Merriam sought to broaden the principle to include collaboration among scientists of different disciplines and/or different institutions. The voluntaristic ideals of individuals like Hale and Merriam fit in well with the political assumptions of Herbert Hoover's associative state, ensuring the appeal of "cooperative" enterprises of various stripes and scales.

Depending on who was employing the term, "cooperative" research might mean little more than the occasional collaboration of physicists with chemists, or as much as the application to scientific "men" of principles of discipline and organization learned in the army and the modern corporation. Such ambiguity enhanced rather than detracted from the appeal of "cooperative research," broadening the ideological base of support for such ventures.[45]

42 For contemporary idealizations of Ehrlich, see F. H. Garrison, "Ehrlich's Specific Therapeutics in Relation to Scientific Method," *Popular Science Monthly* 78 (March 1911), 209–22; S. J. Meltzer, "The Present Status of Therapeutics and the Significance of Salvarsan," *JAMA* 56 (June 10, 1911), 1709–1713. On Ehrlich's supervision of clinical testing, see Patricia Spain Ward, "The American Reception of Salvarsan," *JHM* (January 1981), 46.

43 On salvarsan, see Ward, "American Reception of Salvarsan" (n. 42); on insulin, see John P. Swann, *Academic Scientists and the Pharmaceutical Industry: Cooperative Research in Twentieth-Century America* (Baltimore: Johns Hopkins University Press, 1988), pp. 133–135, 139–140; on pernicious anemia, see Swann, ibid., pp. 155–162; William B. Castle to William S. Middleton, May 15, 1930, Box 7, William S. Middleton papers, NLM. Other researchers faced similar problems; see Simon Flexner to Arthur S. Loevenhart, November 14, 1923, and December 12, 1923; Wade Brown, "Analysis of the Status of Clinical Work with A 189" [1918]; and Brown to Flexner, March 3, 1919, all in Simon Flexner papers, APS.

44 On the wartime programs of the NRC, see Daniel J. Kevles, "George Ellery Hale, the First World War and the Advancement of Science," *Isis* 59 (1968), 427–437; idem, *The Physicists: The History of a Scientific Community in Modern America* (New York: Vintage Books, 1979), pp. 139–154; and, on the postwar NRC, David F. Noble, *America by Design: Science, Technology and the Rise of Corporate Capitalism* (New York: Alfred A. Knopf, 1977), esp. pp. 153–166. On World War I and organizational reform in medicine, see Rosemary Stevens, *In Sickness and in Wealth: American Hospitals in the Twentieth Century* (New York: Basic Books, 1989), pp. 80–104.

45 On American corporatism, see Ellis Hawley, "Herbert Hoover, the Commerce Secretariat, and the Vision of an Associative State," *Journal of American History* 61 (June 1974), 116–140. On the functions of ambiguity in political language, see JoAnne Brown, *The Definition of a Profession: The*

The majority of working medical researchers held no particular brief for the ideological virtues of cooperation. Rather, cooperative studies seemed to offer an organizational solution to a variety of intellectual problems. Their special appeal was in promising to combine several investigative virtues in one: gathering large numbers of patients, to offset the effects of spontaneous recoveries; bringing the combined judgments of experienced investigators to bear on a problem, to offset the effects of individual bias; and, so far as was possible, specifying in advance the means and techniques for selecting patients, delivering treatment, and evaluating results.

Despite their perceived scientific advantages, cooperative studies proved especially difficult to carry out. Researchers wishing to engage in cooperative therapeutic experiments not only had to develop the necessary financial resources to support their work, but they had to adopt social norms and organizational controls that would ensure that a plan of study, once agreed on, would be carried out according to agreement. Such sacrifices of intellectual autonomy proved especially difficult for researchers raised in a medical culture that prized individual experience and judgment above all else.

The following section examines the experiences of a pioneering venture in organized therapeutic research: the Cooperative Clinical Group study of syphilis treatment.[46]

THE COOPERATIVE CLINICAL GROUP STUDY

In March 1928, John H. Stokes, Professor of Dermatology and Syphilology at the University of Pennsylvania and scientific advisor for the newly organized Committee on Research in Syphilis, invited a small group of colleagues to join him in a multiclinic "attack" on the problems of treating syphilis. The enterprise offered little money but "perhaps a little glory and certainly a wonderful chance to do something in research in syphilis in this country."[47] Stokes's "wonderful chance"

Authority of Metaphor in the History of Intelligence Testing, 1890–1930 (Princeton: Princeton University Press, 1992), pp. 13–14. On the NRC programs in cooperative research, see Glenn E. Bugos, "Managing Cooperative Research and Borderland Science in the NRC, 1922–1942," *Historical Studies in the Physical and Biological Sciences* 20 (1989), 1–32. On Merriam's activities, see Frank F. Bunker, "Cooperative Research: Its Conduct and Interpretation," in *Cooperation in Research by Staff Members and Research Associates of the Carnegie Institution of Washington* (Washington, DC: Carnegie Institution of Washington, 1938), pp. 713–742. For a discussion that links the hospital, clinical research, and organizational reform, see Raymond Pearl, "Modern Methods in Handling Statistics," *Bulletin of the Johns Hopkins Hospital* 32 (1921), 186–193.

46 For prior studies of the Cooperative Clinical Group, see Harry Dowling, "The Emergence of the Cooperative Trial," *Transactions and Studies of the College of Physicians of Philadelphia,* 4th ser., 43 (July 1975), 20–29, and Harry M. Marks, "Notes From the Underground: The Social Organization of Therapeutic Research, 1920–1950," in Russell C. Maulitz and Diana E. Long, eds., *Grand Rounds: One Hundred Years of Internal Medicine* (Philadelphia: University of Pennsylvania Press, 1988), pp. 297–336, from which portions of the following are taken.

47 Stokes to O'Leary, March 26, 1928, F 235, Thomas Parran Jr. papers, University of Pittsburgh [hereafter cited as Parran papers].

was an opportunity to establish a standard for syphilis treatment based on facts rather than opinion.

Apart from Stokes, participants included Udo Wile, Professor of Dermatology and Syphilology at the University of Michigan and Stokes's former mentor; Joseph Earle Moore, a Johns Hopkins professor who, like Stokes, was at work on one of the first textbooks summarizing the "modern" treatment of syphilis; Paul O'Leary, who had taken over from Stokes as head of the Dermatology Section at the Mayo Clinic in 1924; and Harold Cole, a respected dermatologist at Western Reserve and close associate of the therapeutic reformer, Torald Sollman. Thomas Parran Jr., Commissioner of Public Health for New York State and soon to be Surgeon General of the U.S. Public Health Service, served as the public spokesman for the study and the unofficial arbiter among the feuding clinicians.

Distinguished specialists in venereal disease, Stokes and his collaborators saw many more patients, for much longer periods of time, than the average practitioner. If the group could agree on uniform standards for selecting, classifying, treating, and evaluating patients, they might provide a reliable guide among the welter of opinions that bedeviled practicing physicians in choosing among syphilis treatments.[48]

The physician treating syphilis in the late 1920s faced an embarrassment of riches: a diversity of drugs and an even greater diversity of opinions about how to use them. Since the introduction of Paul Ehrlich's salvarsan (arsphenamine) in 1910, pharmaceutical researchers had added neoarsphenamine and a variety of other arsenical compounds designed to potentiate the more toxic effects of Ehrlich's drug. Easier to prepare and safer to administer, the newer arsenicals were especially favored by practitioners who did not specialize in treating syphilis. But their value was doubted in turn by some who had mastered the art of using the more potent drug.[49] Along with development of the arsenicals came improve-

---

48 Committee on Research in Syphilis, Scientific Committee, *Draft Agenda for Session on Clinical Problems,* April 30, 1928, F 220, Parran papers.

49 On medical and public health approaches to syphilis prior to the 1930s, see Allan M. Brandt, *No Magic Bullet: A Social History of Venereal Disease in the United States since 1880* (New York: Oxford University Press, 1985), pp. 4–133. From the outset, specialists advocated that physicians receive hands-on training in administering salvarsan. Henry Eksber, "The New Treatment of Syphilis (Ehrlich-Hata): Observations and Results," *JAMA* 55 (December 10, 1910), 2053. On the difficulties of using the drug, see Oliver S. Ormsby, "Salvarsan and Neosalvarsan in Syphilis," *JAMA* 68 (March 31, 1917), 949–950. On the pros and cons of endorsing the use of neoarsphenamine, see "Abstract of Discussion," *Transactions of the Section on Pharmacology and Therapeutics. A. M. A.* (1920), 217–228. Although various improvements in the manufacture and technique of administering arsphenamine occurred following its introduction, it remained a trickier drug to administer. See Joseph Earle Moore, Harold N. Cole, J. F. Schamberg, H. C. Solomon, Udo J. Wile, and John H. Stokes, "The Management of Syphilis in General Practice," *Venereal Disease Information* 10 (February 29, 1929), 66–73. On the production of arsphenamine in the United States, see Jonathan Michael Liebenau, *Medical Science and Medical Industry, 1898–1929: A Study of Pharmaceutical Manufacturing in Philadelphia* (Ph.D. thesis, University of Pennsylvania, 1981), 313–351, and on the use of sulpharsphenamine and neoarsphenamine relative to arsphenamine, see George H. Bigelow and N. A. Nelson, "The Distribution of Arsenicals by the Massachusetts Department of Public Health," *NEJM* 201 (October 17, 1929), 761–763.

ments in more traditional treatments. Heavy metals, such as mercury, with limited powers to attack the infecting spirochetes, were nonetheless believed to promote local and general resistance to the disease, complementing the arsenicals' specific spirocheticidal effect.[50] Venereal disease specialists, while advocating the superiority of arsphenamine, agreed on little else: schedules of treatment, co-therapies, and the duration of treatment were all up for debate.[51]

The members of the Cooperative Clinical Group, by reviewing the records of their own experiences, meant to provide a more authoritative basis for recommending one syphilis treatment over another. Once successful in their initial endeavors, they hoped to become a national resource for the evaluation of new syphilis remedies as they were developed. Studies conducted by experienced specialists would, they anticipated, be of much greater value than the haphazard evaluations sponsored by the manufacturers of new remedies or the solitary general practitioner.[52]

The simplicity of their objectives masked the complexity of the task. Awaiting the Cooperative Group was a host of unresolved questions: which stages of syphilis, and what combinations of treatment should be studied first? Which patients should be included and which kept out? Who should perform the assessments of outcomes? What constituted a treatment success and what a failure? What kinds of ancillary data, clinical and laboratory, were needed to make sense of the results? Deciding such questions was a necessary stage in any therapeutic study. What made the Cooperative Group unusual was the requirement that the investigators agree on the answers.

From the beginning, the Cooperative Group was plagued with the problem they had set out to resolve: the lack of uniformity among physicians in approaches to treating syphilis. "Astonishing variations between the course pursued by different patients in the same clinic as well as between the practice of individual clinics frequently disclosed themselves."[53] Unlike the majority of physicians, the

---

50 On combination treatments, see John H. Stokes, "The Application and Limitations of Arsphenamine in Therapeutics," *Transactions. Section on Therapeutics and Pharmacology. A. M. A.* (1920), 194–197. The introduction of bismuth, less toxic than mercury, in 1922 further assisted the resurgence of interest in combined treatments. See Carroll S. Wright, "The Effect of Bismuth Alone and in Combination with the Arsenobenzenes on the Wasserman Reaction," *American Journal of Medical Sciences* 173 (February 1927), 232. While few experts recommended treatment with mercury alone, it was still preferred by some physicians as an initial treatment. Jay F. Schamberg and Carroll S. Wright, *Treatment of Syphilis* (New York: D. Appleton, 1932), p. 3.

51 Compare the conclusions of Louis Chargin, favoring the use of intensive therapy with rest periods, with Joseph Moore's advocacy of continuous, alternating, treatment. Louis Chargin, "Early Syphilis: Results," *Archives of Dermatology and Syphilis* 19 (May 1929), 750–763; Joseph Earle Moore and Albert Keidel, "The Treatment of Early Syphilis: I. A Plan of Therapy for Routine Use," *Bulletin of the Johns Hopkins Hospital* 39 (July 1926), 6–8.

52 *Report of the Conference of Clinicians. January 5–6, 1929,* F 226; Parran to O'Leary, May 7, 1929, F 235, Parran papers; Joseph Earle Moore, "Clinical Investigation in Syphilis," *Venereal Disease Information* 9 (December 20, 1928), 529.

53 John H. Stokes, Harold N. Cole, Joseph Earle Moore, Paul A. O'Leary, Udo J. Wile, Taliaferro Clark, Thomas Parran Jr., and Lida J. Usilton, "Cooperative Clinical Studies in the Treatment of Syphilis: Early Syphilis," *Venereal Disease Information* 13 (June 1932), 208.

specialists in the Cooperative Group favored arsphenamine, the original and more difficult to handle arsenical. But a reliance on arsphenamine was all they had in common: how frequently they used it, the preferred dosages, and the choice of co-treatment (mercury or bismuth) varied from clinic to clinic and patient to patient.[54]

Were the difficulties of classifying patients by stage of disease, regimen, and treatment outcome merely technical, they might have been readily resolved. Yet each time a question seemed to be settled, it arose again.[55] Differences of opinion about how to classify patients, treatments and outcomes were at the heart of existing therapeutic controversies: "It seems as if the question of interpretation is an individual matter for every case and accordingly the abstracting of each case would have to be conducted by the head of the department personally and then would reflect to a considerable extent his particular slant on the treatment of syphilis."[56]

Committed to a program of rigorous therapeutic investigations, the senior clinicians involved in the study nonetheless found it difficult to devote the necessary time and attention to the cooperative project. The lure of other research "work of a more spontaneous nature" grew progressively stronger, and the daily work of classifying patients and outcomes accordingly fell to the statistical clerks provided by the Public Health Service.[57] The problem was organizational, the consequences intellectual: without the active participation of experienced clinicians, Joseph Moore deemed the resulting analyses unreliable. The delegation of the abstracting to statisticians, Moore argued, "introduces into the whole study a problematic inaccuracy which . . . may invalidate the whole material."[58]

Cooperative studies were meant to transcend the limited resources of individual institutions. But in the case of the Cooperative Clinical Group, collaboration proved to demand more, not less, of individual researchers: more time, more energy, and more willingness to reach agreement about fundamental issues in the biology and management of human disease, a particularly elusive goal in the case of syphilis. The work of cooperating overloaded clinicians whose efforts were already divided among laboratory and clinical research, patient care, and teaching.

54 Ibid.
55 Lida J. Usilton, Memorandum for Doctor Joseph Earle Moore, January 15, 1935, F 223, Parran papers.
56 Stokes to Parran, August 16, 1929, F 236, Parran papers.
57 Wile to Parran, March 9, 1932, F 231; Moore to Parran, January 21, 1932, F 228. On the difficulties that arose when senior investigators tried to review the statisticians' work, see Joseph Earle Moore to John H. Stokes, April 1, 1932, F 224, and to Thomas Parran Jr., April 2, 1932; Stokes to Moore, April 4, 1932, F 228. See also Stokes to Parran, May 23, 1930, F 230. Experience was no teacher in this regard: the same problem recurred in developing the group's later papers on cardiovascular syphilis. Harold N. Cole to John McMullen [Assistant Surgeon General], April 20, 1935, F 223. All references to Parran papers.
58 Joseph Earle Moore to John H. Stokes, April 6, 1932, PHS, VD Division 1918–1936, Committee on Research in Syphilis, RG 90, Box 326, NA. See also Moore to Stokes, July 25, 1934, F 222, Parran papers.

In organizing its study, the Cooperative Group lacked examples to follow, and it lacked what development economists call an "infrastructure": a network of resources, personnel, and opportunities on which to draw, and the ability to use them productively. The problems to be resolved ranged from issues of intellectual credit (Who were the authors in a cooperative study?) to more mundane questions of financial management (Could the funds intended to pay for a nurse and an automobile be used to keep a doctor on the study payroll instead?).[59] Most serious were those circumstances – intellectual and material – directly preventing the principal investigators from accomplishing their scientific aims. The ideological barriers that kept them from leaving nonmedical personnel in charge of the data analysis were every bit as real as the material lack of time available for the principals to complete the work on their own. Together, they made the already difficult intellectual questions about measuring the outcomes of treatment or the severity of disease practically impossible to resolve.

At the Public Health Service's request, the group's initial studies were published in *Venereal Disease Information*, the house organ of the service's Venereal Disease Division.[60] Two years after publication, Surgeon General Thomas Parran expressed concern that "the detailed reports have made very little impression upon the medical profession. . . . I think a large part of the practical value of our studies will be lost unless a concerted effort is planned and put into practice for persistent propagandizing of the medical profession with the facts elicited by the studies."[61] Publishing their findings in an obscure journal, further concealed by the detailed presentation of the methodology, did not help. But for all their careful work, members of the Cooperative Group did not have much to show: "we found ourselves in the unique situation of measuring one type of treatment, namely that administered in high type clinics, while in this country at least, a large part of the syphilis treatment is in the hands of private practitioners using quite another type of treatment."[62]

The study clinics principally used arsphenamine, a drug "too complex for the practicing physician" to handle. Meanwhile, they had produced little or no data on the merits of the most commonly used treatments – neoarsphenamine, silver arsphenamine, or bismarsen – much less how they compared with arsphenamine.[63] Arsphenamine was, in the opinion of specialists, the treatment of choice, and

59 On questions of intellectual credit, see Harry M. Marks, "Notes from the Underground" (n. 46), 304; on the budgeting issue, see Harold Cole to Thomas Parran, November 24, 1930, F 228, Parran papers.
60 Moore was especially reluctant to "smothering" his paper in *VDI*. Taliaferro Clark to Parran, October 29, 1931, F 221, Parran papers; Stokes strongly objected when the Public Health Service indicated it would be unable to provide substantial numbers of reprints at a subsidized price, which "seems to me to be one unintentional method of blanketing the work so far as its popularization and dissemination among the medical profession is concerned." See Stokes to Clark, June 21, 1932, F 230, Parran papers.
61 Parran to John McMullen, May 9, 1934, F 222, Parran papers.
62 *Minutes of the Fourth Meeting of the Cooperative Clinical Group,* May 6, 1931, F 220, Parran papers.
63 Moore to Parran, December 20, 1930, F 228, Parran papers.

establishing more precisely its therapeutic value remained a desirable objective from the Cooperative Group's point of view. Officials of the Public Health Service, which had supported and assisted the study, felt otherwise:

All health officers know that few physicians in private practice will go to the trouble of making up old arsphenamine even though they are qualified to do so. If we are to succeed in our campaign to encourage physicians to administer intravenous treatment for syphilis, I believe it is necessary that we recommend neo-arsphenamine because of its simplicity of administration until some drug of much greater efficacy is discovered.[64]

The Cooperative Group had planned to examine the relative merits of simpler, if less effective, treatments, which "would enable us to outline for the vast army of physicians who treat the majority of patients with early syphilis, if not the ideal treatment scheme, at least the best treatment scheme which they are capable of carrying through."[65] But its plans for more comprehensive, prospective, therapeutic research into the merits of new syphilis treatments foundered repeatedly on an inability to find a stable source of funding.[66]

In an era when laboratory research received the lion's share of philanthropic largesse, obtaining stable funds for clinical studies was difficult.[67] If finding interested money was difficult, getting money from sources that were interested *and* respectable was even more problematic. Thomas Parran, who did not operate a clinic of his own, objected to various proposals from the investigators to solicit funds from "responsible" drug manufacturers: "I have always thought that manufacturers of pharmaceuticals are the least desirable of all possible sources of funds for syphilis research."[68] Even if corporate sponsors did not exploit the group's research in subsequent promotions, as Parran and Stokes feared, they lacked the necessary appearance of impartiality. Research into the value of syphilis

---

64 R. A. Vonderlehr to Moore, February 29, 1936, F 223, Parran papers.

65 Moore to Parran, January 21, 1932, F 228, Parran papers.

66 The account that follows draws on the more detailed discussion in Marks, "Notes from the Underground" (n. 46), pp. 306–307.

67 On lack of support for clinical investigation, see Harold Cole to Parran, January 29 and February 18, 1929, F 227; O'Leary to Edward L. Keyes, April 16, 1929, F 235; Stokes to Moore, February 8, 1929, F 228; Moore to Parran, October 7, 1931, F 222, all Parran papers. The lack of stable funding was a generic problem in medical research prior to 1930, with short-term grants predominating. See Richard H. Shryock, *American Medical Research* (New York: Commonwealth Fund, 1947), p. 107.

68 Parran to Moore, October 13, 1931, F 222, Parran papers. Harold Cole was similarly suspicious of subsidies from commercial firms. In this he was probably following the lead of his mentor, Torald Sollman, who, as the leading figure of AMA's Council on Pharmacy and Chemistry, had ample reason to suspect the motives of individual firms. See Cole's objections to accepting a subvention from Abbott Laboratories to publishing the Cooperative Group's studies under its auspices: Cole to O'Leary, February 16, 1935, and to John McMullen [Assistant Surgeon General], PHS, Venereal Disease Division, 1918–1936, RG 90, Box 325, NA. For proposals, see *Report of the Conference of Clinicians. January 5–6, 1929,* F 226, Parran papers; Moore to Parran, January 21, 1932, Venereal Disease Division, 1918–1936, RG 90, Box 324, NA; and Stokes to Parran, December 18, 1930, F 236, and Moore to Parran, January 3, 1932, F 228, Parran papers.

treatments not only had to be disinterested, it had to appear disinterested.[69] The Cooperative Group limped along, with support from the Milbank Fund and a starting grant from H. M. Timkin of "Timkin Roller Bearing" fame, but its more expansive plans for prospective testing of syphilis treatments had to be curtailed.[70]

When the Cooperative Group was first getting underway, Joseph Earle Moore had worried that, with Public Health Service sponsorship, the study might prove *too* influential: the service's "prestige . . . in this country was so great" that if it endorsed "incomplete or erroneous conclusions it might take years to remove the impression created on the medical profession."[71] Moore need not have worried. With the publication of studies on syphilis in pregnancy and cardiovascular syphilis, the active phase of the Cooperative Group began to wind down.[72]

Its reports did not take the medical world by storm. Outside of a few specialized areas, its therapeutic pronouncements contained few surprises. The uniqueness of the enterprise was nonetheless duly noted, and over the years the group's results became a benchmark against which other studies could compare themselves.[73] Clinicians who relied on the Cooperative Group as an authoritative source were sometimes "surprised," on closer examination, "to see what a relatively small number of cases the [critical conclusions about] neoarsphenamine are based on."[74]

As the Cooperative Clinical Group study was getting underway, another group of researchers was confronting head on the difficulties of getting community practitioners to trust a treatment that, decades of experience had taught them, could only be used safely and effectively by experienced specialists with access to the latest hospital laboratory facilities. In the Commonwealth Fund's field studies of serum treatment for lobar pneumonia, therapeutic reformers encountered the

69 See the extensive correspondence between Stokes and Parran in the fall of 1929 regarding the misrepresentation of some of Harold Cole's work by Loeser Laboratory, manufacturer of a bismuth solution for treating syphilis in F 221; see also Parran to Stokes, December 31, 1930, F 230, both Parran papers.

70 On Timkin, see O'Leary to Parran, March 27, 1929, and February 27, March 8, and April 26, 1929, F 221. Parran obtained funding from the Milbank Fund in part by emphasizing the public health importance of evaluating syphilis treatments. See Parran to John A. Kingsbury, January 12, 1931, F 222. All Parran papers.

71 Moore to Stokes, November 16, 1928, F 228, Parran papers.

72 Harold N. Cole with Lida J. Usilton, Joseph Earle Moore, Paul A. O'Leary, John H. Stokes, Udo J. Wile, Thomas Parran Jr., and R. A. Vonderlehr, "Syphilis in Pregnancy," *Venereal Disease Information* 17 (February 1936), 39–46; idem, "Cardiovascular Syphilis," *Venereal Disease Information* 17 (April 1936), 91–118.

73 Louis Chargin, William Leifer, and Theodore Rosenthal, "Marpharsen in the Treatment of Early Syphilis: Comparison of Results in One Hundred and Eighty-Eight Cases with Those of the Cooperative Clinical Group," *Archives of Dermatology and Syphilology* 40 (August 1939), 208–217.

74 [Cornell] Conferences on Therapy, "Evaluation of Drugs Used in the Treatment of Syphilis," *JAMA* 112 (June 10, 1939), 2417. As late as 1937, even PHS officials were skeptical about the strength of the evidence on which claims for the superiority of arsphenamine rested. R. A. Vonderlehr to Joseph Earle Moore, August 21, 1937, PHS, General Classified Files, 1936–1944, RG 90, Box 53, NA.

ultimate barrier to a rational therapeutics: the practitioner's concern to do nothing which would jeopardize the loyalty of his patients.

PNEUMONIA: FROM THE LABORATORY TO THE BEDSIDE

In 1913, the Rockefeller Institute's Rufus Cole introduced what was arguably the first successful serum treatment for pneumococcal pneumonia. The object of over twenty years' laboratory research, serum therapy for pneumonia relied on serum from intentionally infected animals, which, when injected in patients with pneumonia, appeared to lower mortality. Cole's serum was based on the recent observation that there were several "types" of pneumococci, and that a serum developed from one such type had no effect on pneumonias caused by another.[75] Just how the serum worked, no one knew, but by 1917, Cole and his co-workers were reporting mortality of 7.5 percent in serum-treated patients, well below the case fatalities of 30 percent or more generally experienced. Cole's results remained exceptional, however, even among advocates of the serum.[76]

The use of Cole's serum was inhibited less by doubts about its potential value than by its numerous practical disadvantages. It was injected intravenously, then an unfamiliar procedure to many physicians. A successful course of treatment could require repeated administration of serum over one or more days, easier to accomplish in the large urban hospitals than in community practice. More important, the horse-based serum produced reactions in many patients, ranging from severe chills to the potentially life-threatening allergic response experienced by a small proportion of a patients. To guard against such reactions, Cole advocated "day and night" supervision of the patient over the course of treatment.[77] Although

75 Rufus Cole, "Treatment of Pneumonia by Means of Specific Serums," *JAMA* 61 (August 30, 1913), 663–666; for an overview of serum therapy, and the development of pneumonia serums, see Harry Dowling, *Fighting Infection: Conquests of the Twentieth Century* (Cambridge: Harvard University Press, 1977), pp. 36–49; idem, "Frustration and Foundation: Management of Pneumonia before Antibiotics," *JAMA* 220 (June 5, 1972), 1341–1345. I have found no satisfactory historical account of the earliest work on pneumonia serum, or of the relation between the German and American research in the 1910s. For a comparative account of British and American reactions to serum treatments in the 1920s and 1930s, which in my view overemphasizes U.S. enthusiasm for the therapy, see Michael Worboys, "Treatments for Pneumonia in Britain, 1910–1940," in Ilana Löwy, ed., *Medicine and Change: Historical and Sociological Studies of Medical Innovation* (Paris: Editions John Libbey Eurotext, 1993), pp. 317–336.

76 Oswald T. Avery, H. T. Chickering, Rufus Cole, and A. R. Dochez, *Acute Lobar Pneumonia: Prevention and Serum Treatment* (New York: Rockefeller Institute for Medical Research, 1917), p. 79. For comparative results, see Augustus K. Wadsworth, "Review of Recently Published Reports on the Serum Treatment of Type I Pneumonia, Together with a Report of 445 Additional Cases," *American Journal of Hygiene* 4 (March 1924), 119–33; Edwin A. Locke, "The Treatment of Type I Pneumococcus Lobar Pneumonia with Specific Serum," *JAMA* 80 (May 26, 1923), 1510–1511. Although Locke thought the serum would eventually prove itself useful, he was extremely critical of Cole's observations, and his failure to use simultaneous untreated controls; see ibid., 1508–1509.

77 Avery et al., *Acute Lobar Pneumonia* (n. 76), pp. 60–74 (quotation from p. 69); William S. Thomas, "Type I Pneumonia and Its Serum Treatment," *JAMA* 77 (December 31, 1921), 2102–2103.

improvements in the serum and increased experience with its clinical use reduced the frequency and hazards of the injections required, the potential of adverse patient reactions to serum remained a powerful deterrent to its use by the inexperienced practitioner.[78]

While the hazards and inconveniences of serum treatment loomed large, its benefits were diminished by the requirement for type-specific serum. Cole claimed results only for patients infected with Type I pneumonia. By the end of the decade, other researchers reported successes with Type II pneumonias.[79] A patient treated with the wrong serum would not respond to treatment. Selecting the correct serum meant sending a sputum sample to one of the few laboratories equipped for pneumococcal typing. Moreover, as specialists soon discovered, the serum worked best when given early in the disease, underscoring the need to establish "the diagnosis of [pneumococcal] type ... at the earliest possible moment."[80]

In the fifteen years following its introduction, serum therapy for pneumonia was used by only a handful of practitioners with access to hospital and laboratory facilities, and considerable experience in administering serum.[81] The majority of physicians steered clear of serum treatment, deterred by the practical impediments to its use, including its high cost.[82] To Cole (and other serum advocates), money was a poor excuse for depriving patients of the therapeutic benefits: "if it could

78 On the persistence of reactions with the improved serums, see Horace S. Baldwin and Russell L. Cecil, "The Rationale of Specific Therapy in Pneumococcus Pneumonia," *JAMA* 87 (November 20, 1926), 1715; Frederick T. Lord to Russell L. Cecil, June 15, 1928, Frederick T. Lord papers, Countway Library [hereafter Lord papers].

79 Russell L. Cecil, "The Treatment of Lobar Pneumonia with Pneumococcus Antibody Solution," *New York State Journal of Medicine* 25 (March 6, 1925), 355–358; F. M. Huntoon, "Treatment of Pneumonia with Pneumococcus Antibody Solution," *Transactions of the American Therapeutic Society* 27 (1926), 206–207; William H. Park, Jesse G. M. Bullowa, Milton Rosenbluth, "The Treatment of Lobar Penumonia with Refined Specific Antibacterial Serum," *JAMA* 91 (November 17, 1928), 1503–1507; Rufus Cole, "Serum Treatment in Type I Lobar Pneumonia," *JAMA* 93 (September 7, 1929), 741–742.

80 Frederick T. Lord, "The Serum Treatment of Type I Pneumococcus Pneumonia," *Medical Clinics of North America* 7 (November 1923), 778–780 (quotation from 779); Locke, "The Treatment of Type I Pneumococcus Lobar Pneumonia" (n. 76), 1507.

81 On the difficulties of using serum for the general practitioner without access to laboratory facilities, see L. L. Powell, "Treatment of Pneumonia Based upon Clinical, Bacteriological and Pathological Findings," *Journal of the Maine Medical Association* 10 (January 1920), 164; F. C. Rinker, "The Care and Treatment of Pneumonia," *Virginia Medical Monthly* 48 (April 1921), 37; W. W. Herrick, "Serum Treatment and Management of Lobar Pneumonia," *Medical Record* 99 (June 4, 1921), 950; Blodgett, [Remarks in Discussion at Vermont Medical Society], *NEJM* 202 (May 22, 1930), 994.

82 Little used, the costs of serum treatment remained high, unlike that of other biological products. See George H. Bigelow, "The Serum Treatment of Pneumonia," *NEJM* 206 (July 30, 1931), 245. Cost estimates at the end of the decade are available in *Pneumonia Mortality and Health Department Facilities for Typing Pneumococci,* prepared by Kenneth McGill, National Institutes of Health, General Records 1930–1948, RG 443, Box 14, F 0425, NA. For expressions of concern over cost, see Doctor Kirkbride to Doctor Parran, February 4, 1935, F 147, Parran papers.

be demonstrated that it was effective, the matter of expense and labor involved should not be a serious matter. After all most of the procedures carried out by the surgeons are expensive and laborious, but nevertheless they are widely employed."[83]

Demonstrating efficacy was not a simple matter. As with arsphenamine, experts agreed in general about the value of the treatment but disagreed about the dosages to be used, how late in an illness treatment could start and still be effective, the necessity for typing before beginning treatment, and the type of serum to be used. In 1924, Harvard Medical School's Lloyd Felton had introduced a "concentrated serum" that was said to be easier and safer to use than Cole's original serum. By the end of the decade, New York pneumonia specialists who had studied Felton's serum over several pneumonia seasons pronounced it safe and effective, while others, including Cole and his former student, Francis Blake, regarded it as still "experimental."[84] Cole's skepticism regarding Felton's serum was largely based on the difficulties of obtaining a standard measure of potency for Felton's serum without further laboratory research. Lacking such a measure, effective dosages would vary from lot to lot. Unless units of standard potency were used, Cole maintained, one never knew whether a treatment failure was due to underdosing, or to a more basic inadequacy of the serum. To Cole, premature advocacy of Felton's serum in clinical practice violated the orderly progression of therapeutic knowledge from laboratory to clinic, threatening to "discredit a therapeutic measure that is apparently of value."[85]

With the high death toll from pneumonia largely unaltered, public health specialists and other clinicians were less cautious than Cole. In 1928, the Massa-

83 Rufus Cole to Fred Neufeld, April 26, 1922, Cole papers, APS. Cole was not alone in contrasting the willingness to invest in surgery with the unwillingness to pay for (medically supervised) serum treatment. See Harold D. Levine, "The Opportunity for the Modern Treatment of Lobar Pneumonia in General Practice," *NEJM* 219 (October 27, 1938), 647. See also C. N. B. Camac, "Antipneumococcus Serum in Lobar Pneumonia: A Clinical Report," *American Journal of Medical Sciences* 166 (December 1923), 541.

84 William H. Park, Jesse G. M. Bullowa, and Milton Rosenbluth, "The Treatment of Lobar Pneumonia . . . ," *JAMA* 91 (November 17, 1928), 1503–1507; Jesse Bullowa, "The Serum Treatment and Its Evaluation in Lobar Pneumonia," *Bulletin of the New York Academy of Medicine* 5 (1928), 328–362; Russell L. Cecil and Norman Plummer, "Pneumococcus Type I Pneumonia: A Study of Eleven Hundred and Sixty-One Cases, with Especial Reference to Specific Therapy," *JAMA* 95 (November 22, 1930), 1548–53; Russell L. Cecil, "The Prevention and Treatment of Pneumonia," *New York State Medical Journal* 30 (February 15, 1930), 210–214; Francis G. Blake, "The Diagnosis and Treatment of Pneumonia," *NEJM* 262 (May 22, 1930), 994; Rufus Cole to G. W. McCoy, May 31, 1929, Cole papers, APS.

85 For reservations about the value of Felton's serum, see Rufus Cole, "Serum Treatment in Type I Lobar Pneumonia," *JAMA* 93 (September 7, 1929), 746–747; Blake, "Diagnosis and Treatment" (n. 84), 94; George McCoy [Director, Hygienic Laboratory] to C. W. White, January 5, 1929, National Institutes of Health, 1930–1948, General Records, RG 443, Box 27, F 0470, NA. See also Rufus Cole to Augustus B. Wadsworth, February 7, 1930, and Cole to G. W. McCoy, February 28, 1933, Cole papers, APS. Felton's advocates were publicly dismissive of Cole's arcane concern. For Cole's concerns at an earlier stage of serum development about disrupting evaluation of serum through premature clinical dissemination, see Rufus Cole, in "Discussion," *Transactions of Congress of American Surgeons and Physicians* 10 (1916), 140.

chusetts Department of Public Health had begun distributing Felton's serum to a select group of hospitals. The high costs of serum production led Commissioner George H. Bigelow to initiate a study "to determine once and for all whether the State should undertake the manufacture and distribution of such a serum on a state-wide basis."[86] Incorporated in this succinct statement of the problem were several, sometimes conflicting, objectives: Was Felton's serum "effective"? Could community practitioners be induced to use serum in both a clinically and economically effective manner? Could the serum itself be made more potent and less dangerous?[87]

To the Commonwealth Fund, which financed the Massachusetts study, and to the pneumonia specialists who served on its advisory committee, the study's main objective was clear: to promote the safe and effective use of pneumonia serum by general practitioners.[88] If general practitioners would not bring their pneumonia patients to the hospital for serum treatment, public health authorities would bring the hospital's laboratory facilities (and free serum) to them.

But along with free serum came the culture of rational therapeutics, and an elaborate system of controls to ensure that the serum was appropriately used. To obtain serum, a practitioner had first to call in one of several designated "clinical consultants," who had received special training in using the serum. After confirming the clinical diagnosis and assuring themselves that the pneumonia was less than four days old, the consultants would provide the serum or, "if the doctor requests it," administer the treatment themselves. At the same time, the consultant would dispatch a sputum sample for typing to one of twenty designated hospital laboratories. Subsequent serum treatment would be discontinued unless Type I or II pneumonia was diagnosed.[89] In return for all this assistance, the "only thing" expected of participating doctors was that they provide "a case record properly filed out for each patient so treated."[90]

To Roderick Heffron, the study's director, controls on the distribution of serum were necessary, to ensure reliable data about the benefits of serum, and justifiable:

86 Roderick Heffron, "Massachusetts Pneumonia Program," *NEJM* 206 (February 18, 1932), 328; Bigelow, "Serum Treatment of Pneumonia" (n. 82), 244–245. On Bigelow's career and tenure as commissioner, see Rosenkrantz, *Public Health and the State* (n. 22), pp. 172–174.

87 Dr. Anderson to Dr. Bigelow, "Proposed Plan for the Use of Pneumonia Serum," April 13, 1933, Lord papers; George H. Bigelow to Barbara S. Quin, *Proposed Pneumonia Study and Service to Be Undertaken by the Massachusetts Department of Public Health,* September 9, 1930, Box GT 184, Commonwealth Fund records, RAC [hereafter Commonwealth Fund records]; Roderick Heffron, "A Study of Lobar Pneumonia in Massachusetts. Preliminary Report," *NEJM* 207 (July 28, 1932), 153–157. In addition, the DPH conducted several epidemiological studies of the incidence of pneumonia around the state, the prevalence and infectiousness of pneumococcal carriers (discussed in Heffron, ibid.).

88 See the remarks of Frederick T. Lord and Edwin A. Locke in "Discussion [of Heffron's paper]," *NEJM* 207 (July 28, 1932), 157–159. For evidence of the Commonwealth Fund's interest, see Barbara S. Quin to Roger I. Lee, November 20, 1930; George H. Bigelow to Barbara Quin, December 22, 1930, Box GT 184, Commonwealth Fund Records.

89 Heffron, "A Study of Lobar Pneumonia" (n. 87), 155–156.

90 Heffron, "Massachusetts Pneumonia Program" (n. 86), 329.

reliable data were what the Commonwealth Fund was paying for.[91] But practitioners remained leery, not only of the serum's side effects but of the consultants, "feeling" that to call in a consultant "will tend to belittle themselves in the eyes of the patient."[92] That the consultants were permitted to charge for their services was yet another irritant in the eye of practitioners whose incomes were suffering from the Depression. The availability of a small fund to reimburse consultants called in to see indigent patients apparently provided little comfort to Massachusetts physicians.[93]

The consultants, Department of Public Health officials realized, would have to go. Their use in the study had been

> justified from the fact that the basic purpose was to obtain accurate data as to the efficacy of the serum under controlled conditions. It is extremely doubtful whether or no [*sic*] it the State would ever be justified in permanently limiting the use of serum to specially designated consultants. In the eyes of the state which licenses the physicians, all must be considered alike. . . . To continue to distribute the serum through a group of consultants would be to limit the use of the serum in such a fashion as to defeat the main purposes of its distribution. It would furthermore stimulate a growing resentment among the medical profession.[94]

With the consultants removed, the only remaining problem was the serum itself. And that, Massachusetts officials assured the Commonwealth Fund, was a "very real problem which is best solved by improving the quality of the serum" – in a word, by returning to the laboratory.[95]

On the question of serum efficacy, the Massachusetts pneumonia study added to the growing body of favorable reports on Felton's serum, while supporting the view that the earlier cases were treated, the better the outcome.[96] As a vehicle for placing serum treatment in the hands of the general practitioner, results were mixed. During the course of the study, the use of laboratory facilities for pneumococcal typing increased eightfold, and serum treatment became readily available outside of Boston, at least in the eastern third of the state. Of the cases treated

---

91 See Heffron, "A Study of Lobar Pneumonia" (n. 87), and idem, "Massachusetts Pneumonia Program" (n. 86). To some extent, the Commonwealth Fund was a convenient scapegoat for Heffron to blame for a consensus policy which originated with the various groups involved in the study: the fund, the Department of Public Health, and the local advisory committee.

92 *Plan of Pneumonia Study for 1934 and 1935* [n.d.]. See also *Memo, Pneumonia Project, Conference with Dr. George Bigelow, Department of Public Health, Massachusetts,* August 16, 1933. On local practitioners' fear of side effects, see *The Massachusetts Pneumonia Program: Progress Report to the Commonwealth Foundation,* October 17, 1934. All Box GT 184, Commonwealth Fund records.

93 Heffron, "Massachusetts Pneumonia Program" (n. 86), 329.

94 *Plan of Pneumonia Study for 1934 and 1935* [n.d.]. On the removal of the consultants, see Henry Chadwick to Barbara S. Quin, October 11, 1934, Box GT 184, Commonwealth Fund records.

95 *The Massachusetts Pneumonia Program: Progress Report to the Commonwealth Foundation,* October 17, 1934, Box GT 184, Commonwealth Fund records.

96 Roderick Heffron and Elliott S. Robinson, "Final Report of the Massachusetts Pneumonia Study and Service," *The Commonhealth* 27 (January–March 1937), 40–42. Results in Type 2 cases were far less dramatic, even in the cases treated early (ibid., 44–47).

through the program, 22 percent were managed at home, without hospitalization.[97] Nonetheless, specialists judged, "not more than 10% of Type 1 and 2 pneumonias" in the state were getting serum treatment, and the vast majority of that (90 percent) continued to be administered by consultants or by hospital-based physicians.[98]

Just what the Massachusetts program demonstrated was unclear.[99] To Benjamin White, director of the Department of Public Health's Laboratories, it showed the need to improve the serum still further, to make it safer and easier to use.[100] To the Commonwealth Fund, it showed the need to get the word about serum therapy out to practitioners in "useable, understandable" form, by getting Heffron to produce a suitably "dogmatic" handbook on serum therapy.[101] And to New York pneumonia specialists, in the process of organizing their own program to distribute serum, it apparently demonstrated the importance of keeping control over serum out of the hands of the public health department.

In the spring of 1935, Russell Cecil, a prominent New York pneumonia specialist and a longtime advocate of serum, approached Thomas Parran, New York State's Commissioner of Public Health, in the name of the State Medical Society with a request to distribute pneumonia serum more widely. With support from the Commonwealth Fund, Metropolitan Life Insurance, and a state appropriation for serum production, the program was soon under way.[102] Under Medical

97 On specimens typed, see ibid., 38–39; on the number of home cases, see 40. Most of the study consultants and hospitals were located in the eastern third of the state, and especially in the Boston metropolitan area. In the remainder of the state, the program was established in Worcester, Pittsfield, Springfield, and Great Barrington. With the exception of Great Barrington, these are the major population centers in the central and western portions of the state. Only in the last six months of the study was the number of participating hospitals and communities increased to cover the rest of the state effectively. Ibid., 32, 71–72. Unfortunately, accrual and participation rates by area are not available.

98 Dr. Evans to Ms. Quin, April 4, 1935 [quoting the opinions of Frederick Lord], Box GT 184, Commonwealth Fund records; Heffron and Robinson, "Final Report" (n. 96), 52.

99 For a far more positive assessment of the Massachusetts pneumonia program (and its successors), see Harry F. Dowling, "The Rise and Fall of Pneumonia-Control Programs," *Journal of Infectious Disease* 127 (February 1971), 201–206.

100 *The Massachusetts Pneumonia Program, Progress Report to the Commonwealth Fund,* October 17, 1934, Box GT 184, Commonwealth Fund records; see also the material from Benjamin White advising the Commonwealth Fund to emphasize improvements in serum production in its Michigan program. Box GT 202, Commonwealth Fund records.

101 Barbara S. Quin to Benjamin White, October 31, 1931, Box GT 184, Commonwealth Fund records. On the continued difficulties of getting the study's expert specialists to produce such a book, see Dr. Scamman to Miss Quin, June 13, 1932; *Heffron Manuscript, Interview with Walter W. Palmer,* June 26, 1934; and *The Massachusetts Pneumonia Program, Progress Report to the Commonwealth Fund,* October 17, 1934, all Box GT 184, Commonwealth Fund records; and Roderick Heffron to Frederick T. Lord, July 27, 1934, Lord papers.

102 *Memo, Preliminary Discussion on New Pneumonia Program,* May 1, 1935; *Telephone Conversation with Dr. Thomas Parran,* May 17, 1935; Thomas Parran to Barry Smith, June 25, 1935. All Box GT 249, Commonwealth Fund records. See also Thomas P. Farmer to The Honorable Herbert H. Lehman, February 13, 1935, F 137, Parran papers. On Cecil's career, see "Russell Lafayette Cecil," in David Reisman, ed., *History of the Interurban Clinical Club, 1905–1937* (Philadelphia: John C. Winston, 1937), pp. 100–103.

Society direction, the watchword of the New York program proved to be voluntarism. Determining the pneumococcal type before treatment was desirable, but requiring typing was inadvisable.[103] Practitioners would be allowed to initiate serum treatment as much as four days after diagnosis, despite a consistent record of poor results in "late" cases.[104] Educational materials distributed to the physician, the Medical Society's consultants advised, should "avoid anything which would have the appearance of trying to direct or otherwise force physicians to use any given form of treatment."[105] While the program's laissez-faire policies originated with pneumonia experts eager to obtain widespread physician participation, State Health Department officials were similarly reluctant to establish policies that might antagonize either ordinary practitioners or the Medical Society's experts.[106] State deference to the experts allowed them to delay use of Type II serum in the program, leaving Roderick Heffron to comment that "the Type II pneumococcus cares not a whit what the powers in New York State think [about Type II serum] and will go merrily on its way killing 40% or more of all the persons having pneumonia due to it."[107]

In Massachusetts, Commonwealth Fund representatives had repeatedly found themselves reminding state officials that adding to the science of pneumonia was not their main purpose. After a mere six months of living with New York medical politics, the scientific scruples of Massachusetts officials began to seem extremely attractive.[108] Although experts and public health authorities had become increas-

103 Summary Record of Meeting of the Advisory Board on Pneumonia Control, December 18, 1936; *New York State Pneumonia Program, Interview with Doctors Godfrey, Ramsey and Rogers*, September 3, 1936; Barbara S. Quin to George H. Ramsey, September 25, 1936. Mandatory typing was adopted only when the Commonwealth Fund threatened not to renew the grant: see *Interview*, Dr. Ramsey, August 19, 1937; Dr. Godfrey to Ms. Quin, September 23, 1937. All Box GT 249, Commonwealth Fund records.

104 *Memo, New York State Pneumonia Program*, January 29, 1939; Edward Rogers to B. S. Quin, May 17, 1937. Both Box GT 249, Commonwealth Fund records.

105 *Record of Meeting of General Advisory Committee on Pneumonia Control, December 20, 1935.* There was repeated discussion about whether the State Health Department or other groups outside the profession (such as the Metropolitan Life Company) should be allowed to prepare educational materials for physicians: *Sub-committee Meeting on Pneumonia of the New York State Medical Society,* October 18, 1935; Interview with Dr. Edward S. Rogers, Director of the New York State Pneumonia Control, January 10, 1936; *Memo New York State Pneumonia Program,* January 39, 1936; *Record of Meeting of General Advisory Committee on Pneumonia Control,* October 18, 1935. All box GT 249, Commonwealth Fund records.

106 *Report of Attendance at New York State Pneumonia Committee Meeting at Saratoga Springs,* C. L. Scamman, June 23, 1936; *New York State Pneumonia Program, Interview with Doctors Godfrey, Ramsey and Rogers,* September 3, 1936; George H. Ramsey to Barbara Quin, September 24, 1936; Quin to Ramsey, September 25, 1936. All Box GT 249, Commonwealth Fund records.

107 Roderick Heffron to Barry Smith, January 30, 1936. For discussions of Type II serum, see Barbara Quin to Benjamin White, November 20, 1935; Roderick Heffron to Edward Rogers, January 30, 1936; and Rogers to Heffron, February 2, 1936. All Box GT 249, Commonwealth Fund records. In 1938, 238 patients in New York received Type II serum, as compared with 151 the previous year. See State of New York, Department of Health, *Fifty-Ninth Annual Report* (1938), vol. 1, p. 145.

108 See Barbara S. Quin to Benjamin White, November 20, 1935, Box GT 249, Commonwealth Fund records.

ingly convinced of the merits of serum therapy, the New Yorkers' cautious politics proved no more capable of getting community practitioners to use pneumonia serum readily. Even when "the doctor knew he had Type I, that the serum was available . . . he postponed use of it hoping that the patient would improve."[109]

Despite laboratory advances in the 1930s that made pneumonia serum technically easier to use, physicians remained skeptical about the wisdom of using serum therapy in community practice.[110] Serum therapy remained a treatment conceived in and for the well-equipped urban hospital. The Commonwealth Fund's largesse could bring the hospital's technical facilities to the community, but they could not so readily change the physicians who practiced there. Practitioners' fears of serum therapy were ultimately rooted in the economics of medical practice. Using serum remained a tricky business not only because of the potential danger to the patient, but because of the potential injury to the physician's reputation, should the patient react badly to serum or the expensive treatment fail. Serum therapy for pneumonia might be rational therapeutics but the prudent physician might do best to avoid it.[111]

The advent of a drug treatment for pneumonia – sulfapyridine – in 1939 gradually put an end to the Commonwealth Fund's interest in pneumonia treatment, although not to state pneumonia programs or to debates about the merits of serum therapy.[112] The Commonwealth Fund, although willing to engineer physicians' use of proven therapies, was not in the business of attempting "to evaluate clinically a new drug" – a task best left to others.[113]

---

109 C. L. Scamman to Barbara S. Quin, March 14, 1936, Box GT 249, Commonwealth Fund records. See also the discussion in E. S. Rogers, "Type I Pneumococcus Pneumonia: Observations from Study of Two Thousand Cases Treated with Specific Serum," *New York State Journal of Medicine* 38 (November 1, 1938), 1369–1375, esp. 1370. As late as 1937, a report of over 1,200 cases treated at Buffalo City Hospital noted in passing that serum was "used in such a small number of cases that any clinical deductions are unwarranted." Frederick Painton and Herbert J. Ulrich, "Lobar Pneumonia: An Analysis of 1298 Cases," *Ann Int Med* 10 (March 1937), 1345–1364 (quotation from 1363).

110 The advent of rapid typing, introduced in this country around 1932, and the 1937 development of a rabbit-based serum each facilitated serum use. See Dowling, *Fighting Infection* (n. 75), p. 50; A. B. Sabin, "Immediate Pneumococcus Typing from Sputum by Neufeld Reaction," *JAMA* 100 (May 20, 1933), 1584–1586.

111 The most thorough analysis of serum treatment from the practitioners' point of view is Levine, "The Modern Treatment of Lobar Pneumonia" (n. 83), 644–649. See also the objections voiced by the AMA's Olin West who emphasized the "cost" and "waste" of serum treatment, quoted in a letter from Donald Armstrong to Thomas Parran, March 5, 1937, National Institutes of Health, 1930–1948, RG 443, Box 14, 0425P, NA.

112 As late as 1942, the Commonwealth Fund was still supporting pneumonia control programs in Michigan, although the emphasis was on improvements in serum production. See Dr. Heffron to Miss Quin, May 25, 1942, Box 203, Commonwealth Fund records. On the demise of the serum pneumonia programs, see Dowling, "The Rise and Fall of Pneumonia-Control Programs" (n. 99), 201–206. On drug treatments for pneumonia more generally, see the following chapter and Worboys, "Pneumonia in Britain" (n. 75), pp. 326–329.

113 Roderick Heffron to Elliott S. Robinson, November 1, 1939; and Michigan Department of

THE LIMITS OF ORGANIZATION

Over the past two decades, American historians have emphasized "large-scale organizations as the centerpiece of recent U.S. history." Taking the modern corporation as the paradigmatic example, historians have discussed the importance of bureaucratic organizations, both public and private, to twentieth-century U.S. history.[114] By and large, they have not discussed the many settings where organizations failed to take hold, or those where, despite their evident importance, organizations were unable to bring significant actors into the organizational fold. Medicine, in general, and the complex terrain of drug evaluation and practice, in particular, were one such domain in which organizations failed in reshaping the landscape more often than they succeeded.

Corporate research and development of new drugs, not surprisingly, was a prime arena for organizational success. To a growing in-house research capacity, drug firms added a variety of cooperative agreements with university researchers. University–business ties were strongest in laboratory disciplines such as pharmacology with no other visible means of support.[115] Nonetheless, industry's reputation for exploiting clinical research in subsequent promotions made them suspect to many physicians engaged in therapeutic research.[116] Cooperative research among drug firms marked another boundary of organizational success, as the failure of several efforts to organize research consortia among a group of firms demonstrated.[117]

Health Pneumonia Study, Comments on Progress Report and Visit to Project by Drs. Robinson and Heffron, June 22, 1940, both Box GT 203, Commonwealth Fund records. (The latter document concerns Michigan's interest in testing sulfathiazole, a newer sulfa drug.)

114 Louis Galambos, "The Emerging Organizational Synthesis in Modern American History," *Business History Review* 44 (Autumn 1970), 279–290; idem, "Technology, Political Economy and Professionalization: Central Themes of the Organizational Synthesis," *Business History Review* 57 (Winter 1983), 471–493; Brian Balogh, "Reorganizing the Organizational Synthesis: Federal-Professional Relations in Modern America," *Studies in American Political Development* 5 (Spring 1991), 119–172.

115 On the development of industrial research in pharmacology, see John Parascandola, *The Development of American Pharmacology: John J. Abel and the Shaping of a Discipline* (Baltimore: Johns Hopkins University Press, 1992), pp. 103–125; Louis Galambos and Jeffrey Sturchio, *The Origins of An Innovative Organization: Merck and Co, Inc, 1891–1960,* a paper presented to the History Department, Johns Hopkins University, October 5, 1992; Louis Galambos with Jane Eliot Sewell, *Networks of Innovation: Vaccine Development at Merck, Sharpe & Dohme, and Mulford, 1895–1995* (Cambridge: Cambridge University Press, 1995). On the corporate ties of university researchers, see Swann, *Academic Scientists and the Pharmaceutical Industry* (n. 43).

116 See Eugene F. DuBois to Linsley R. Williams, April 13, 1933, Box 2, Morris Fishbein papers, Regenstein Library, University of Chicago; Parascandola, *Development of American Pharmacology* (n. 115), pp. 115–125. Objections to corporate patenting policies of medical discoveries were also crucial in shaping academic resistance to corporate influence. See Howard Poillon to Isaiah Bowman, June 15, 1936, RG 02.001, Series 1, Box 112, President's Papers, Johns Hopkins University Archives. On the general animus against corporate support of medical research, see Shryock, *American Medical Research* (n. 67), pp. 141–146.

117 For a detailed analysis of one such venture, see John Parascandola, "Charles Holmes Herty and the Effort to Establish an Institute for Drug Research in Post World War I America," in John

Philanthropic foundations represented a second class of influential organizations interested in medical knowledge. Historians of science differ as to just how much foresight and influence foundation managers had in shaping the direction of medical research.[118] But in general, foundations interested in research steered clear of therapeutic investigations, something they expected corporations to do (or pay for) themselves.

The Commonwealth Fund's efforts with pneumonia treatment belonged to a different philanthropic tradition – the field experiment – in which foundations provided seed money in the hopes of convincing communities to devote their energies and resources to proven interventions.[119] The problem with serum treatment, as with other therapeutic innovations, was that each community within medicine had its own ideas about what it meant to "prove" a new therapy worthwhile. Even the experts disagreed about the relative weights of experimental reasoning and clinical observation in assessing the value of serum treatment.[120] Differences of opinion among experts, however, diminished by comparison with the gap separating them from physicians in private practice, who measured therapeutic value as much by a therapy's effects on the size of their practice as by any evidence experts could marshal.[121] Moreover, foundation officials generally had difficulty understanding, much less changing, the motives of practicing physicians.[122]

The legacy of the pneumonia studies, like that of the Cooperative Clinical Group, lay less in the realm of therapeutic practice than in therapeutic research. Cooperative studies would enjoy a considerable vogue during and immediately

Parascandola and James C. Whorton, eds., *Chemistry and Modern Society* (Washington, DC: American Chemical Society, 1983), pp. 94–96. Parascandola's account is supplemented by Harden, *Inventing the NIH* (n. 24), pp. 83–91.

Other abortive NRC efforts to organize industry support are charted in the reports of the committees on internal antisepsis and on organic arsenicals, *Minutes of the Annual Meeting of the Division of Chemistry and Chemical Technology,* April 10, 1925, NRC: Div Chem: Meetings, NAS. See also Stanhope Bayne-Jones's discussion in Council on Pharmacy and Chemistry, *Bulletin* 59 (September 6, 1933), 18–19; Morris Fishbein to Eugene F. DuBois, April 27, 1933, Box 2, Morris Fishbein papers, Regenstein Library, University of Chicago. Corporate efforts to establish a consortium for drug evaluation on the model of the British Medical Council were not successful until after World War II; industry interest in the British example is documented in the letter and accompanying documents from George W. Merck to Thomas Parran, October 18, 1938, F 19, Parran papers.

118 Robert E. Kohler, "A Policy for the Advancement of Science: The Rockefeller Foundation, 1924–1929" *Minerva* 16 (Winter 1978), 480–515; Pnina Abir-Am, "The Discourse of Physical Power and Biological Knowledge in the 1930's: A Reappraisal of the Rockefeller Foundation's 'Policy' in Molecular Biology," *Social Studies of Science* 12 (August 1982), 341–382.

119 Edgar Sydenstricker, "The Measurement of Results of Public Health Work: An Introductory Discussion" [1927], reprinted in Richard V. Kasius, ed., *The Challenge of Facts: Selected Public Health Papers of Edgar Sydenstricker* (New York: Prodist, 1974), 51–52.

120 Rufus Cole, "Immune Serum in the Treatment of Pneumonia," *Transactions of the Association of American Physicians* 44 (1929), 194–200.

121 For a similar analysis regarding polio treatments, see Rogers, *Dirt and Disease* (n. 18), pp. 74–75.

122 Peter Buck, "Why Not the Best? Some Reasons and Examples from Child Health and Rural Hospitals," *Journal of Social History* 18 (1985), 413–429.

after World War II, a development discussed in Chapter 4. As a solution to the problem of therapeutic authority in the interwar years, however, cooperative studies failed to provide a secure foundation for regulating therapeutic practice. Those who undertook cooperative studies were unable to escape the cultural and institutional milieu in which such studies were conceived. And the divide between that milieu and the environment of private practice ultimately proved too great to bridge. Meanwhile, therapeutic reformers found themselves in a position of unprecedented influence, as the U.S. Congress authorized the U.S. Food and Drug Administration to begin reviewing therapeutic products before their release on the open market.

3

Playing it safe: The Federal Food, Drug and Cosmetic Act of 1938

It is a well recognized scientific fact that a drug may be useful under certain conditions, useless under other conditions, or detrimental under still other conditions, and in coming to a decision with respect to the safety of a drug it is necessary to take into account the use to which the drug is put. . . . Safety as applied to a drug in the Act is unquestionably a relative term. Absolute safety is very difficult to obtain.[1]

What we are seeking to do here is to put the courts on notice . . . that it is the purpose of Congress to have consideration given therapeutic claims.[2]

On June 25, 1938, after five years of failed attempts, Congress enacted legislation authorizing the U.S. Food and Drug Administration (FDA) to review the safety and composition of new drugs. Passed in the wake of an episode of mass poisoning from an untested drug, the Federal Food, Drug and Cosmetic Act of 1938 granted the FDA authority to act before, not after, the hazards of a drug were revealed through distribution on the open market.[3] The new law required drug firms to demonstrate that drugs were "safe for use under the conditions prescribed, recommended or suggested in the proposed labeling thereof."[4]

---

1 J. J. Durrett, "Some of the Implications of Section 505(b) (1) of the Food, Drug and Cosmetic Act," American Drug Manufacturers Association, *Proceedings,* 28th Annual Meeting (1939), 98.

2 Testimony of W. G. Campbell [FDA], U.S. Senate, Committee on Commerce, *Hearings on S. 2800. Food, Drugs and Cosmetics. February 27 to March 3, 1934,* p. 557, 73rd Congress, 2nd Session.

3 Public Law 717, Federal Food, Drug and Cosmetic Act, 75th Congress, 3rd Session. The best source on the legislative history of the 1938 law remains David F. Cavers, "The Food, Drug and Cosmetic Act of 1938: Its Legislative History and Its Substantive Provisions," *Law and Contemporary Problems* 6 (Winter 1939), 2–42. See also James Harvey Young, *The Medical Messiahs: A Social History of Health Quackery in Twentieth Century America* (Princeton: Princeton University Press, 1967), pp. 158–190. Charles O. Jackson's *Food and Drug Legislation in the New Deal* (Princeton: Princeton University Press, 1970) describes the lobbying process in excruciating detail; it is rather short on analysis, however.

4 Federal Food, Drug and Cosmetic Act, chap. 5, sec. 505 (d). This clause sets the standards for new drugs; sec. 502 (j) authorized the secretary to treat as misbranded *any* drug that was dangerous to health when used in the dosage and conditions recommended in the labeling.

This statutory language reflected the long-standing view of therapeutic reformers that no drug is absolutely safe, and that many drugs are, in fact, quite dangerous. In determining a drug's safety, FDA officials would apply a utilitarian calculus: a "safe" drug was one whose proposed use would benefit patients more than it harmed them.[5] A drug that was unsafe for treating colds might be safe for treating pneumonia or influenza. In the view of FDA officials, such assessments required an evaluation of therapeutic merit. Even an inert but ineffective drug allowed on the market would do harm if it kept the patient from treatment with a more effective, albeit more toxic, drug.

Readers familiar with the history of federal drug regulation will be surprised by the claim that considerations of drug efficacy played an important role in the 1938 law. The 1938 law is regarded as allowing the FDA to regulate the safety of new drugs, and no more.[6] The narrow construction such interpretations place on the notion of drug safety is an artifact that, in large part, results from reading subsequent regulatory and judicial history into the original legislation. Before 1945, there is little evidence that anyone, even members of the regulated industry, questioned the FDA's interpretation of the act. Meanwhile, the FDA operated on the presumption that the determination of drug safety necessarily entailed making judgments about therapeutic merit.

In formulating policies, FDA officials were only following the lead of therapeutic reformers in the medical profession. To advocates of a rational therapeutics, assessing a drug's dangers and identifying its therapeutic limitations were part of the same task.[7] Passage of the 1938 law marked the end of a long effort to put these convictions to work in federal drug regulation. It was not reformers' assumptions about drug safety but the power to act on them that forms the novelty of the 1938 legislation.

FDA officials adopted as well the evidentiary procedures and standards fashioned by therapeutic reformers. Although laboratory procedures were used to screen out some drugs either as inert or too toxic, final judgments were arrived at on the basis of clinical evidence. In formulating judgments about therapeutic merit, the FDA relied on a system of expert consultants not unlike that developed by the AMA's Council on Pharmacy and Chemistry. Decisions in difficult cases were arrived at by a consultative process in which the opinions and values of clinical specialists as well as their data were elicited and deliberated.

5 On the nineteenth-century origins of the utilitarian calculus in clinical medicine, see especially Martin S. Pernick, *A Calculus of Suffering: Pain, Professionalism and Anesthesia in Nineteenth-Century America* (New York: Columbia University Press, 1985).
6 See Peter Temin, *Taking Your Medicine: Drug Regulation in the United States* (Cambridge: Harvard University Press, 1980), pp. 38–57.
7 A. J. Carlson to Mr. Virgil Chapman, February 21, 1938, Record Group 88, Accession no. 52A-89, Box 124, Folder 062 (Food and Drug Act A, March–April), W-NRC. [All FDA records hereafter cited by listing Record Group followed by accession number, as in "88-52A-89."] Chapman was the sponsor of new drug legislation in the House of Representatives. See also testimony of W. G. Campbell [FDA], U.S. Senate, Committee on Commerce, *Hearings on S. 2800. Food, Drugs and Cosmetics. February 27 to March 3, 1934*, pp. 550–552, 73rd Congress, 2nd Session; Joseph A. Capps, "Irrational Tendencies in Modern Therapy," *JAMA* 83 (July 5, 1924), 1–3.

My argument here is that governmental drug regulation in the late 1930s and 1940s was profoundly shaped by the experiences and values of therapeutic reformers. But the policies and practices of the FDA were also shaped by the culture of government. In a decade when federal authorities unceasingly refashioned their relation to private economic activity, the choice of regulatory instruments and the scope of bureaucratic ambitions for federal power took on heightened political meaning. FDA officials adopted a regulatory policy that seemed – to them – minimally intrusive on the prerogatives of practicing physicians and drug manufacturers. The FDA would contribute to the public good largely by regulating what manufacturers *said* about drugs, while leaving other efforts to improve the use of drugs to medicine's scientific and professional authorities.

The following section provides a quick overview of federal law and policy on drug regulation before 1938. I then describe the procedures elaborated by FDA officials to evaluate existing and new drugs under the 1938 law, examining in detail the case of sulfapyridine, the first novel therapeutic compound evaluated by the FDA. The chapter ends with an analysis of the roles of medical researchers, practicing physicians, and the drug trade in the system of drug regulation created under the 1938 act.

DRUG REGULATION, 1900–1938

The history of drug regulation in this century reflects a central tenet of therapeutic reformers: the more potent the drug and the more serious the disease for which it was intended, the greater the importance of regulating the therapeutic claims made on its behalf. As Jonathan Liebenau has emphasized, federal efforts at drug regulation in this century began with the Biologics Control Act of 1902, which mandated the Public Health Service's Hygienic Laboratory to regulate the interstate commerce of "viruses, serums, toxins and analogous products." The act authorized the Hygienic Laboratory (later the National Institute of Health) to license manufacturers producing mandated products, to set standards and to test for the potency of approved items, to inspect manufacturers' facilities before and after licensing, and, to a limited extent, to evaluate manufacturers' claims concerning the therapeutic value of their products.[8]

---

8 Responsibility for biologics regulation remained with the Public Health Service until 1972, when it was transferred to the FDA. The Hygienic Laboratory supervised the production not only of biologic products such as serums and vaccines but, as of 1919, the chemically produced antisyphilis drugs such as arsphenamine. On their regulatory activities, see Laurence F. Schmeckbeier, *The Public Health Service: Its History, Activities and Organization* (Baltimore: Johns Hopkins University Press, 1923), pp. 27, 129–133; Ramunas Kondratas, "The Biologics Control Act of 1902," in James Harvey Young, ed., *The Early Years of Federal Food and Drug Control* (Madison, WI: American Institute of the History of Pharmacy, 1982), pp. 8–27, and Jonathan Liebenau, *Medical Science and Medical Industry, 1890–1929: A Study of Pharmaceutical Manufacturing in Philadelphia* (Ph.D. thesis, University of Pennsylvania, 1981), pp. 254–258, 269–270. Liebenau correctly stresses the extent to which the activities of the Hygienic Laboratory under the 1902 legislation were a more significant model for subsequent approaches to drug development and evaluation than the 1906 food and drug legislation.

Questions of therapeutic merit that could be resolved in the laboratory were actionable: a license need not be granted to inactive or subtherapeutic products.[9] But beyond laboratory tests, Hygienic Laboratory officials tread cautiously. Like the members of the AMA Council on Pharmacy and Chemistry, they found proof positive that a product lacked clinical value the most difficult of claims to establish. George McCoy, the Hygienic Laboratory's director, was especially reluctant to impose his views on practicing physicians in cases where experts disagreed. When it came to scientific questions, McCoy was a strong believer in pluralism. Given the fallibility of all human judgments, he argued, it was better to allow some individuals to err than to lead everyone astray by insisting that they all follow the conclusions of a central authority. Official pronouncements were particularly loaded, if only because most citizens were inclined to forget that government officials were as fallible as anyone else.[10]

The 1906 Food and Drug Act, while covering a greater range of products, granted even fewer powers. The act gave the federal government no right to screen drugs before their commercial introduction. It merely authorized the Bureau of Chemistry to seize "adulterated" or "misbranded" products.[11] From the reformers' point of view, the law had many defects: only claims that physically accompanied the product label were actionable; claims made in advertising the product were not. Producers who elected not to specify the contents of their products on their labeling could not be prosecuted for misrepresenting them, nor could producers whose labeling acknowledged the presence of a small number of mandated dangerous substances. The law's greatest flaw was that it was remedial but not preventive: the Bureau of Chemistry could act only after a drug was distributed and harm done.[12]

9 Under the 1902 law, the Hygienic Laboratory regularly tested new products for their "therapeutic or prophylactic value" in the laboratory. See Schmeckbeier, *The Public Health Service* (n. 8), p. 130.

10 On the agency's policies, see G. W. McCoy, "Official Methods of Control of Remedial Agents for Human Use," *JAMA* 74 (June 5, 1920), 1554. See also "Report of the Committee on Sera and Vaccines," Council on Pharmacy and Chemistry, *Bulletin* (August 20, 1908), 88–89, American Medical Association Archives; [George M. McCoy], *Memorandum to the Surgeon General, U.S. Public Health Service on H.R. 5845* [1924], Public Health Service (PHS), General Files, 1924–1935, RG 90, Box 70, NA. McCoy's views did not prevent him from acting against certain products, most notably vaccines intended for the treatment of tuberculosis. For more on McCoy's philosophy, see Victor H. Kramer, *The National Institute of Health: A Study in Public Administration* (New Haven: Quinnipiack Press, 1937), pp. 31–37. My thanks to Dr. Ramunas Kondratas for calling this reference to my attention.

11 The 1906 act was administered by the Bureau of Chemistry in the Department of Agriculture until 1927, when its regulatory functions were established in the Food, Drug and Insecticide Administration (after 1930, the Food and Drug Administration). See Young, *Medical Messiahs* (n. 3), p. 98. The diversity of nomenclature obscures a strong continuity of personnel. See Temin, *Taking Your Medicine* (n. 6), pp. 7, 40. On the legislative origins of the 1906 act, see James Harvey Young, *Pure Food: Securing the Federal Food and Drugs Act of 1906* (Princeton: Princeton University Press, 1989).

12 The limits of the labeling provision, and its failure to contain comparable abuses in freestanding advertising, were singled out for criticism by Bureau Chemist Carl L. Alsberg in an otherwise positive ten-year review of the act. See Gustavus A. Weber, *The Food, Drug and Insecticide Administration: Its History, Activities and Organization* (Baltimore: Johns Hopkins University Press, 1928), p. 27. While the 1906 law required that certain narcotic or otherwise hazardous components be identified

Even under the limited authority of the 1906 act, the Bureau of Chemistry tried to regulate therapeutic efficacy, by confiscating as "misbranded" products that made grossly inflated or misleading therapeutic claims. From the regulators' perspective, even a nontoxic but ineffective drug represented "a definite public health menace . . . because its use may cause delay in resorting to rational methods of treatment."[13] As interpreted by the courts, however, the law required that the bureau demonstrate not merely the falsity of a manufacturer's claims but that he knew the claims to be false. Such demonstrations were costly, time consuming, and hampered by the legal difficulties of proving fraudulent intent. The bureau's aspirations to regulate therapeutic claims foundered on the courts' reluctance to accept scientific and medical authority as prima facie grounds for establishing a standard of knowledge in this area. The courts did not always recognize the distinction, embraced by the bureau, between the opinions of experts, backed by laboratory studies of drug action and a critical review of the clinical literature, and the testimony of physicians and patients, grounded on uncontrolled personal experience. Proving fraud under these conditions was onerous.[14]

Unlike the Hygienic Laboratory's George McCoy, FDA officials actively sought expanded authority over drug regulation. In 1933, Rexford Tugwell, President Roosevelt's newly appointed Assistant Secretary of Agriculture, offered FDA officials a long-sought opportunity to extend their powers.[15] When Senator Royal Copeland introduced legislation to replace the 1906 law, FDA chief Walter G. Campbell urged Congress to "put the courts on notice" that evaluating therapeutic claims was part of their job.[16] The subject of extensive congressional hearings,

when used, it was no crime to employ them. The labeling requirement, moreover, did not cover a longer list of equally dangerous substances. See Young, *Medical Messiahs* (n. 3), p. 54.

13 *Report of the Food and Drug Administration. 1930,* 11; see also *Report of the Food and Drug Administration. 1931,* 15–16. On the congressional support for this view, see House Report 1138, 62nd Congress, 2nd Session, 1912, cited in Ashley Sellars and Nathan D. Grundstein, *Administrative Procedure and Practice in the Department of Agriculture under the Federal Food, Drug and Cosmetic Act of 1938* (Washington, DC: U.S. Department of Agriculture, 1940), part I, p. 14.

14 Contrast Peter Temin's reading of the legislative and judicial history of drug regulation, which emphasizes judicial doubts about the authority of medical opinion, with the interpretation of James Harvey Young, which places greater emphasis on the opportunity costs legal precedent imposed on the bureau's regulatory strategy, and the consequent emphasis on obtaining the industry's voluntary compliance. See Temin, *Taking Your Medicine* (n. 6), pp. 32–34; Young, *Medical Messiahs* (n. 3), chaps. 1, 3, and 5, esp. pp. 53–54, 56–59, 92–96, 99–101, 104–106, 111–112. For a more detailed discussion of the judicial history, see Harry M. Marks, *Ideas As Reforms: Therapeutic Experiments and Medical Practice, 1900–1980* (Ph.D. thesis, Massachusetts Institute of Technology, 1987), pp. 57–58.

15 Jackson, *Food and Drug Legislation* (n. 3), pp. 3–5, 24–29.

16 Testimony of W. G. Campbell [FDA], U.S. Senate, Committee on Commerce, *Hearings on S. 2800. Food, Drugs and Cosmetics. February 27 to March 3, 1934,* p. 557, 73rd Congress, 2nd Session. Copeland had earlier attempted to extend the scope of federal authority regarding drugs by amending the 1902 Biologics Act to regulate therapeutic claims. His attempts were rebuffed by Public Health Service officials and the director of the Hygienic Laboratory. Royal S. Copeland to H. S. Cumming, February 12, 1924; G. W. McCoy to A. H. Stimson, January 29, 1924, PHS, General Files, 1924–1935, RG 90, Box 70, NA. The Hygienic Laboratory's reticence in these matters contrasts with that of FDA officials, who had made an earlier attempt, in 1912, to revise the drug statute on the model of the 1902 Biologics Act. See Sellars and Grundstein, *Administrative Procedure and Practice* (n. 13), part I, pp. 82–83.

the proposed legislation underwent numerous revisions in response to industry and consumer criticisms. Some legislative initiatives foundered because consumer groups or administration officials thought them too weak. Others were blocked by industry objections that they gave too much power to the FDA. Whether a new drug law should address the truth of therapeutic claims was not a central issue in these legislative maneuvers. To the extent the subject was discussed, attention focused on the choice of means for accomplishing this end.

One option was to model the new statute on the Biologics Control Act of 1902, authorizing the FDA to "license" new products after reviewing the claims and evidence submitted by manufacturers. Industry opponents, conjuring up the specter of federal abuses of authority, effectively foreclosed this option.[17] The AMA's Council on Pharmacy and Chemistry similarly opposed a licensing system because "it would involve a guarantee by the Government of the integrity of all drugs and might give a false sense of security."[18] Instead, reformers proposed to vest powers in a scientific board of experts to advise the FDA.[19]

Both AMA and industry lawyers expressed reservations about any apparent delegation of governmental powers to nongovernmental groups, lest excessive delegation of federal authority lead the courts to invalidate the proposed new law. These concerns about the constitutionality of delegating federal powers could only have been reinforced by the subsequent Supreme Court decision in 1935, invalidating the National Recovery Administration statute on similar grounds.[20] In subsequent drafts, the idea of a formal consultative body was abandoned, along with any language that evoked the bar of "medical opinion" to which judicial attention had been drawn.[21]

17 On industry opposition, see "Appendix A. Preliminary Conferences" [1933], in Charles Wesley Dunn, *Federal Food, Drug and Cosmetic Act: A Statement of Its Legislative Record* (New York: G. E. Stechert, 1938), pp. 1040–1041; "Report of the Committee on Legislation," American Drug Manufacturers' Association, *Proceedings, 27th Annual Meeting* (1938), 44–45. Some firms took a more aggressive stance: Eli Lilly, for example, opposed equally granting the FDA licensure powers or the power to review new drugs: Eli Lilly to Clarence Lea, March 15, 1938, Food and Drug Administration (FDA), Office of the Commissioner, Legislation (1927–1940), RG 88, Box 10, NA.

18 J. C. Clarke to W. G. Campbell, November 26, 1937, FDA, Office of the Commissioner, Legislation (1927–1940), RG 88, Box 12, NA.

19 On the proposal for a body of experts to advise the FDA, see AMA Council on Pharmacy and Chemistry, *Bulletin* 58 (May 3, 1933), 11–13; *Bulletin* 60 (February 21, 1934), 432; A. J. Carlson to Mr. Virgil Chapman [House of Representatives], February 21, 1938, 88-52A-89, Box 124, F 062 (Food and Drug Act A, March–April), W-NRC; Stephan Wilson, *Food and Drug Regulation* (Washington, DC: American Council on Public Affairs, 1942), p. 105.

20 For industry opposition to this provision, see Charles Wesley Dunn, *The Revision of the Federal Food and Drugs Act* (n.p., [1934]), pp. 5–6. For AMA concerns about delegation, see the remarks of Paul Nicholas Leech, Council on Pharmacy and Chemistry, *Bulletin* 62 (November 7, 1934), 577; Olin West, "Verbatim Report on Special Meeting of the Council with Board of Trustees" [November 15, 1934], *Bulletin* 62 (December 6, 1934), a48, a57–a58. On the NRA decision, see Ellis W. Hawley, *The New Deal and the Problem of Monopoly* (Princeton: Princeton University Press, 1966), pp. 127–129.

21 The testimony of W. G. Campbell [FDA] and the ensuing discussion by Senators Copeland and Herbert emphasize the importance of finding a legally defensible procedure for incorporating the views of experts. See U.S. Senate, Committee on Commerce, *Hearings on S. 2800. Food, Drugs and*

The new law ultimately placed its confidence in the FDA, which was to decide "by all methods reasonably applicable" whether a new drug was "safe for use" under the conditions proposed by the producer.[22] But repeated objections to expanded federal authority left their mark, both in the statutory language and in the FDA's approach to implementing the act. The FDA was not authorized to "approve" new drugs but, in the statute's torturous language, the FDA could "refuse to permit [an] application to become effective."[23] The agency's approach to reviewing new drug applications was similarly circumspect: it was the applicant's "responsibility" to withdraw a deficient application, once these deficiencies "become entirely apparent to him."[24]

Behind the FDA's caution lay a pluralist philosophy of governance and of science. FDA officials deemed the scientific community at large wiser than any member of it, including the FDA's professional staff. If FDA officials were to "dictate in any great detail the type of investigation which should be made" of new drugs, they might only "discourage or prevent [its] proper investigation."[25] With industry and medical researchers looking on eagerly to see how they would interpret their new powers, FDA officials opted for reaction over proaction, preferring to make policy on a case-by-case basis rather than promulgate broad general rules.[26]

Cosmetics. February 27–March 3, 1934, pp. 548–558, 73rd Congress, 2nd Session. The AMA proposed that "competent medical witnesses" or the authority of "reputable" journals be specified and defined in the legislation, to avoid the ambiguity in terms like "substantial medical opinion." Testimony of William C. Woodward, ibid., p. 376. See also Bureau of Legal Medicine and Legislation, AMA, "Food, Drug, Therapeutic Device and Cosmetic Legislation Pending in Congress," *JAMA* 105 (December 21, 1935), 2055–2062. Even representatives of industry were agreed in the importance of recognizing "substantial medical or scientific opinion" in determining the truth of drug claims. See testimony of James F. Hoge, Proprietary Manufacturers Association, *Hearings before a Subcommittee of the Committee on Commerce on S. 5. March, 1935*, in U.S. Food and Drug Administration, *A Legislative History of the Federal Food, Drug and Cosmetic Act and Its Amendments* (Washington, DC: FDA, n.d), vol. 3, p. 325; Charles Wesley Dunn, *Revision of the Federal Food and Drugs Act* (n. 20), pp. 7, 18.

22 Public Law 717, Federal Food and Drug Act, 75th Congress, 3rd Session, sec. 505 (d), vesting legal authority in the administrator of the Federal Security Agency, under whose jurisdiction the Food and Drug Administration operated.

23 Public Law 717, Federal Food and Drug Act, 75th Congress, 3rd Session, sec. 505 (e).

24 J. J. Durrett to Arthur C. DeGraaf, March 22, 1940, 88-59A-2736, Box 24, F 505.1–508.2, W-NRC.

25 Walton van Winkle to William Deichmann, July 6, 1944, 88-59A-2736, Box 166, F 505.1–505.6; see also H. F. Kennedy, *Memorandum of Interview with Warren M. Cox, Jr.*, September 4, 1942, 88-59A-2736, Box 107, F 511.07 (August). Other instances of self-imposed restraint include the FDA's refusal (prior to 1942) to rule generally on what constitutes a "new drug," leaving it up to manufacturers to determine whether they had a new drug. See Theodore Klumpp to Arthur DeGraaf, March 22, 1940, 88-59A-2736, Box 24, F 505.1–508.2; H. F. Kennedy, *Memorandum of Telephone Conversation with James Burch*, July 1, 1942, 88-59A-2736, Box 107, F 505.1–510.67. All W-NRC.

26 For more on the "dance of regulation" under the FDA, see Harry M. Marks, "Revisiting 'The Origins of Compulsory Drug Prescriptions,'" *AJPH* 85 (January 1995), 109–115.

IMPLEMENTATION: "DANGEROUS" DRUGS

Potent drugs, containing large amounts of acetanilid and bromide, should not be sold over the ice cream counter, as if they were just another fizz concoction in the same class as ice cream soda.[27]

The average layman little realizes ... the serious consequences which may follow indiscriminate and ignorant use of potent ethical preparations whose administration the manufacturer has tried to limit to professional supervision.[28]

The 1938 law required the FDA to see that drugs were "safe for use . . . under the conditions recommended." But according to clinical specialists, any drug was potentially unsafe: "I do not know what the word 'dangerous' means in the way he uses it. I am sure it is at least grossly undesirable for people to take indefinitely 9 grains of acetanilid or 20 grains of bromide."[29] In a regulatory context, such ambiguity might lead to legal challenges and, possibly, defeats. One of the first tasks facing FDA officials was to translate reformers' opinions into defensible policies.

The majority of drugs presented to the FDA posed few problems. The rank fraud and the known poison were easy to identify. As with the AMA Council on Pharmacy and Chemistry, either the laboratory or the library sufficed in many cases to evaluate minor variations on relatively innocuous compounds. By requiring adequate documentation of a drug's composition and extensive screening on animals for toxicological effects, the FDA readily disposed of most applications. The more difficult problem was posed by drugs whose potency was not in doubt, but whose benefit depended on the precautions taken in their use.

The men in charge of the Drug Division, Theodore Klumpp and J. J. Durrett, came to the FDA from backgrounds in academic medicine. Durrett, a graduate of Harvard Medical School in 1914, had spent much of his career in government service at the FDA. Klumpp, a more recent graduate of Harvard (1928), had come to the FDA in 1936 from a teaching post at Yale Medical School.[30] Of the two, Klumpp was the more zealous, but both men were familiar with the contention

27 Theodore G. Klumpp, "The Work of the Federal Food and Drug Administration," *Journal of the Medical Association of Georgia* 28 (July 1939), 280.
28 *Memorandum Submitted by Winthrop Chemical Company . . . With Respect to Proposed Regulations for the Enforcement of the Federal Food, Drug and Cosmetic Act,* p. 7, 88–52A-89, Box 144, F 603 (Proposed Regulations), Book 3, W to Z, W-NRC.
29 George Minot to Soma Weiss, October 3, 1939, Soma Weiss papers, Countway Library.
30 Apart from a brief excursion to industry (in 1935), Durrett had been responsible for drug control at the U.S. Department of Agriculture since 1928. Shortly after passage of the new law, Durrett was kicked upstairs, to serve as a technical advisor to W. G. Campbell on administration of the new law. His post as chief of the Drug Division at FDA was taken over by Theodore Klumpp. See Jacques Cattell, ed., *American Men of Science,* 10th ed. (Tempe, AZ: Jacques Cattell Press, 1960–1962), vol. I, p. 1021; Council on Pharmacy and Chemistry, *Bulletin* 65 (December 4, 1935), 774; "Changes in the Food and Drug Administration," *JAMA* 111 (September 17, 1938), 1116; *Who's Who in America, 1982–1983,* 42nd ed. (Chicago: Marquis Publishing, 1982), vol. I, p. 1838.

of reformers that many worthwhile drugs were causing problems because of "inappropriate" use. They soon put their academic contacts to work to document the hazards of such use.[31] Among the drugs on which they focused attention was a powerful new antiinfective agent, sulfanilamide.

The first of a new class of compounds known as sulfonamides, sulfanilamide was introduced into the United States in 1936. Almost overnight, it established a reputation as a "truly remarkable" drug in treating otherwise fatal infections. Its dramatic successes in treating advanced streptococcal infections were followed by evidence of its value in meningococcal, gonococcal, and other infections.[32] One of the first clinical uses of the drug in this country was on Franklin Roosevelt Jr., whose dramatic recovery was widely reported in the general press.[33]

Among clinical investigators, however, enthusiasm for sulfanilamide's healing potential was soon tempered by knowledge of the drug's toxicity. Initial reports of mild reactions were supplemented by the fall of 1937 with studies associating its use with anemias, depressed white-cell counts, and a variety of other serious blood disorders.[34] Sulfanilamide thereby joined a long list of drugs whose value depended on the intelligence and skill with which it was used. When employed to treat the life-threatening conditions for which it was effective, under conditions

31 Dr. George Dobbs and Dr. James Q. Gant, *Memorandum of Interview. Dr. DuBois. October 4, 1938*, 88-52A-89, Box 137, F 512.1.10–512.6, W-NRC; George Minot to Soma Weiss, October 3, 1939, Soma Weiss papers, Countway Library. In addition to prominent clinicians, surveyed for their experience with particular drugs, superintendents at large, prestigious hospitals were asked to report adverse drug reactions on specific drugs. For a list of individuals surveyed in March 1939, see 88-58A-277, Box 38, F 511.07–512, W-NRC. On Klumpp's more aggressive use of the FDA's new powers to guide therapeutic practice, see Theodore Klumpp to J. J. Durrett, November 9, 1938, and Durrett's annotated reply, NDA 131 (Estradiol), 88-69A-2099, Box 2; Theodore Klumpp to J. J. Durrett, October 10, 1938, NDA 2 (Neoprontosil), 88-72A-2335, Box 1, both at W-NRC.

32 A handful of American investigators tried out samples of the drug in 1935, but "serious laboratory and clinical investigations" here did not begin until 1936. Perrin H. Long and Eleanor A. Bliss, *The Clinical and Experimental Use of Sulfanilamide, Sulfapyridine and Allied Compounds* (New York: Macmillan, 1939), p. 9. For a full discussion of the range of conditions treatable with sulfanilamide, and a critical evaluation of the evidence upon which such claims were based as of 1939, see Long and Bliss, pp. 147-229. For general background on the development and early use of sulfanilamide, see Harry Dowling, *Fighting Infection: Conquests of the Twentieth Century* (Cambridge: Harvard University Press, 1977), chap. 8.

33 James Harvey Young, "Sulfanilamide and Diethylene Glycol," in John Parascandola and James C. Whorton, eds., *Chemistry and Modern Society* (Washington, DC: American Chemical Society, 1983), p. 107. In addition to the sources cited by Young, see "Prontosil," *Time* (December 28, 1936), 21; "Again, Sulfanilamide," *Time* (August 30, 1937), 61.

34 Perrin H. Long and Eleanor Bliss, "Para-Amino-Benzene-Sulfonamide and Its Derivatives: Experimental and Clinical Observations on Their Use in the Treatment of Beta-Hemolytic Streptococcic Infection: A Preliminary Report," *JAMA* 108 (January 2, 1937), 37. For early rumors of acute hemolytic anemia and agranulocytosis, see Council on Pharmacy and Chemistry, "Report of the Council: Sulfanilamide and Related Compounds," *JAMA* 108 (May 29, 1937), 1889. Subsequent reports, more adequately documented, include A. M. Harvey and C. A. Janeway, "The Development of Acute Hemolytic Anemia during the Administration of Sulfanilamide," *JAMA* 109 (July 3, 1937), 12–16; S. E. Kohn, "Acute Hemolytic Anemia during Treatment with Sulfanilamide," *JAMA* 109 (September 25, 1937), 1005–1006; Perrin H. Long and Eleanor A. Bliss, "Clinical Use of Sulphanilamide and Its Derivatives in the Treatment of Infectious Disease," *Ann Int Med* 11 (October 1937), 584–585.

that allowed for the close monitoring of drug reactions, sulfanilamide's contribution was welcome. But until more was known about the drug's toxic properties and the manner in which the body used the drug, reformers advised caution and discouraged indiscriminate use. "It is not," the AMA's Council on Pharmacy and Chemistry urged, "a panacea."[35]

By spring 1938, evidence of sulfanilamide's potential toxicity was well established. Whether the more severe reactions associated with the drug were due to the "idiosyncrasies" of individual patients was still under investigation. But FDA officials found little disagreement among the experts they consulted that sulfanilamide, employed without awareness of its potential to cause such reactions, was a dangerous drug. Patients being treated with sulfanilamide, authorities agreed, were best handled under close medical supervision.[36]

On August 26, 1938, the FDA announced that marketing of sulfanilamide that allowed for "indiscriminate use by the general public" would be "actionable" under the new law. Manufacturers would be liable to prosecution, unless they attached to packages of sulfanilamide a "warning so conspicuous as to certainly attract attention" that the drug was dangerous unless used under "appropriate medical supervision."[37] The notice on sulfanilamide was soon followed in September by similar announcements on aminopyrine and cinchophen, drugs whose toxic properties had long been noted in the literature.[38]

35 Council on Pharmacy and Chemistry, "Report of the Council: Sulfanilamide and Related Compounds," *JAMA* 108 (May 29, 1937), 1889. The council's cautions were echoed by the other investigators reporting on the drug. See references in note 34. See also W. G. Campbell, J. J. Durrett, and A. G. Murray, *Memorandum of Interview with Charles E. Vanderkleed and Carson P. Frailey*, November 2, 1937, 88-52A-89, Box 135, F Combined Contact Committee, W-NRC, warning them of the dangers to industry of continuing to distribute in subtherapeutic amounts drugs "known to be deadly" like Elixir Sulfanilamide.

36 On the issue of individual idiosyncrasy, see "Sulfanilamide and the Leukocytes," *JAMA* 110 (January 29, 1938), 372–373, and the studies cited therein. The most detailed work was being done at Johns Hopkins. See E. K. Marshall Jr., W. C. Cutting, and Kendall Emerson Jr., "The Toxicity of Sulfanilamide," *JAMA* 110 (January 22, 1938), 252–257.

37 Charles Wesley Dunn and Vincent A. Kleinfeld, *Federal Food, Drug and Cosmetic Act: Judicial and Administrative Record, 1939–1949* (New York: Commerce Clearing House, 1949), Trade Correspondences 1, 4.

38 See Dunn and Kleinfeld, *Federal Food, Drug and Cosmetic Act, 1939–1949* (n. 37), Trade Correspondences 2, 3. The AMA Council on Pharmacy and Chemistry had similarly developed a "warnings" and informational approach to cinchophen and aminopyrine. On cinchophen, see Council on Pharmacy and Chemistry, *Bulletin* 50 (November 13, 1929), 414; *Bulletin* 58 (June 14, 21, 28, 1933), 248, 289, 332, 342; *Bulletin* 60 (March 14, 1934), 546. For aminopyrine, see *Bulletin* 61 (June 6, 1934), 195.
   Decisions were made on a case by case basis. The dangers of some drugs proved especially difficult to establish, owing to differences of medical opinion about the relative risk–benefit ratios. The use of thyroid substances for weight reduction were one such difficult case. See the correspondence in 88-58A-277, Box 22, F 512.1.10–512.631, W-NRC, especially Fuller Albright to Theodore G. Klumpp, January 28, 1939. See also Theodore G. Klumpp to Ephraim Shorr, October 22, 1938, 88-52A-89, Box 137, F 512.1, and Theodore G. Klumpp to Arthur G. Sullivan, June 4, 1940, 88-59A-2736, Box 27, F 511.06, W-NRC. For a general account of the thyroid campaign, see Young, *Medical Messiahs* (n. 3), pp. 210–215.

The new law said nothing about the FDA's right to control the way drugs were used; its authority was vested in the right to regulate what manufacturers *said* about a drug. But the idea of restricting the sale of sulfanilamide to physicians did not trouble manufacturers.[39] What bothered them was the possibility of being held accountable for the acts of others: the distributors, licensees, and purchasers of their products.[40] The manufacturers proposed a compromise: require detailed labeling except in cases where the product was distributed only to professionals, when companies would be allowed to label the actual product "for professional use only." Such labeling would substitute for the detailed warnings otherwise called for.[41] With minor modifications, the FDA accepted the industry proposal.[42] That "solved" the "problem" of "indiscriminate" use by the lay public.[43] Regulating unintelligent practices by the medical profession proved to be another problem.

Over the course of the 1920s, therapeutic reformers had continued their researches into the pharmacological principles that underlay effective therapeutic practice. The growth of knowledge about the proper use of familiar drugs such as

39 In at least one draft of the proposed new law, industry spokesmen had themselves proposed that products sold to physicians be exempted from the bill's labeling requirements. James F. Hoge, *A Bill for a Food, Drug and Cosmetic Act* [1935], Food and Drug Administration, Office of the Commissioner, Legislation, 1927–1940, RG 88, Box 10, NA. After the bill's passage, one manufacturer objected, not to the requirement that certain drugs be used under medical supervision but to the possibility that they might not be so used. According to Winthrop Chemical Company, the proposed labeling requirements were tantamount to granting a "correspondence course in medicine" to laymen who were unqualified to understand, much less evaluate, the dangers of using such drugs. *Memorandum Submitted by Winthrop Chemical Co, Inc.,* November 25, 1938, 88-52A-89, Box 144, F 603 (Proposed Regulations, Book 3, W to Z), W-NRC.

40 J. J. Durrett, *Memorandum of Interview with Mr. David Rasch,* September 16, 1938, 88-72A-2335, Box 1, NDA 2 (Neoprontosil), W-NRC. "Testimony of James F. Hoge," *Hearings on Proposed Regulations. November 17 & 18, 1938,* pp. 70–96, 88-52A-89, Box 144, F 603 (Proposed Regulations, Book 1), W-NRC. See also Hoge's remarks as reported in "Drug Law Hearing Shows Labeling Opposition," *Oil Paint and Drug Reporter* 134 (November 21, 1938), 32A.

41 *Memorandum Submitted by Winthrop Chemical Co, Inc.,* November 25, 1938, 88-52A-89, Box 144, F 603 (Proposed Regulations, Book 3, W to Z); Charles Wesley Dunn [General Counsel, American Pharmaceutical Manufacturers' Association] to Members, *Bulletin No. 261,* March 3, 1939, 88-58A-277, Box 22, F 512.1 (General Correspondence January–March), W-NRC. For more on the history of "professional labeling," as it was termed, see Marks, "Revisiting 'The Origins of Compulsory Drug Prescriptions' " (n. 26), 109–115.

42 "Professional labeling" would be permitted and the companies would not be liable if the products were misused. They would, however, lose the right to continue shipping the drug under the "professional" exemption. The question of liability continued to concern manufacturers, however. See the discussion in J. J. Durrett, "Some of the Implications of Section 505(b) (1) of the Food, Drug and Cosmetic Act," American Drug Manufacturers Association, *Proceedings. 28th Annual Meeting* (1939), 105–112.

43 On the difficulties of policing the marketing of drugs with a restricted labeling, both before and after the formal promulgation of the regulations, see O. Olsen to George P. Larrick, December 27, 1938, 88-58A-277, Box 22, F 512.1, W-NRC; J. J. Durrett to Assistant General Counsel [FDA], October 24, 1940, 88-59A-2736, Box 24, F 505.1–508.2, W-NRC. Compliance was highly variable, from year to year and depending on the drug in question. Food and Drug Administration, *Annual Report 1941,* 17; *Annual Report 1942–1943,* 39–40.

digitalis, arsenical compounds, and the barbiturates enhanced reformers' awareness of the dangers inherent in inappropriate medical use.[44]

The Elixir Sulfanilamide episode only reinforced this concern. By 1937, more than 100 firms were marketing variants of sulfanilamide. One such company, S. E. Massengill, hit upon the ingenious idea of manufacturing sulfanilamide in syrup form. The substance they chose as a buffer, ethyl diglycerol, was an antifreeze additive whose toxic properties were well known, except to Massengill's chemist. Distribution on the open market led to 106 deaths, and the subsequent passage of the 1938 drug act.[45]

The job of tracking down the victims and reporting on the circumstances of their deaths fell to the FDA. While putting the new law to work, the FDA's Klumpp was also writing up an analysis of the tragedy that led to its passage:

> I think you will be interested in some of the implications that arise from the observations recorded. I refer particularly to the fact that of 105 deaths associated with the consumption of the drug and, to the best of our knowledge, attributable to the drug, in a hundred instances the drug was administered on a physician's prescription. The physician's diagnoses . . . are also of some interest.[46]

Among the questionable conditions for which the drug was prescribed, Klumpp noted "Bright's disease, bichloride of mercury poisoning, renal colic and back-ache," none with the remotest connection to the infectious diseases for which sulfanilamide was known to work. Moreover, in "most cases" the recommended blood tests used to monitor patients on sulfanilamide "were not made."[47] If Klumpp and his colleagues needed additional grounds for believing that physicians too needed more guidance in selecting drugs, the Elixir Sulfanilamide episode provided it.[48]

44 On digitalis, see the remarks by Henry Christian in "Abstract of Discussion," *JAMA* 75 (August 14, 1920), 465. On the arsenicals, see Council on Pharmacy and Chemistry, *Bulletin* 55 (April 6, 1932), 450. For inappropriate physician uses of other dangerous drugs, see Council on Pharmacy and Chemistry, *Bulletin* 58 (June 14, 1933), 248; *Bulletin* 64 (June 26, 1935), 379 (cinchophen). On the barbituates, see W. C. Ashworth, "Injurious Effect of Veronal and Related Drugs, and Suggestions for More Restricted Use," *Southern Medical Journal* 22 (1929), 813–817; H. M. Walker, "Barbital: Its Uses and Misuses," *U.S. Naval Medical Bulletin* 28 (March–April, 1930), 327–335; Soma Weiss, "The Indications and Dangers of Sedatives and Hypnotics with Special Reference to the Barbituric Acid Derivatives," *International Clinics* 46 (1936), 47–61. For a more optimistic view of barbiturate abuses, see Otto Lowy, "A Comparative Study of the Habitual Use of Barbituates and Coal-Tar Derivatives As Furnished by Reports from Various Hospitals throughout the United States," *Canadian Medical Association Journal* 31 (December 1934), 638–641. For a similar story on dinitrophenol, see John Parascandola, "Dinitrophenol and Bioenergetics: An Historical Perspective," *Molecular and Cellular Biochemistry* 5 (1974), 69–77.
45 Young, "Sulfanilamide and Diethylene Glycol" (n. 33), 105–126.
46 Theodore G. Klumpp to John P. Peters, December 29, 1939, 88-58A-277, Box 38, F 511.07–512, W-NRC.
47 Herbert O. Calvery and Theodore G. Klumpp, "The Toxicity for Human Beings of Diethylene Glycol with Sulfanilamide," *Southern Medical Journal* 32 (November 1939), 1106–1107.
48 For additional expressions of FDA skepticism regarding physicians' knowledge of drugs, see the remarks of J. J. Durrett, addressing members of the drug industry: "Some of the Implications of Section 505(b) (1) of the Food, Drug and Cosmetic Act," American Drug Manufacturers Associa-

NEW DRUGS: THE CASE OF SULFAPYRIDINE

> If the drug that killed one person in 10,000 was of only minor use therapeutically it might still be judged to be unsafe, whereas the drug which killed one in a thousand persons if it had marked and undisputed therapeutic value, such as the drug under question, it would still be a safe and valuable drug.[49]

> The clinical information submitted with the application is usually the ultimate basis upon which a decision regarding the product is reached. . . . The appraisal of the clinical work is not easy.[50]

Notwithstanding their dangers, the therapeutic promise of the sulfonamides was substantial. By 1937, numerous chemical compounds related to sulfanilamide were under development. Such variants, researchers counseled, must be tested carefully in controlled laboratory and clinical settings before their introduction into clinical practice.[51]

Therapeutic reformers had issued such warnings before, but now they had the opportunity to put the force of law behind them. The new legislation not only enabled the FDA to regulate the hazards of existing drugs, it authorized the agency to rule on the safety of novel compounds before their introduction into general use. The announcement of a new sulfonamide product in the spring of 1938 gave FDA officials an opportunity to define the standards they would use in evaluating new drugs.

In May 1938, shortly before enactment of the new law, British investigators reported on a new sulfonamide compound, 2-para-aminobenzene sulfonamide pyridine (sulfapyridine), which appeared to be extremely effective in a variety of experimental infections. Claims that the drug showed low toxicity in mice led to speculation that it might prove to be a safer and more beneficial drug than sulfanilamide: "Dose for dose, the drug appears more efficient than sulphanilamide, and, in low dose, it is very definitely superior."[52] The prospect of a drug

tion, *Proceedings. 28th Annual Meeting* (1939), 104. See also Theodore Klumpp to J. J. Durrett, October 10, 1938, 88-72A-2335, Box 1, NDA 2 (Neoprontosil), W-NRC.

49 J. J. Durrett, *Memorandum of Interview with Perrin H. Long and E. Kennerly Marshall* [Johns Hopkins], December 5, 1938, 88-69A-2099, Box 1, NDA 90, vol. 1, W-NRC.

50 Walton Van Winkle Jr. to Paul Dunbar and Robert Herwick, January 30, 1946, 88-59A-2736, Box 220, F 505.1074–509, W-NRC.

51 References to variant compounds under development may be found in "Sulfanilamide – A Warning," *JAMA* 109 (October 2, 1937), 1128. Lionel Whitby makes reference to over 1,000 "such compounds" by the following year: "Chemotherapy of Bacterial Infections," *Lancet* ii (November 12, 1938), 1095.

52 Lionel Whitby, "Chemotherapy of Pneumococcal and Other Infections with 2-(p-Aminobenzenesulphonamido) Pyridine," *Lancet* i (May 28 1938), 1212. The initial British clinical studies were reported by G. M. Evans and Wilfrid F. Gaisford, "Treatment of Pneumonia with 2-(p-aminobenzenesulphonamido) Pyridine," *Lancet* ii (July 2, 1938), 14–19. On comparative toxicity relative to sulfanilamide, see letter of J. B. Ravdin [University of Pennsylvania] to D. F. Robertson [Merck], September 3, 1938, 88-69A-2099, Box 1, NDA 90, vol. 1, W-NRC. On the British response to the drug, see Michael Worboys, "Treatments for Pneumonia in Britain, 1910–1940," in

that might be beneficial, when used safely, made sulfapyridine an ideal test case for putting the new law to work.

On October 7, 1938, representatives of Merck & Company submitted their application for sulfapyridine to the FDA. Along with copies of the published British literature and preliminary clinical reports from investigators in this country, the Merck representatives noted that "great demand had [already] arisen for the article" owing to advance publicity. Review by the AMA's Council on Pharmacy and Chemistry, they added, was imminent.[53] The FDA was not persuaded: the toxicological data submitted were quite "meagre," the manner in which humans metabolized the drug was undocumented, and clinical reports from investigators in this country were few in number. The firm would have to present more data before the FDA would rule on its application.[54]

On scientific and economic grounds, the most promising use of sulfapyridine appeared to be for pneumonia. Existing serum treatments of pneumonia were, as we have seen, expensive, required special facilities and experience to use effectively, and only worked on certain strains of pneumococci. Sulfanilamide was of limited use in treating pneumonias. The idea of a cheap, effective drug for pneumonia that could be used readily by the average physician had great appeal.[55] The clinical investigators to whom Merck entrusted sulfapyridine therefore focused their attention on pneumonia cases.

During the fall, the FDA continued to accumulate clinical and laboratory data favorable to sulfapyridine. Apart from material submitted through Merck, FDA officials actively solicited the opinions and reports of investigators known to be using the drug.[56] By December, the initial deficiencies in the animal toxicological data had been remedied.[57] The FDA had decided to approve sulfapyridine, but

Ilana Löwy, ed., *Medicine and Change: Historical and Sociological Studies of Medical Innovation* (Paris: Editions John Libbey Eurotext, 1993), pp. 317–335.

53 J. J. Durrett, *Memorandum of Interview with Joseph Rosin and R. E. Gruber,* October 7, 1938; Joseph Rosin to Henry Wallace, October 7, 1938. Preliminary clinical data from A. R. Dochez, Columbia College of Physicians and Surgeons, and J. B. Ravdin, University of Pennsylvania, were presented with the application. Though finding the drug useful in pneumonia and systemic infections, Dochez noted that the number of cases "are still too small to draw any conclusions based on statistics." Dochez to D. F. Robertson, September 26, 1938. All references 88-69A-2099, Box 1, NDA 90, vol. 1, W-NRC.

54 W. G. Campbell to Joseph Rosin, Merck and Company, Inc., October 28, 1938. Perrin H. Long, who was to act as the FDA's advisor on this drug, had already expressed some skepticism about the "very enthusiastic reports" appearing in the British literature, and advised getting "really good detailed clinical work" from "reputable hospitals" in the United States. Perrin H. Long to Theodore Klumpp, September 28, 1938. Both references 88-69A-2099, Box 1, NDA 90, vol. 1, W-NRC. See also J. J. Durrett, *Memorandum of Interview with R. E. Gruber* [Merck], October 14, 1938, 63A-292, Box 374, AF 12-611, vol. 1, W-NRC.

55 J. J. Durrett, *Memorandum of Interview with Perrin H. Long and E. Kennerly Marshall* [Johns Hopkins], December 5, 1938, 88-69A-2099, Box 1, NDA 90, vol. 1, W-NRC. On the complexities of serum treatment, see Chapter 2.

56 Harrison F. Flippin to J. M. Carlisle, November 28, 1938; J. J. Durrett, *Memorandum of Interview with A. R. Dochez, Dr. Cook,* November 28, 1938; J. J. Durrett to M. A. Blankenhorn and to W. C. Davison, December 9, 1938. All 88-69A-2099, Box 1, NDA 90, vol. 1. W-NRC.

57 Herbert E. Stokinger, *Absorption, Acetylation and Excretion of 2-sulfanilamide (Dagenan, M & B 693),*

had not yet decided under what restrictions. Determining sulfapyridine's "safety" depended as much on its value in treating specific clinical conditions as on any toxicological data. Safety, according to this philosophy, was "a relative term and its exact meaning for each preparation would, on the basis of the facts, have to be determined."[58]

Investigators agreed that the drug was likely to prove of considerable benefit in treating pneumonias. Questions remained, however, about when and how it was safest to use. Clearly, "the drug was not killing many people" but at the same time, there was "no uniformity of opinion with respect to the harm which the drug might be capable of doing from one investigator to another."[59] Some researchers reported extensive vomiting and nausea among their patients; others did not. The differences might be due either to variations in manufacturing routine, or to differences in the dosages used by different investigators.[60] Before approving the drug, the FDA would require additional clinical data, a demand to which Merck representatives readily agreed.[61]

Some clinical investigators were not as patient. With the next pneumonia season imminent, and the data favorable to sulfapyridine mounting, several researchers began to urge release to the medical profession at large, if not to the lay public.[62] Others placed less confidence in their peers: even the medical profession might abuse the drug if it was released before more was known about appropriate dosage. Some pneumonia specialists feared that sulfapyridine's premature release

November 11, 1938, and Hans Molitor, *Preliminary Report: Toxicity of 2-sulphanilyl-aminopyridine*, November 28, 1938, 88-69A-2099, Box 1, NDA 90, vol. 1, W-NRC. Stokinger was a biochemist in Michael Heidelberger's lab at Columbia; Molitor worked for Merck.

58 J. J. Durrett, *Memorandum of Interview with Perrin H. Long and E. Kennerly Marshall* [Johns Hopkins], December 5, 1938, 88-69A-2099, Box 1, NDA 90, vol. 1, W-NRC. Marshall, a supporter of the 1938 act, expressed himself pleasantly surprised with the FDA's philosophy. See also J. J. Durrett to W. C. Davison, December 9, 1938, 88-63A-292, AF 12-611 [Merck], vol. 1, Box 374, W-NRC.

59 J. J. Durrett, *Memorandum of Interview with Dr. Joseph Rosin* [Merck] *and D. W. Richards* [Columbia University], December 1, 1938; in Durrett's view, "there was no way to dispute the value of this drug." See J. J. Durrett, *Memorandum of Interview with Perrin H. Long and E. Kennerly Marshall* [Johns Hopkins], December 5, 1938. All references 88-69A-2099, Box 1, NDA 90, vol. 1, W-NRC.

60 J. J. Durrett, *Memorandum of Interview with Perrin H. Long and E. Kennerly Marshall* [Johns Hopkins], December 5, 1938, 88-69A-2099, Box 1, NDA 90, vol. 1, W-NRC. By the end of the month, it appeared as if manufacturing variations did not account for the variation in such reactions: J. J. Durrett to Perrin H. Long, December 22, 1938, 88-69A-2099, Box 1, NDA 90, vol. 2, W-NRC.

61 On being informed of the FDA's position, the firm's representative expressed its "sympathy with it." See J. J. Durrett, *Memorandum of Interview with Dr. Joseph Rosin* [Merck] *and D. W. Richards* [Columbia University], December 1, 1938, 88-69A-2099, Box 1, NDA 90, vol. 1, W-NRC. By this time, an additional application had been filed by Calco Chemical Co., 88-69A-2099, Box 2, NDA 160, W-NRC. Three additional firms filed in January: see 88-69A-2099, Box 3, NDA 422 (E. R. Squibb), and NDA 469 (Sharp & Dohme), and 88-68A-1292, Box 1, NDA 476 (Abbott Laboratories), W-NRC.

62 J. J. Durrett, *Memorandum of Interview with E. K. Marshall and Perrin H. Long*, December 30, 1938, 88-69A-2099, Box 1, NDA 90, vol. 2, W-NRC. By the end of the month, Marshall and Long had reversed their position of December 5, and become advocates for immediate release. Compare the following discussion with Worboys, "Treatments for Pneumonia in Britain" (n. 52), pp. 326–328, who emphasizes the comparative reluctance of U.S. researchers to abandon serum therapy for the new drug.

might lead physicians to abandon a proven remedy, serum therapy, even for those cases where it was best suited.[63]

Faced with conflicting advice, FDA officials took their dilemma to the leaders in the field. In a series of interviews, they polled the group of investigators who had been working with sulfapyridine: Should the drug be released now for use by physicians, or should its distribution be limited to qualified investigators while additional research continued?[64] The answers they got depended largely on how the question (and the law) was read.

Proponents of delay were concerned about having the drug released to general practitioners before sufficient information was available on its safe and optimal use. A few months delay would have several advantages: (1) additional data on the use of sulfapyridine would be accumulated, enabling physicians to assess its merits in specific types of pneumonias; (2) by the end of the pneumonia season, sufficient reports of the drug's side effects would be in print to chasten and instruct physicians' use of the drug; (3) more would be known about safe and effective dosage, an issue that was growing increasingly complex.[65] Some researchers feared losing the opportunity to study the drug on sufficient numbers of patients if it was released immediately: "Putting this drug on the market right now will make it difficult to get the data which will make it possible to evaluate the action of this drug alone and in combination with serum."[66]

By contrast, advocates of early release thought that the FDA already had enough data to act. The ultimate determination of the new drug's toxicity, like that of

---

63 Some, but not all, of this opposition came from advocates of serum therapy, including Rufus Cole, who had initially developed the serum treatment. For Cole's position on sulfapyridine, see John L. Rice [New York City Commissioner of Health] to Thomas Parran, [U.S. Surgeon General], December 22, 1938, and the accompanying resolution of New York State's Advisory Committee on Pneumonia Control, 88-69A-2099, Box 1, NDA 90, vol. 2, W-NRC. For other advocates of further study, see J. J. Durrett, *Memorandum of Interview with Sanford M. Rosenthal and Carl Voegtlin,* December 5, 1938, 88-62A-292, Box 374, AF 12-611 [Merck], vol. 1, W-NRC.

64 W. G. Campbell to M. A. Blankenhorn, January 5, 1939. For a list of those surveyed, see W. G. Campbell to Paul Leech, [AMA Council on Pharmacy and Chemistry], January 5, 1939, 88-69A-2099, Box 1, NDA 90, vol. 2, W-NRC.

65 Walter Grady Reddick to W. G. Campbell, January 13, 1939; Charles McKhann to W. G. Campbell, January 7, 1939. Alphonse Dochez, one of the more careful and reflective investigators, while he did not oppose immediate distribution, noted two intellectual/practical problems with the current state of knowledge: (1) because individuals reacted to the drug differently, and acetylation rates between individuals were highly variable, controlling dosage required measuring actual serum concentrations directly at frequent intervals, rather than simply regulating the amount administered by units; (2) the East Coast was experiencing a wave of nonpneumococcal pneumonia on which the drug was useless, and at present "we find ourselves considerably confused from a clinical and laboratory standpoint, with what kind of pneumonia we are dealing and a decision whether or not to use the drug becomes difficult." A. R. Dochez to W. G. Campbell, January 11, 1939. For other reports of variability in acetylation/absorption of drug, see the remarks of Jesse M. Bullowa and H. E. Stokinger, reported at the New York Academy of Medicine meeting, January 17, 1939; and C. A. Hermann [Chief Eastern District] to Food and Drug Administration, January 18, 1939. All references 88-69A-2099, Box 1, NDA 90, vol. 2, W-NRC.

66 John T. Cain and R. W. Weilerstein, *Memorandum of Interview with Norman Plummer and Dr. Henning,* and *Memorandum of Interview with Dr. Colin McLeod,* January 27, 1939, 88-69A-2099, Box 1, NDA 90, vol. 2, W-NRC.

sulfanilamide, would be a long time in coming. Hopkins's Perrin H. Long urged release despite his speculation that the more serious toxicities experienced with sulfanilamide – hemolytic anemia and agranulocytosis – would eventually show up with sulfapyridine, even though he had not yet seen any such cases. For the treatment of pneumonia, where sulfanilamide had little effect, Long argued, the merits of sulfapyridine were already established.[67]

The press was already convinced. The *New York Times* found the prospect of saving money as well as lives irresistible: "before long we shall swallow tablets of a complex chemical instead of resorting to expensive injections of serum and thus deal with all 32 types of pneumonia."[68] Opposition to release, several investigators charged, was simply an effort on the part of specialists in serum treatment to protect their investment in knowledge and equipment for pneumococcal typing and serum production.[69]

To accumulate more data without excessive delay, the FDA contacted the two principal manufacturers for a list of all investigators to whom they had distributed the drug. On February 1, 1939, they began surveying an additional forty-five physicians having research experience with the drug. The individuals contacted constitute a virtual who's who of clinical investigators and infectious disease specialists.[70] More reasons for caution began to emerge. Even under current arrangements, which restricted the drug to investigational use, it was hard to confine its uses to pneumococci. Some researchers feared that preliminary reports of its use in gonococcal infections would trigger premature and uninformed use by physicians unless the FDA somehow held the floodgates. Surely there was some way, researchers wrote, to release it for pneumonias only, or perhaps limit distribution to "qualified clinicians in many centers . . . as an intermediate step."[71] Holding on to the drug until the spring might cost the lives of a few patients, but

67 See P. H. Long to David Bryce, January 13, 1939, 88-69A-2099, Box 2, NDA 160, W-NRC; J. J. Durrett, *Memorandum of Interview with E. K. Marshall and Perrin H. Long,* December 30, 1938, 88-69A-2099, Box 1, NDA 90, vol. 2, W-NRC. See also I. S. Ravdin to J. J. Durrett, January 4, 1939, and January 9, 1939; Perrin H. Long to W. G. Campbell, January 9, 1939; and John T. Cain and R. W. Weilerstein, *Memorandum of Interview with Evan Evans,* January 27, 1939, all 88-69A-2099, Box 1, NDA 90, vol. 2, W-NRC. For one drug company's representation, see David A. Bryce to W. G. Campbell, January 25, 1939, 88-69A-2099, Box 2, NDA 160, W-NRC.
68 "The Fight against Pneumonia," *New York Times,* January 19, 1939, 18. See also J. D. Ratcliff, "Death to the Killer," *Colliers* 102 (December 24, 1938), 18, 52–53.
69 R. W. Weilerstein and John T. Cain, *Memorandum of Interview with M. H. Dawson* and *Memorandum of Interview with Harold Thomas Hyman,* January 27, 1939, 88-69A-2099, Box 1, NDA 90, vol. 2, W-NRC.
70 John T. Cain and R. W. Weilerstein, *Memorandum of Interview with J. M. Carlisle, Mr. Anderson, Miss Person* [Merck], January 25, 1939; and John T. Cain and R. W. Weilerstein, *Memorandum of Interview with David A. Bryce* [Calco], January 25, 1939, 88-69A-2099, Box 1, NDA 90, vol. 2, W-NRC. Additional letters went out the following week.
71 M. A. Blankenhorn to W. G. Campbell, February 2, 1939; Hugh Morgan to W. G. Campbell, February 6, 1939; *Memorandum of Interview with Harris S. Johnson,* February 3, 1939; O. H. Robertson to W. G. Campbell, February 7, 1939; David D. Rutstein to W. G. Campbell, February 7, 1939; W. H. Carroll to W. G. Campbell, February 9, 1939; L. H. Schmidt to W. G. Campbell, February 9, 1939. All 88-69A-2099, Box 1, NDA 90, vol. 3, W-NRC.

many more would benefit in the long run by the knowledge obtained of how best to use the drug. The greatest benefit, advocates of restraint urged, would come from controlled evaluations on large numbers of patients, by experienced investigators willing to alternate patient assignment between serum and sulfapyridine.[72] The AMA's Council on Pharmacy and Chemistry and Morris Fishbein, editor of *JAMA*, each counseled patience while additional research was completed under suitable conditions.[73]

Whatever the reservations of skeptics, press reports accentuated the positive. News of favorable investigations reached the public overnight.[74] While continuing to gather data, the FDA was coming under pressure from friend and foe alike to release sulfapyridine. By February, E. K. Marshall, who had initially endorsed the agency's caution about sulfapyridine, wrote: "I was very much interested and did what little I could to promote the passage of the present Food, Drug and Cosmetic Bill. I do not want to feel that I was mistaken in doing this but cannot help occasionally wondering if the present lack of the drug for seriously ill patients is not worse than operating under the old Food and Drug Act."[75]

As the six-month statutory deadline for acting on the original application approached, additional calls to release the drug came from former skeptics.[76] Reviewing the evidence from months of interviewing and data collection, the FDA's Theodore Klumpp, by then chief of the Drug Division, concluded that the majority of investigators consulted approved of release:

72 John T. Cain and R. W. Weilerstein, *Memorandum of Interview with Jesse G. M. Bullowa, and Dr. Holle,* January 26, 1939, 88-69A-2099, Box 1, NDA 90, vol. 2, W-NRC. To guard against the multiple problems of spontaneous remission, differential response to treatment by age, seasonal variability in infectiousness, and investigator bias, Bullowa wanted to study a minimum of thirty persons for each of several age groups, over the course of at least one pneumonia season, with automatic treatment assignment to serum, drug, or serum plus drug to guard against investigators biasing treatment selection. See Jesse G. M. Bullowa, Norman Plummer, and Maxwell Finland, "Sulfapyridine in the Treatment of Pneumonia," *JAMA* 112 (February 11, 1939), 570, and Maxwell Finland to W. G. Campbell, February 8, 1939, 88-69A-2099, Box 1, NDA 90, vol. 3, W-NRC.

73 Council on Pharmacy and Chemistry, "Preliminary Report of the Council," *JAMA* 112 (February 11, 1939), 538; "Sulfapyridine – The New Sulfanilamide Derivative," *JAMA* 112 (February 11, 1939), 541. The council's recommendation was a curious one: Long, the author of the council's report, was by this time urging release, but the other members felt that the drug should be retained on "experimental status." See Council on Pharmacy and Chemistry, *Bulletin* (January 18 and 25, 1939), and Paul Nicholas Leech to W. G. Campbell, February 1, 1939, 88-69A-2099, Box 1, NDA 90, vol. 3, W-NRC. Fishbein was apparently collecting information on sulfapyridine from his own sources, who reported both "spectacular results" and the absence of any opportunity to conduct the necessary controlled observations as yet. See William S. Middleton to Morris Fishbein, March 11, 1939, William S. Middleton papers, Box 8, MS C 206, NLM.

74 "New Drug Is Hailed As Pneumonia Cure," *New York Times* (January 18, 1939), 21.

75 E. K. Marshall to W. G. Campbell, February 3, 1939, 88-69A-2099, Box 1, NDA 90, vol. 3, W-NRC.

76 The New York State and New York City Advisory Committees for Pneumonia Control, which in December had opposed release, endorsed release of the drug in late February. Russell L. Cecil to Theodore G. Klumpp, February 27, 1939, 88-69A-2099, Box 1, NDA 90, vol. 3, W-NRC. The change of heart was noted at the time by the FDA's Klumpp. See his *Memorandum for Mr. Campbell,* February 23, 1939, 88-69A-2099, Box 1, NDA 90, vol. 3, W-NRC.

While a few investigators recommended that the drug be withheld from the market, such recommendations upon analysis do not appear to rest upon considerations of the intrinsic safety or danger of the drug. Principally those workers were concerned with the orderly development of medical scientific knowledge concerning the therapeutic efficacy of the drug and the relation of this drug to other available forms of therapy in pneumonia.

While these are important considerations from the point of view of research and medicine, they do not constitute, in our judgment, a substantial basis for withholding this application under the provisions of section 505.[77]

On March 9, 1939, letters went out to each of six firms, indicating that the FDA would not deny their applications for sulfapyridine, provided the manufacturers ensure, through labeling and advertising, that the drug be used "under close, continuous observation of a qualified practitioner of medicine." It was the manufacturers' responsibility to warn physicians of the drug's toxicity, and instruct them in managing such cases.[78] But neither the FDA nor the industry could take responsibility for the likelihood that sulfapyridine "will undoubtedly be abused by the unwise and ill-informed whenever it is put on the market." This was a "problem of medical practice" and not of drug regulation.[79]

THE BURDEN OF REGULATION

This was the first time in the history of American medicine that I know of where it was possible for the medical profession to have opportunity to be informed about a new drug before the detail man was around at his door importuning him to use a drug about which he knew little.[80]

In their handling of the sulfapyridine case, FDA officials established procedures and enunciated a philosophy of drug regulation that, with minor changes, would govern the agency's behavior and that of the regulated industry until after World War II. The law mandated the FDA to prevent the sale of "unsafe" drugs. But the idea of an unsafe drug covered a multitude of sins. The toxicity of some drugs could be readily established in the laboratory. The standards imposed by the FDA's toxicologists enabled the agency to screen out demonstrably unsafe drugs, or compounds whose safety for clinical testing had not yet been established. In the first year of operation under the new law, more than half of the applications

77 Theodore G. Klumpp, *Memorandum for Mr. Campbell,* February 23, 1939, 88-69A-2099, Box 1, NDA 90, vol. 3, W-NRC.
78 W. G. Campbell to Dr. Joseph Rosin [Merck], March 9, 1939, 88-69A-2099, Box 1, NDA 90, vol. 3, W-NRC.
79 Theodore G. Klumpp, *Memorandum for Mr. Campbell,* February 23, 1939, 88-69A-2099, Box 1, NDA 90, vol. 3, W-NRC.
80 Paul Nicholas Leech, "Relation of the Food, Drug and Cosmetic Act to the Work of the Council on Pharmacy and Chemistry and Manufacturing Pharmacy," American Drug Manufacturers Association, *Proceedings. 28th Annual Meeting* (1938), 119.

submitted were withdrawn without prejudice, many of these for insufficient data.[81]

Drugs such as sulfapyridine presented a different problem. There was no question that it was toxic and little question either that it was of considerable benefit. Only clinical evidence could determine whether it would do more harm to ban the drug or release it. With nearly 1,700 applications filed during the first eighteen months of the act, the FDA was in no position to do its own research on each drug.[82] Nor, even if it were possible, did the FDA wish to do so:

> In our judgement, the question of safety is so important that it is ordinarily desirable to have a number of independent investigators study the question. From this standpoint, then, we go to the literature and study the reports of investigations contained therein, as well as those submitted by the manufacturer. In many cases these are sufficient to establish a prima facie case of safety and then it is unnecessary to go further. In the instances such as, for instance, sulfapyridine, where the problem is a very difficult one, we obtain from the manufacturer a list of all the investigators who have studied the drug and communicate with them, visit them, go over their records, and on the basis of the sum total of experiments with the drug we are in a much better position to arrive at a correct conclusion than if we made tests ourselves.[83]

The work of one group of scientists, no matter how eminent, was always subject to error. The scientific community, in the view of FDA officials, was far less likely to err. To evaluate drugs like sulfapyridine, the physicians responsible for administering the 1938 legislation turned to their peers and mentors.

In considering the applications for sulfapyridine, the FDA reviewed over 2,000 cases.[84] For drugs known to produce reactions, like the sulfonamides or the arsenicals used in the treatment of syphilis, "a very large series of cases is necessary" for weighing the severity and frequency of hazards against the therapeutic benefits obtained.[85] But numbers alone were not enough: "Sheer volume of

81 For an example of the FDA's requirements on toxicological data, see the testimony of Robert P. Herwick, *Hearings on Quinimid. 1939*, 51–59, 88–58A-277, Box 19, F 505.7, W-NRC. For approval rates, see Carl M. Anderson, "The 'New Drug' Section," *Food Drug Cosmetic Law Quarterly* (March 1946), 84; Theodore G. Klumpp to Arthur DeGraaf, February 17, 1940, 88–59A-2736, Box 24, F 505.1–508.2, W-NRC.

82 Theodore Klumpp to Arthur DeGraaf, September 27, 1939, 88–58A-277, Box 38, F 511 (General, September–December), W-NRC.

83 Ibid. See also Jack M. Curtis, Theodore G. Klumpp, *Memorandum of Interview with A. Stanley Cook,* April 8, 1938, 88–52A-89, Box 138, F 520–32G; testimony of Theodore Klumpp, *Transcript of Hearing. Quinimide Corporation. 1939*, 228–230, 88–58A-277, Box 19, F 505; Walton Van Winkle Jr. to William Deichmann, July 6, 1944, 88–59A-2736, Box 166, F 505.1–505.6, W-NRC.

84 Theodore G. Klumpp, *Memorandum for Mr. Campbell,* February 23, 1939, 88–69A-2099, Box 1, NDA 90, vol. 3, W-NRC.

85 J. J. Durrett to Bruce Webster, February 6, 1940, 88–59A-2736, Box 24, F 505.1–508.2, W-NRC. Interestingly, only a handful of the 280 individuals who received "investigational" shipments of sulfapyridine treated more than 100 cases. Of the 98 investigators reporting results to the FDA, only 20 based their arguments on more than 35 patients. As noted already, obtaining multiple "takes" on the data appears to have been more important than the number of cases seen by any

clinical reports or large numbers of cases are not sufficient in themselves to be decisive. Attention must be directed to the character of the investigations and the quality of the investigators."[86] "Qualified investigators" provided the most valuable data: "We are always delighted to receive the kind of well-controlled, qualified reports that emanate from our better institutions."[87]

To those whose work showed little appreciation of experimental rigor, the FDA's scientists emphasized the basic elements of therapeutic research: the importance of controls and the need for a sufficient number of cases.[88] In this, they shared the views of the Council on Pharmacy and Chemistry: "the word 'control' isn't the only thing. You have to have fair controls and adequate controls, just as much so in clinical work as in pharmacological work."[89] But good methods alone did not provide good decisions. Where a detailed review of the available evidence did not produce a clear recommendation, then the strategy developed in the sulfapyridine case was called for: "Choosing those investigators with the greatest experience, or those known to be critical in their approach to investigative problems, personal visits should be made to these men and the doubtful points discussed."[90] Francis Blake's endorsement of sulfapyridine, for example, was "significant" because Blake was "recognized throughout the country as one of the most critical and conservative therapeutists."[91]

Translating the convictions of academic physicians into directives for regulatory policy was not always an easy matter. In the absence of formal criteria, determinations of safety were bound to be complex judgments, dependent upon the beliefs of those consulted as well as the available data. In deciding when to release

one group. On the importance of numbers in other cases, see J. J. Durrett to Joseph Rosin, March 29, 1940; J. J. Durrett, *Memorandum of Interview with Perrin H. Long and E. K. Marshall*, April 3, 1940, 88-69A-2009, Box 7, NDA 2076, W-NRC.

86 Walton Van Winkle Jr. to Paul Dunbar and Robert Herwick, January 30, 1946, 88-59A-2736, Box 220, F 505.1074–509, W-NRC.

87 Theodore G. Klumpp to Arthur DeGraaf, October 28, 1939, 88-58A-277, Box 38, F 511 (General, September–December), W-NRC. FDA physicians were at pains to convince reluctant specialists that the problems of therapeutic evaluation deserved their attention. Theodore G. Klumpp to Fuller Albright, February 4, 1939, 88-58A-277, Box 22, F 512.1.10–512.6.31, W-NRC.

88 On the importance of controls, see the testimony of Sanford M. Rosenthal, B. J. Vos, and Ernest King, *Transcript of Hearing. Teotisil Labs Corporation. 1940*, 56–58, 339, 349–350; testimony of George Bobbs, *Transcript of Hearings. The Dominion Laboratories. "Sunica." 1940*. Both transcripts in 88-59A-2736, Box 24, W-NRC. See also Walton Van Winkle Jr. to Paul Dunbar and Robert Herwick, January 30, 1946, 88-59A-2736, Box 220, F 505.1074–509, W-NRC.

89 Leech, "Relation of the Food, Drug and Cosmetic Act to the Work of the Council" (n. 80), 121.

90 Walton Van Winkle Jr. to Paul Dunbar and Robert Herwick, January 30, 1946, 88-59A-2736, Box 220, F 505.1. 074–509; Sulfaguanidine, NDA 3911, vol. 1, p. 12, 88-76-89, Box 2, W-NRC.

91 Theodore G. Klumpp, *Memorandum of Interview with Francis G. Blake*, February 2, 1939, 88-69A-2099, Box 1, NDA 90, vol. 3. Klumpp came to the FDA from Yale, where Blake had been a senior colleague. E. K. Marshall made a similar remark about the acuity of the clinical observations made by his colleague, Perrin Long. Ernest Q. King, *Memorandum of Interview with E. K. Marshall, Jr.*, April 26, 1941, 88-59A-2736, Box 71, F 511.07 (January–July), W-NRC. See also NDA 3911, Sulfaguanidine, 88-76-69, Box 2, vol. 1, 12; Theodore G. Klumpp, Fred W. Irish, and Ernest Q. King, *Memorandum of Interview with Perrin H. Long*, March 19, 1941, 88-80-22, Box 1, NDA 3726, Sulamyd, vol. 1, W-NRC.

sulfapyridine, the key question was whether to delay approval until the research community could establish a scientific basis for rational use of the drug. One group of experts felt that thorough therapeutic evaluation of sulfapyridine, like that of any drug, was a matter of years, not months. In the meantime, individual physicians would be better off learning to live with a degree of uncertainty about the drug's toxic effects. Provided they used the drugs intelligently, physicians need not fear harming their patients.[92] Other researchers held that even a brief delay would produce valuable information about the safest and most appropriate use of the drug, benefiting patients and practitioners alike.

Those most reluctant to release the drug immediately were especially skeptical about the ability of general practitioners to use drugs intelligently and safely. Their comments indicate a desire that the FDA not only anticipate but prevent the potential misuse of new drugs by the profession at large. The question was, how far could the FDA go in this direction? Klumpp and his colleagues decided they had gone far enough. In determining drug safety, the FDA would require proof of a drug's clinical value and insist that manufacturers pay careful attention to the therapeutic claims that accompanied their products. Such literature would, where possible, instruct physicians in when and how to use a drug.[93] Sulfapyridine was approved for the treatment of pneumonia, and nothing else. Proposed new uses would require a new review.[94] But whether physicians went on to use the drugs as they were intended was not the FDA's problem.

The principles and procedures adopted in the sulfapyridine case served as the

---

92 On the notion that thorough drug evaluation was a matter of years, not months, see University of Chicago physiologist A. J. Carlson to Mr. Virgil Chapman, February 21, 1938, citing the examples of insulin and the arsenicals, 88-52A-89, Box 124, F 062 (F&D Act. March–April), W-NRC; S. L. Christian [Hospital Division, Public Health Service], *Memorandum for Medical Officers,* May 6, 1935, PHS General Classified Files, 1924–1935, RG 90, Box 67, F 0470, NA. See also the general remarks of E. K. Marshall Jr. on the recent tendencies to abandon "time honored slow and laborious method[s] of reaching conclusions" in "An Unfortunate Situation in the Field of Bacterial Chemotherapy," *JAMA* 112 (January 28, 1939), 352–353. On the need for physicians to accustom themselves to managing the toxic effects of the sulfa drugs, see Perrin H. Long and James Haviland, "A Clinical Evaluation of the Use of Sulfanilamide, Sulfapyridine and Sulfathiazole in the Treatment of Bacterial Infections," American Drug Manufacturers Association, *Proceedings. 29th Annual Meeting* (1940), 91.

93 The FDA frequently monitored the nature and extent of therapeutic claims made on behalf of products, though apparently with limited effect in some cases. See J. J. Durrett to Hoffman La Roche, April 20, 1940, and Ernest Q. King, *Memorandum for Dr. Durrett,* June 4, 1940, 88A-68A-1292, Box 1, NDA 776; Ernest Q. King, *Memorandum to Dr. Herwick,* May 26, 1941, 88-80-22, Box 1, NDA 3726, vol. 1; R. P. Herwick to Lederle Laboratories, September 29, 1942, 88-59A-2736, Box 107, F 511.07 (August); and Walton Van Winkle Jr. to Lederle Laboratories, Inc., April 13, 1943, 88-59A-2736, Box 142, F 511.07 (January–April), W-NRC.

94 When sulfapyridine was subsequently presented for use in treating gonorrhea, manufacturers were asked to provide "supporting scientific reports" for the new claims, although not as extensive as for the initial review. FDA officials were, if anything, more concerned, that the average physician lacked the information to use the drug safely for the new indication. It was up to the manufacturer to provide that information. George W. Merck to J. J. Durrett, March 13, 1940, and J. J. Durrett to Paul N. Leech, March 28, 1940, 88-69A-2099, Box 1, NDA 90, vol. 3, W-NRC.

basis for the FDA's approach to drug regulation into the postwar era.[95] In translating the statutory language of the 1938 drug law into a viable system of drug regulation, the FDA relied heavily on the cooperation of three groups: the regulated industry, the medical–scientific community, and practicing physicians. The FDA's success in obtaining this cooperation depended on two conditions: that each group shared the assumptions on which the FDA premised its philosophy of drug regulation, and that the actions to which this philosophy led did not conflict with the more fundamental desires and purposes of any group.

On the first condition, there was widespread agreement. All three groups accepted that the safety of new drugs could not be determined in the abstract but depended, as the statute indicated, on the way in which a drug was meant to be used. The viability of the FDA's approach to drug regulation therefore depended ultimately on the burdens it imposed on each of the affected groups.

The medical–scientific community, which originated the principles under which the FDA operated, found little to quarrel with in the agency's adoption of their credo.[96] FDA officials expected research physicians to divert energy and attention from their scientific work to provide data and advice on the therapeutic consequences of new drugs. Some, if not all, investigators complied.[97] Much of the work submitted in support of new drug applications, however, did not come from experienced researchers. But lacking defensible criteria to identify the "line

---

95 In the case of certain compounds recommended by civilian experts for military use, the FDA expedited approval by reducing the volume of cases required. See the letters by Perrin H. Long on behalf of the National Research Council to J. J. Durrett, and Dr. Paul Nicholas Leech (AMA Council on Pharmacy and Chemistry), June 5, 1940, requesting approval for sulfathiazole. Two months previously, Long and his colleagues had recommended that the FDA require analysis of 2,000 to 3,000 cases before approval. J. J. Durrett, *Memorandum of Interview with Perrin H. Long and E. K. Marshall, Jr.*, April 3, 1940. All documents in NDA 2076 (Sulfathiazole), 69A-2099, Box 7, W-NRC. Similar expedited handling was arranged for sulfaguanidine: W. G. Campbell to David A. Bryce, May 1, 1941, NDA 3911, 88-76-79, Box 2, vol. 1, W-NRC.

96 By and large, dissents from this community regarding the FDA's policies are confined to technical disagreements about specific decisions or rules of evidence. See, for example, Hunter F. Kennedy to Perrin H. Long, August 27, 1942, 88-59A-2736, Box 107, F 511.07 (August), W-NRC. The most substantial criticism of the FDA's practices I have found is the commentary of several prominent toxicologists that the FDA's approach to toxicity testing may be too standardized and retarding the appearance of new drugs on the market. Chauncey D. Leake, Raymond Gregory, Paul L. Ewing, and George A. Emerson, "Appraisal of New Drugs," *JAMA* 127 (January 27, 1945), 244. To my knowledge, this letter represents the first appearance in print of the induced "drug lag" hypothesis, which has achieved ideological popularity in recent years. In practice, the FDA's approach to new drug application review appears to have been far less standardized than the critique by Leake et al., implies. See the letter of Walton Van Winkle Jr. to Richard K. Richards, December 19, 1944, 88-59A-2736, Box 166, F 505.1–505.6, W-NRC, which discusses many of the issues in the Leake critique.

97 Some individuals found greater appeal in their own researches than in the questions inspired by the FDA; others were reluctant to challenge the work of colleagues and mentors even when they disagreed with them. See A. DeGraaf to T. G. Klumpp, October 3, 1939, 88-58A-277, Box 38, F 511 (General, September–December); Fuller Albright to T. Klumpp, January 26, 1939, 88-58A-277, Box 22, F 512.1.10–512.66; Jack M. Curtis, *Memorandum of Interview with William M. Allen, G. W. Corner, Harold C. Hodge,* January 16, 1939, 88-58A-277, Box 23, F 520.32G, W-NRC.

of demarcation between ordinary physicians and those obviously devoting a major portion of their time to investigative work," the agency could only judge the work, not the worker.[98] FDA officials complained frequently about the quality of scientific and clinical work presented to them, but apart from educational efforts, did little about it. For the individual physician, producing adequate therapeutic research was a moral, not a legal, obligation. No unpleasant consequences followed for the individuals who elected not to comply.[99]

The FDA's policies could not avoid "impinging" on the practicing physician.[100] Like other therapeutic reformers, FDA officials remained skeptical of practitioners' diligence in informing themselves about drugs. Such concern lay behind the FDA's proposal to adopt so-called prescription labeling which would permit the agency to routinely regulate the information manufacturers provided physicians about their products.[101] By monitoring the information practicing physicians received about new drugs, FDA officials hoped to improve the quality of therapeutic practice. The more direction the FDA's reviews could provide about the relative merits of different drugs, the safer the therapeutic practices that might be observed. But for long-term assessments of therapeutic merit, the FDA deferred to the scientific community and the AMA's Council on Pharmacy and Chemistry. By and large, FDA officials offered no challenges to physicians who used drugs without regard to agency approved indications: the prospect of physicians using drugs "contrary to the recommendations in the labelling is unfortunately a matter

---

98 Walton Van Winkle Jr. to Paul Dunbar and Robert Herrick, January 30, 1946, 88-59A-2736, Box 220, F 505.1074–509, W-NRC; on the moral "obligations" of medical experts, see J. J. Durrett to Stanley P. Reimann, January 28, 1939, 88-58A-277, Box 38, F 511 (General, January–February); Theodore G. Klumpp to Arthur DeGraaf, October 28, 1939, 88-58A-277, Box 38, F 511 (General, September–December), W-NRC.

99 For the FDA's assessment of the quality of work submitted in the initial years of operation under the 1938 act, see Theodore G. Klumpp [Address], American Pharmaceutical Manufacturers, *Proceedings* (1941), 51–55; and J. J. Durrett to Arthur C. Degraaf, March 22, 1940, 88-59A-2736, Box 24, F 505.1–508.2, W-NRC.

On the continued inadequacy of the clinical and laboratory data submitted to the FDA, see Walton Van Winkle Jr. to Richard K. Richards, December 19, 1944, 88-59A-2736, Box 166, F 505.1–505, W-NRC; and Food and Drug Administration, *Annual Report. 1944* (Washington, DC: Food and Drug Administration, n.d.), 50. While the FDA did not take action against investigators whose work was not up to par, firms that attempted to market drugs under the guise of distributing them for investigative purposes were considered fair game. Los Angeles District, Division of Regulatory Management, New Drugs, *Memorandum, Spicer-Gerhart Company,* July 27, 1950, 88-63A-292, Box 55, F 501.2–510, W-NRC.

100 Walter G. Campbell, "Administration of New Federal Food, Drug and Cosmetic Law," *Oil, Paint and Drug Reporter* 134 (October 31, 1938), 41.

101 For evidence of the continuing skepticism of FDA officials toward the scientific awareness and therapeutic capabilities of most physicians, see Durrett, "Some of the Implications of Section 505(b) (1)" (n. 1), 104; Ernest Q. King, *Memorandum to Dr. Herwick,* May 26, 1941, 88-80-22, Box 1, NDA 3726, vol. 1; P. B. Dunbar, *Memorandum of Interview with Dr. Austin Smith,* May 26, 1947, 88-59A-2736, Box 234, F 045.91–046.5; and McKay McKinnon Jr. to Chief, Baltimore Station, February 3, 1942, 88-57A-2736, Box 108, F 511.07 (January–February), W-NRC. On "prescription labeling" regulations, see J. J. Durrett to the Assistant General Counsel, October 24, 1940, 88-59A-2736, Box 24, F 505.1–508.2, W-NRC.

which we are not permitted to consider in connection with the new drug applications."[102]

At times, reformers thought the FDA should go further. For some potent yet dangerous drugs, individual physicians suggested, perhaps the FDA should restrict their use to experienced, hospital-based, clinicians.[103] Here, too, FDA officials demurred:

Used by experts in hospitals, [a new spinal anesthetic] may be reasonably safe. But we are concerned about what may happen if it is used in the general practice of obstetrics. Personally, I do not feel that the Congress intended the Act to cover a discrimination between the anesthetists of the large hospital and [the] general practitioner. There is no reason, however, why you [the Council on Pharmacy and Chemistry] should not discriminate between them.[104]

Improving therapeutic practice was, in the final analysis, a task for the profession and not the government.[105]

The FDA's emphasis on regulating drugs, not medical practice, placed the heaviest burden of regulation on the industry. Given the costs the 1938 drug Act imposed on manufacturers, their initial response to the law was surprising. Numerous firms could agree with the representative of Lederle Laboratories who welcomed the FDA's inclination "to tell us things we ourselves didn't fully appreciate about our drug and to improve the directions that were to be put thereon." Although the FDA required firms to provide extensive laboratory and clinical information on the merits (and disadvantages) of new drugs, and restricted the conditions for which those drugs should be marketed, industry generally responded favorably to the burden.[106]

So long as the FDA confined itself to policing the claims that accompanied

102 Hunter F. Kennedy to Perrin H. Long, August 27, 1942, 88-59A-2736, Box 107, F 511.07 (August), W-NRC.
103 *Memorandum to Walton van Winkle,* February 15, 1945; *Memorandum of Interview with Dr. Elmer C. Bartels and Dr. Brissard,* March 17, 1945; and *Memorandum of Interview with Dr. Abraham Cantarow and Dr. A. E. Pashkis,* March 12, 1945, vol. 1, NDA 5627 [Thiouracil], 72A-2335, Box 68, W-NRC.
104 Erwin Nelson and Ernest Q. King to Walton van Winkle Jr., August 4, 1947, 88-59A-2736, Box 247, F 510C, W-NRC.
105 In general, the FDA proposed to handle the question of potential inappropriate use by carefully managing the terms of the product-labeling statement. See W. G. Campbell to Merck & Co., Inc., November 3, 1941, 88-64A-314, Box 374, AF 12-6111, vol. 2, W-NRC. See also R. A. Vonderlehr, W. T. Harrison, M. I. Smith, and S. M. Rosenthal to the Surgeon General, September 16, 1940, Public Health Service, General Classified Records, 1936–1944, RG 90, Box 57, NA.
106 See the remarks of R. S. Childs [Lederle Laboratories] in discussion of J. J. Durrett's "New Drug Application Requisites," *Oil, Paint and Drug Reporter* (May 22, 1939), 46. For an opposing point of view, see James F. Hoge, "An Appraisal of the New Drug and Cosmetic Legislation from the Viewpoint of Those Industries," *Law and Contemporary Problems* 6 (Winter 1939), 121. In general, however, "the trade has accepted [the] decision" to regulate the distribution of drugs by controlling the labeling for the use. "Drug Enforcement Reviewed in Campbell Report," *Oil, Paint and Drug Reporter* 136 (December 25, 1939), 3.

approved drugs, industry spokesmen acknowledged the FDA's right to consider the benefits, as well as the hazards, of new drugs. FDA determinations based on the risk–benefit criterion and even, on occasion, considerations of risk–benefit relative to existing products went unchallenged.[107] But when the FDA attempted to remove products from the market, on the grounds that they were without therapeutic merit, individual firms and industry representatives began challenging not only the FDA's decisions in individual cases but the premises on which the FDA's entire approach to drug regulation was based.[108]

One of the FDA's initial moves came against the labeling of ovarian substances: "physicians who use such products are entitled to know that there is no scientific evidence that such products when administered orally possess any therapeutic activity." In the view of the trade press, the FDA's dictum was tantamount to telling "the manufacturer that he must undertake to educate the physicians."[109]

The real confrontation did not come, however, until 1948 when the FDA decided that *no* labeling for inert glandular substances could satisfy the terms of the law, since it was impossible to write instructions for the safe use of a drug that was without effect.[110] According to industry spokesmen, the ruling set a dangerous precedent by usurping the physician's therapeutic judgment, a sentiment echoed by congressional physician George Calver, who reported himself embarrassed because he was now unable to "fill [such] prescriptions for the wives of my Congressional group."[111] The skirmish over glandular substances was one of

---

For examples of FDA requests for additional data to accompany new drug applications and/or modifications of therapeutic claims, see J. J. Durrett to Hoffman-LaRoche, Inc., March 26, 1940, 68A-1292, Box 1, NDA 776; Walton Van Winkle to R. J. Strassenburgh, March 11, 1943, 88-59A-2736, Box 142, F 511.07 (January–April), W-NRC.

107 See, for example, J. J. Durrett, *Memorandum of Interview with Perrin Long and E. K. Marshall,* April 3, 1940; and J. J. Durrett to Joseph Rosin, July 19, 1940, 88-69A-2099, Box 7, NDA 2076, W-NRC. Similar discussions of comparative benefit–risk occurred in correspondence with clinicians concerning this drug: see 88-68A-1292, Box 6, NDA 2701, vol. 1, W-NRC. Owing to conflicting opinions among investigators, the FDA ruled that "comparative statements with respect to sulfathiazole and sulfapyridine" should not be included in the labeling. J. J. Durrett to H. G. Bertram, July 19, 1940, 88-68A-1292, Box 8, NDA 2712, vol. 1. For other instances of relative risk–benefit reasoning, see Walton Van Winkle Jr. to David A. Bryce [Lederle Laboratories], January 11, 1946, 88-69A-2099, Box 20, NDA 5656, vol. 1; Theodore G. Klumpp, Fred W. Irish, and Ernest Q. King, *Memorandum of Interview with Perrin H. Long,* March 19, 1941, 88-80-22, Box 1, NDA 3726, Sulamyd, vol. 1.; Ernest Q. King, *Memorandum of Interview with Charles B. Huggins and Ronald E. Stevens,* May 5, 1941, and Ernest Q. King, *Memorandum of Interview with E. K. Marshall, Jr.,* April 25, 1941, both in 88-59A-2736, Box 71, F 511.07 (January–June), W-NRC.

108 Any confrontation with industry was postponed until 1940 when the FDA's legal authority to move against companies that made exaggerated therapeutic claims on existing products kicked into effect. After 1940, the FDA no longer had to prove fraudulent intent to regulate such claims. "Drug Law Enforcement Reviewed in Campbell Report," *Oil, Paint and Drug Reporter* 136 (December 25, 1939), 42.

109 "Ovarian Substance Abased by F.D.A.," *Oil, Paint and Drug Reporter* 138 (December 30, 1940), 3. On the FDA's reluctance to act as late as 1947, see A. G. Murray to Central District, July 11, 1947, 88A-59A-2736, Box 250, F 523.4, W-NRC.

110 Dunn and Kleinfeld, *Federal Food, Drug and Cosmetic Act* (n. 36), 756–757.

111 George W. Calver to the Pure Food and Drug Administration, July 1, 1948 and C. W. Crawford to Calver, July 9, 1948, 88-59A-2736, Box 582, F 526-13, W-NRC. See also George R. Hazel,

several in the postwar period in which the FDA's right to examine the therapeutic value of new drugs came increasingly under attack.[112]

So long as regulators and regulated shared the same beliefs, the FDA could make case decisions that seemed both valid and just. Once those principles were challenged, FDA officials looked to higher authority to define the rules of the game. Reviewing eight years of operation under the new law, Walton Van Winkle Jr., chief of the FDA's drug division, concluded that "it would be of great assistance . . . if there were a background of judicial opinion" regarding the weight to be accorded efficacy in considering "the 'relative safety' of a new drug" and the role considerations of "relative efficacy" could play in assessing newer products.[113] By 1950, Van Winkle's successor, Robert Stormont, reported that the FDA no longer felt it possible to consider evidence of efficacy in ruling on new drugs. The industry's challenge did not alter the intellectual commitment of agency officials to the principle of efficacy but they reinforced officials' perception that considerations of efficacy could not be given the deciding weight in reviewing new drug applications.[114] The FDA's circumspection meant that, in the postwar period, reformers would turn once again to the profession's scientific elite to take the lead in reforming therapeutic practice.

"Report of the Medical Section," American Drug Manufacturers Association, *Proceedings. 37th Annual Meeting* (1949), 37; W. W. Wheeler Jr. "Interference with the Practice of Medicine," *Food, Drug and Cosmetic Law Quarterly* (September 1948), 365–375; A. G. Murray, *Memorandum of Interview with Mr. Karl Bambach* [American Drug Manufacturer's Association], March 30, 1948, 88-59A-2736, Box 582, F 526.13, W-NRC.

112 For more on the postwar industry campaign against the FDA, which covered policies ranging from factory inspection to the FDA's right to designate prescription drugs, see Marks, "Revisiting 'The Origins' " (n. 26).

113 Walton Van Winkle Jr. to Paul Dunbar and Robert Herrick, January 30, 1946, 88-59A-2736, Box 220, F 505.1074-509, W-NRC. See also Morris L. Yakowitz to Scientific and Chemical Industries Company, October 23, 1950, 88-63A-292, Box 59, F 534.1, W-NRC; A. Altmeyer [Acting Administrator, FSA] to Senator Forrest C. Donnell, January 19, 1950, Federal Security Administration, General Classified Records (1944–1950), RG 235, Box 311, F 950, NA.

114 Although Stormont's account is probably an exaggeration of actual practice, it suggests a growing consciousness on the FDA's part that it lacked the authority to give primacy to considerations of efficacy. The FDA's desire to seek new statutory authority for efficacy decisions probably stems in part from its changed perception of the legal situation. See Robert T. Stormont, "Our Mutual Responsibilities in the Regulatory Control of Drugs," American Drug Manufacturers Association, *Proceedings. 38th Annual Meeting* (1950), 139–144. Stormont had left the FDA at the time of this address.

4

War and peace

> Both in industry and in war men are regimented. Everywhere there is a system –
> system in reconnoitering from the air, firing shells from a battery, building an
> airplane, preparing and packaging a breakfast food.[1]

During World War II, the cause of organized therapeutic investigation received a
substantial boost. The war provided an unprecedented opportunity for the nation's
scientific elite to direct the conduct and organization of scientific research. In
medicine, clinical investigators from the country's leading medical schools turned
to cooperative studies to guide them in instructing the nation's physicians on how
and when the newest wonder drugs – penicillin and streptomycin – should be
used.

Like many in wartime Washington, medical scientists found themselves awash in
an alphabetic sea of agencies, replete with overlapping jurisdictions and competing
agendas. On June 24, 1941, President Roosevelt vested control over federal
research money and policy in the hands of Vannevar Bush, head of the newly
created Office of Scientific Research and Development (OSRD).[2] In the case of
medicine, Bush relied heavily on an existing network of committees at the
National Research Council's Division of Medical Sciences. Created in World War
I to provide scientific and technological advice to the military, the National
Research Council (NRC) had developed an elaborate system of committees
representing university scientists from multiple disciplines. Engaged during peace-
time in advising corporations and foundations on questions of scientific research,
the NRC returned to advising the military on medical affairs in mid-1940. By the
time OSRD was created, the NRC's Division of Medical Sciences had eight

---

1 Waldemar Kaemffert, "War and Technology," *American Journal of Sociology* 46 (January 1941), 442.
2 On the organization of World War II science, see Daniel J. Kevles, *The Physicists: The History of a
Scientific Community in Modern America* (New York: Vintage Books, 1979), pp. 296–301; Carroll
Pursell, "Science Agencies in World War II: The OSRD and Its Challengers," in Nathan Reingold,
ed., *The Sciences in the American Context: New Perspectives* (Washington, DC: Smithsonian Institution
Press, 1979), pp. 359–378; Irvin G. Stewart, *Organizing Scientific Research for War: The Administrative
History of OSRD* (Boston: Little Brown, 1948), pp. 34–45. On the multiplicity of wartime planning
agencies more generally, see Otis L. Graham Jr., *Towards a Planned Society: From Roosevelt to Nixon*
(Oxford: Oxford University Press, 1976), pp. 79–86.

major committees and thirty-three subcommittees reviewing problems of military medicine.[3]

At OSRD, Vannevar Bush created a Committee for Medical Research (CMR) to oversee government planning and contracting for medical research. At its first meeting, the committee decided to rely heavily on the NRC: Lewis Weed, chairman of the NRC's Division of Medical Sciences, was appointed vice-chairman of the Committee on Medical Research, and the head of each of the NRC's major medical subject committees was appointed a consultant to the Committee on Medical Research. As a nongovernmental body, the NRC could not legally allocate government funds, but its recommendations on investigators and projects usually governed CMR funding decisions.[4]

The NRC's committees had never suffered from a lack of eminent and capable scientists. Having the resources to carry out their plans was another matter.[5] Bush's decision to place the management of medical research in NRC's hands offered academic physicians the opportunity to put prewar ideals of clinical research into practice. For the first time in its history, medicine's intellectual elite had the opportunity not only to set an example for the rest of the profession but actually to direct the conduct of therapeutic research on a national scale. In each area of medicine, NRC's committees selected the topics to be studied and the best means of attack. Investigators willing to research the designated problems received ample funds.[6]

Researchers' prewar convictions regarding cooperative studies dovetailed neatly with military exigencies: putting a group of specialists to work on well-defined problems was deemed both efficient and scientific. For innovative treatments – the newer sulfa drugs or penicillin – the NRC's committees regarded centrally planned cooperative studies as ideal. Such studies, by virtue of their ability to accumulate large numbers of patients treated according to a common regimen, were thought to yield the most reliable answers in the shortest time. But although

3 On the World War I origins of the NRC, see Kevles, *The Physicists* (n. 2), pp. 109–118. Nathan Reingold discusses the origins and interwar years of the NRC in "The Case of the Disappearing Laboratory," *American Quarterly* 29 (Spring 1977), 79–101. See also Glenn E. Bugos, "Managing Cooperative Research and Borderline Science in the NRC, 1924–1942," *Historical Studies in the Physical and Biological Sciences* 20 (1989), 1–32. For World War II, the NRC was largely, though not exclusively, preempted by other organizations in areas outside of medicine. On medical planning for World War II, see Stewart, *Organizing Scientific Research* (n. 2), pp. 99–100; Nathan Reingold, "Vannevar Bush's New Deal for Research: or The Triumph of the Old Order," *Historical Studies in the Physical and Biological Sciences* 17 (1987), 313–314.
4 A. N. Richards, "Foreword," in E. C. Andrus et al., *Advances in Military Medicine* (Boston: Little, Brown, 1948), vol. I, pp. xliii–xliv, 45–46, 98–101; Stewart, *Organizing Scientific Research for War* (n. 2), p. 103. Two exceptions to this pattern were the projects to develop penicillin and to test antimalarial agents, where CMR took a controlling role.
5 Stanhope Bayne-Jones, "A History of the National Research Council, 1919–1933: VI. Division of Medical Sciences," *Science* 78 (July 14, 1933), 26–29.
6 Between 1941 and 1947, CMR spent over $25 million in research funds; by contrast, the National Institutes of Health over this period spent only $5.8 million, $4 million of it in 1947 when CMR had virtually closed up shop. See Stephen Strickland, *Politics, Science and Dread Disease: A Short History of United States Medical Research Policy* (Cambridge: Harvard University Press, 1972), p. 16; *NIH Factbook* (New York: Marquis Academic Publishing, 1972), p. 98.

wartime circumstances favored the organization of cooperative studies, they provided no guarantees that medical researchers would execute their well-designed studies according to plan.

A SCIENTIFIC ETHIC

> Human experimentation is not only desirable but necessary in the study of many of the problems of war medicine which confront us.[7]

Among the many problems identified by the Committee on Medical Research, finding improved ways to treat or, ideally, to prevent venereal disease ranked high on the list. During World War I, syphilis and gonorrhea in the military services caused the loss of nearly seven million days of active duty. Giving up on efforts to "stifle the instincts of man" or "legislate his appetite," the army turned to chemistry and medicine for "adequate preventive measures."[8]

Existing medical methods of prevention were imperfect, and dependent on soldiers' willingness to come forth for "chemical prophylaxis" after exposure. Newer methods, such as providing self-administered prophylactic doses of the newer sulfonamide drugs, carried less of a stigma, but the risks these treatments posed to military operations were unknown. Potential liabilities included adverse drug reactions; sensitization, which would affect subsequent use in more serious medical circumstances; and the possibility of producing undiagnosed gonorrhea carriers who might transmit the disease to other soldiers.[9] The military accordingly focused on increasing the efficiency of existing preventive measures and treatments. Meanwhile, with CMR's support, civilian researchers began the search for more effective medical treatments.

Of the two diseases, syphilis and gonorrhea, the latter posed the greater scientific problem. In the case of syphilis, the immediate challenge was to adapt existing treatments to military circumstances. If new remedies arose, researchers had developed viable animal models for assessing the benefits and risks of treatment. Notwithstanding some difficulties in extrapolating animal studies to humans, systematic exploratory research could proceed. No such animal models existed for gonorrhea: developing a vehicle for experimental infections was CMR's first order of business. In February 1942, the NRC's committee on venereal disease endorsed Justina Hill, a bacteriologist at the Johns Hopkins Hospital, to begin work on such a model.[10] Meanwhile, human studies provided the only means to evaluate treatment.

7 A. N. Richards to J. E. Moore, October 9, 1942, OSRD/CMR, RG 227, Box 36, F Human Experimentation, VD, NA.
8 Joel T. Boone, quoted in Allan M. Brandt, *No Magic Bullet: A Social History of Venereal Diseases in the United States since 1880* (New York: Oxford University Press, 1985), p. 164. For figures on World War I losses, see ibid., p. 115. For an excellent discussion of the political and cultural problem of managing venereal disease in the two world wars, see ibid., pp. 110–115 and 161–170.
9 J. E. Moore to A. N. Richards, February 1, 1943, NAS–NRC Central File: Division of Medical Sciences: Committee on Medicine, Subcommittee on Venereal Diseases: 1943, NAS.
10 On Hill's scientific career and work, see Thomas B. Turner, *Heritage of Excellence: The Johns Hopkins*

If studies in humans were necessary, the ideal approach from the researchers' point of view was to deliberately infect, then treat, human volunteers. Investigators could thereby control the timing and degree of the infection, and monitor their subjects carefully while under treatment. Army medical officials, however, doubted whether soldiers could be successfully isolated for the length of the study. Even if the logistic difficulties of confining soldiers could be overcome, army representatives were unwilling to subject draftees to "deliberate experimentation."[11] The alternative was to study prophylaxis in "naturally occurring populations": individuals who had already been exposed to gonorrhea. Members of the NRC's committee on venereal disease, long familiar with the difficulties of interpreting such uncontrolled studies, were unwilling to rely on them.[12]

By November 1942, Hill's efforts to induce gonococcal infections in animals were only slightly more advanced than they had been in February.[13] The value of sulfathiazole, the newest sulfonamide, in preventing gonorrhea remained relatively untested. The army meanwhile continued to rely principally on older, less promising unctions. Calomel ointment, issued as a syphilis preventive, had no specific effect on gonococcal infections; silver picrate ointment, introduced in July 1942, was soon abandoned by army physicians, owing to the irritations it caused.[14] At a conference held to acquaint various OSRD researchers with the progress of work on chemical prophylaxis, Charles Carpenter and Alfred Cohn, two research physicians from New York, proposed to evaluate the new drug sulfathiazole on experimentally infected prison volunteers.[15]

Medical Institutions, 1914–1947 (Baltimore: Johns Hopkins University Press, 1974), pp. 418–419; Hugh Hampton Young, *A Surgeon's Autobiography* (New York: Harcourt, Brace, 1940), pp. 255–257, 260–262. On the wartime search for an animal model for gonorrhea, see *Conference on Chemical Prophylaxis of Venereal Diseases. 23 March 1942*, NRC Program Files: DIV NRC: Medical Sciences: CMR, Subcommittee on Venereal Diseases: Conferences: 1941-1943, NAS. On the use of animal models for studying syphilis, see Alan M. Chesney, *Immunity in Syphilis* (Baltimore: Williams and Wilkins, 1927).

11 For a summary of army objections, see Lewis H. Weed to Ross G. Harrison, March 2, 1943, OSRD/CMR, RG 227, Box 36, F Human Experimentation, NA. It may have been more difficult to experiment on an army of draftees than it had been in the volunteer army of the Great War. See Mark H. Leff, "The Politics of Sacrifice on the American Home Front in World War II," *Journal of American History* 77 (March 1991), 1296–1318.

12 *Conference on Chemical Prophylaxis of Venereal Diseases. 23 March 1942*, NRC Program Files: DIV NRC: Medical Sciences: CMR, Subcommittee on Venereal Diseases: Conferences: 1941–1943, NAS.

13 NRC, Subcommittee on Venereal Disease, *Minutes of a Conference on Chemical Prophylaxis. November 18, 1942*, NRC Program Files: DIV NRC: Medical Sciences: Committee on Medicine, Subcommittee on Venereal Diseases: Conferences 1941–1943, NAS. J. E. Moore to A. N. Richards, February 1, 1943, NAS-NRC Central File: DIV NRC: Medical Sciences, Committee on Medicine, Subcommittee on Venereal Diseases: 1943, NAS.

14 Oral sulfathiazole prophylaxis, while widely used in various branches, was opposed by many army physicians; the Surgeon General approved its general use in the summer of 1943. For the history of chemical prophylaxis against gonorrhea in the army, see Thomas H. Sternberg, Ernest B. Howard, Leonard A. Dewey, and Paul Padget, "Venereal Diseases," in United States Army, Medical Department, *Preventive Medicine in World War II*, vol. 5, *Communicable Diseases Transmitted through Contact or by Unknown Means* (Washington, DC: Office of the Surgeon General, 1960), pp. 198–204.

15 NRC, Subcommittee on Venereal Disease, *Minutes of a Conference on Chemical Prophylaxis. November*

Joseph Earle Moore, chair of the NRC's committee on venereal disease, and a veteran of the prewar Cooperative Clinical Group, did not question the arguments put forth on behalf of a prison study. Given the problems with either animal experiments or observational studies, Moore did not doubt the need to conduct a human experiment: "It is believed that military necessity and the impossibility of obtaining the desired results immediately or in the predictable future, in any other manner, justify the use of human volunteers for this purpose."[16] The only remaining question, in the experts' view, was the selection of a suitable population. Any study that deliberately inflicted disease, the NRC's specialists reasoned, must have the best chance possible of providing a valid answer. In their view, only a well-controlled study in which the risks were explained in advance could morally justify the undertaking.[17]

A prison study, proponents argued, would offer safeguards to the subjects, who could be closely monitored for the reactions characteristic of sulfa drugs.[18] Most important, prisoners could be isolated from sexual activity for six months. Years of inconclusive research had convinced the specialists on the NRC committee that only sexual isolation would guarantee the experiment's scientific success. Without such measures, subjects might naturally acquire infections, hopelessly contaminating any evaluation of treatment outcomes. Neither civilian nor military volunteers, they reasoned, would subject themselves to the required degree of control. Moore's committee did not believe that inmates of "institutions for the feeble-minded or insane" could offer meaningful consent to such a study.[19] After considering various alternatives, Moore recommended that the Committee on Medical Research endorse "present" and "possibly future" proposals to study "chemical and chemotherapeutic prophylaxis of gonorrhea" in a controlled study of prison volunteers.[20]

18, 1942, NRC Program Files: DIV NRC: Medical Sciences: Committee on Medicine, Subcommittee on Venereal Diseases: Conferences 1941–1943, NAS. Carpenter's proposal had been under discussion for over a month at this point.

16 J. E. Moore to A. N. Richards, February 1, 1943, NAS-NRC Central File: DIV NRC: Medical Sciences, Committee on Medicine, Subcommittee on Venereal Diseases: 1943, NAS.

17 For details of the experimental design, see *Proposed Plan of Procedure in the Study of Chemical Prophylaxis among Human Volunteers among Prison Inmates. December 19, 1942,* OSRD/CMR, RG 227, Box 36, F Human Experimentation, NA. The consent form attached to the protocol bears favorable comparison with current examples of the genre.

18 On the importance of safeguards for the volunteers, see R. E. Dyer [Director, National Institutes of Health] to A. N. Richards [Chair, Committee on Medical Research], January 18, 1943, CMR/OSRD, RG 227, Box 36, NA. On contemporary debates over the use of prisoners (and other groups) as research subjects, see Susan E. Lederer, *Subjected to Science: Human Experimentation in America before the Second World War* (Baltimore: Johns Hopkins University Press, 1995), pp. 110–121, esp. 110–113.

19 Military prisoners and conscientious objectors were also rejected, as neither group was expected to be fully cooperative. J. E. Moore to A. N. Richards, February 1, 1943, NAS-NRC Central File: DIV NRC: Medical Sciences, Committee on Medicine, Subcommittee on Venereal Diseases: 1943, NAS.

20 Ibid. The arguments in Moore's letter reflect several months of deliberation with NRC and CMR/OSRD officials about the merits of the proposed study, but although this document responds to

Customarily, funding recommendations originating with NRC subcommittees were readily acted on by OSRD's Committee on Medical Research, after a brief technical review within NRC. CMR officials had already established the precedent of using prisoners, in a study to test bovine albumin as a blood substitute. A. N. Richards, CMR chairman, saw no problem in using prisoners again for the gonorrhea study, provided "the risks have been fully explained" to the volunteers.[21]

The engineers and physicists in charge of wartime research were less comfortable than their medical associates with the idea of deliberately inflicting gonorrhea. Science officials desired a more comprehensive assessment, one that took into account the proposal's political ramifications as well its scientific merit. This review soon reached the highest levels of NRC and its parent organization, the National Academy of Sciences.[22]

Senior officials in all three organizations recognized the need for the study to receive a careful and thorough peer review. It *must* be shown to be scientifically necessary for either NRC, the National Academy of Sciences, or OSRD to consider sponsoring it.[23] But for the lay individuals in charge of these organizations, the proposed experiment raised questions that the NRC's medical specialists could not address. For Frank Jewett, President of the National Academy of Sciences, the proposal's political implications transcended the specialists' narrow technical competence: "In an extreme case their scientific opinion might be the most authoritative in the world and yet their opinion on a matter of public policy have no more value than that of any similar group of intelligent laymen."[24]

According to Jewett, whether a human experiment was necessary was a "scientific" question; whether prisoners should be used in such a study was a matter of "public policy." Jewett thought Moore's proposal was "certainly loaded with potential dynamite for those sponsoring it."[25] "My difficulty," Jewett explained,

certain concerns of Moore's superiors, the logic of the argument is reflected in earlier, less formal communications.

21 A. N. Richards to J. E. Moore, October 9, 1942, OSRD/CMR, RG 227, Box 36, NA. On the bovine albumin study, see Andrus, *Advances in Military Medicine* (n. 4), vol. I, pp. 450–453.

22 For a detailed chronology of NRC, OSRD, and NAS communications on this subject, see Harry M. Marks, *Ideas As Reforms: Therapeutic Experiments and Medical Practice, 1900–1980* (Ph.D. thesis, Massachusetts Institute of Technology, 1987), pp. 112–113.

23 On OSRD's views, see A. N. Richards [CMR] to J. E. Moore, January 29, 1943, OSRD/CMR, RG 227, Box 53, NA; on the views of senior NRC and NAS officials, see Frank Jewett to Ross Harrison, February 16, 1943, NAS-NRC Central File: DIV NRC: Medical Sciences: Committee on Medicine, Subcommittee on Venereal Diseases: 1943, NAS, and my discussion which follows.

24 Frank Jewett [President, National Academy of Sciences] to Ross Harrison [Chairman, NRC], February 23, 1943 [hereafter cited as letter 2], NAS-NRC Central File: DIV NRC: Medical Sciences: Committee on Medicine, Subcommittee on Venereal Diseases: 1943, NAS.

25 Frank Jewett to Ross G. Harrison, February 16, 1943; February 23, 1943 [in response to Harrison's letter of February 20: hereafter cited as letter 1], and February 23, 1943 [letter 2], NAS-NRC Central File: DIV NRC: Medical Sciences: Committee on Medicine, Subcommittee on Venereal Diseases: 1943, NAS.

"resides in the fact that prison populations are not free populations and that so-called volunteers from such populations are not true volunteers in the ordinary sense. Their volunteering is or can be alleged to have been brought about by reasons which are entirely absent in a free population."[26]

If local officials or the prisoners themselves subsequently objected to the study, Jewett and his associates would find it difficult to convince "public opinion" that the prisoners had freely volunteered. Before Jewett risked the academy's reputation by endorsing such a project, Moore's committee must demonstrate more conclusively that the alternatives were unworkable.[27] After all, as Jewett confided to Ross Harrison, chairman of the NRC: "If the military with some millions of men at their disposal are not prepared to handle the matter on a truly voluntary basis, it would seem to me to raise a very considerable doubt as to the necessity of performing the experiment at all."[28]

Part of Jewett's concern was that of the Washington veteran, eager to establish a procedural record behind which he and Vannevar Bush, head of OSRD, could hide in the event of a subsequent outcry. Bush and CMR chair Richards were "entitled to a record they can use without question in connection with their final decision."[29] But Jewett also required Moore to justify his scientific conclusion that a prison population offered the best means of conducting a valid and informative experiment. Moore's reasons for rejecting studies with military and civilian volunteers not only had to be documented, they had to persuade.

Jewett's regard for the necessity of the study and its scientific merits appears to have progressively increased.[30] Once convinced of the medical experts' logic as

26 Frank Jewett to Ross G. Harrison, February 16, 1943, NAS-NRC Central File: DIV NRC: Medical Sciences: Committee on Medicine, Subcommittee on Venereal Diseases: 1943, NAS.
27 Frank Jewett to Ross G. Harrison, February 16, 1943; February 23, 1943 [letters 1 and 2], NAS-NRC Central File: DIV NRC: Medical Sciences: Committee on Medicine, Subcommittee on Venereal Diseases: 1943, NAS. Although much of Jewett's concern rested on the fact that he and Harrison would be in the front lines of any subsequent inquiry into the decision, Jewett, once he had reviewed the scientific rankings of the proposal, did not wish to see it sidetracked by taking it to the academy's council or administrative committee, which would, in his opinion, be deadlocked on such an issue.
28 Frank Jewett to Ross G. Harrison, February 16, 1943, NAS-NRC Central File: DIV NRC: Medical Sciences: Committee on Medicine, Subcommittee on Venereal Diseases: 1943, NAS.
29 Frank Jewett to Ross Harrison, February 23, 1943 [letter 2]. See also Jewett's draft of a letter for Ross Harrison to send to Lewis Weed, chairman of the NRC's Division of Medical Sciences, and the accompanying cover letter to Harrison, February 25, 1943, NAS-NRC Central File: DIV NRC: Medical Sciences: Committee on Medicine, Subcommittee on Venereal Diseases: 1943, NAS. For Bush's concern with the public reaction, see A. N. Richards to J. Earle Moore, February 8, 1943, OSRD/CMR, RG 227, Box 36, F Human Experimentation, NA. This folder also contains the various endorsements of the study solicited from military and public health officials at the requests of A. N. Richards, Jewett, and Bush.
30 See especially Jewett to Harrison, March 1, 1943. By mid-February 1943, Ross Harrison was certainly "convinced" of the study's "scientific soundness" and "desirability." See Harrison to Vannevar Bush, February 19, 1943. His subsequent task seems to have been to resolve Jewett's continuing reservations. See Harrison to Jewett, February 20, 1943, NAS-NRC Central File: DIV NRC: Medical Sciences: Committee on Medicine, Subcommittee on Venereal Diseases: 1943, NAS.

well as their facts, Jewett and NRC chair Ross Harrison were prepared to take personal responsibility for endorsing the study:

So far as the risk of adverse public reaction is concerned we realize that opinions differ widely and that the possibility unquestionably exists. It is our mature judgment that in view of the weight of scientific and medical advice and the prospective great and continuing advantage both to the miliary and civil populations, it is a warranted risk.[31]

Nonetheless, Jewett and Harrison advised Vannevar Bush, the risk warranted safeguards: "In view of the duress element of risk and in order to minimize it, it would be our suggestion, if the recommended experiment is undertaken, that the securing of volunteers be placed in the hands of other than prison authorities so far as this is feasible."[32]

Given the extensive deliberations preceding the study, its eventual outcome was anticlimactic. After several months of research on prisoners in the federal penitentiary at Terre Haute, John F. Mahoney reported that the procedure for inducing gonorrhea in humans was too unreliable to enable meaningful tests of prophylactic agents. Following his instructions to abandon the project if it proved "difficult or hazardous" to draw "sound conclusions" from the research, Mahoney stopped the study.[33]

The merits of the gonorrhea research lay elsewhere than in its meager scientific yield, in the rationale for controlled experiments that emerged from negotiations between medical researchers and their lay associates. Research on humans worth doing was worth doing well. A less than adequate study from a methodological point of view was morally unacceptable.[34]

THE WAR AT HOME: PENICILLIN

While plans for investigating gonorrhea treatments were getting underway, CMR officials were beginning a much larger program of clinical investigation, to evaluate

---

31 Ross G. Harrison and Frank Jewett to Vannevar Bush, March 5, 1943, NAS-NRC Central File: DIV NRC: Medical Sciences: Committee on Medicine, Subcommittee on Venereal Diseases: 1943, NAS.

32 Ibid.

33 See *Interim Report. February 9, 1944* and *BiMonthly Progress Report No. 4. May 1, 1944,* OSRD/CMR, RG 227, Project no. M-3169, NA; and John F. Mahoney to A. N. Richards, March 1944, OSRD/CMR, RG227, Correspondence: "Mahoney," NA.

34 David J. Rothman, in a different account of these experiments, discounted the ethical concerns of participants, arguing that their ethical perspective was simply "frankly and unashamedly utilitarian." See David J. Rothman, "Ethics and Human Experimentation: Henry Beecher Revisited," *NEJM* 317 (November 5, 1987), 1195–1199 (quotation from 1198). Since publication of this article, Rothman appears to have changed his mind, adopting a view much closer to that of my own (see Marks, *Ideas As Reforms* [n. 22], pp. 107–116). He now describes the CMR as having "conducted a remarkably thorough and sensitive discussion of the ethics of research and adopt[ing] procedures that satisfied the principles of voluntary and informed consent." David J. Rothman, *Strangers at the Bedside: A History of How Law and Bioethics Transformed Medical Decision Making* (New York: Basic Books, 1991), pp. 42–48 (quotation from pp. 42–43).

the therapeutic potential of penicillin. As early as 1940, British and American researchers had begun to demonstrate penicillin's remarkable abilities in uncontrolled staphylococcal and streptococcal infections.[35] Under normal circumstances, these initial reports would be followed by a series of pharmacological and therapeutic studies conducted at various research centers around the country. Results, possibly conflicting, about the effects of penicillin in treating various conditions would slowly accumulate, and, over a period of years, academic specialists in surgery and infectious disease would formulate "official" medical opinion about the drug's optimal uses.

Wartime circumstances provided academic physicians with the unusual opportunity to determine, more systematically and efficiently, when and how penicillin was best used. In the fall of 1941, Vannevar Bush and CMR chair A. N. Richards had initiated a crash program to develop industrial production of penicillin. In January 1942, Richards asked Perrin H. Long, the widely respected clinical expert on the sulfa drugs, to organize a research program under NRC auspices to evaluate the clinical uses of penicillin. By the summer of 1943 production capacity had expanded, but there was still far too little of the precious drug. In July, officials of the War Production Board placed Chester Keefer, Long's successor at the NRC, in charge of all domestic supplies of the drug. The War Production Board action made Keefer virtual "penicillin czar" for the duration of the war.[36]

Professor of Medicine at Boston University, Chester Keefer was a member in good standing with the academic elite of clinical investigators. A product of Hopkins and Harvard, Keefer turned naturally to organized cooperative investigations to study penicillin.[37] He supplied the drug only to a handful of "experienced investigators" who agreed in return to work "under [CMR's] direction and supervision."[38] As historian David Adams notes, rationing penicillin in the name

35 See Gladys L. Hobby's excellent *Penicillin: Meeting the Challenge* (New Haven: Yale University Press, 1985), pp. 69–77. A participant in the earliest United States studies of penicillin, Dr. Hobby has complemented her personal knowledge with extensive archival research, producing the best general account of penicillin's history.

36 On the origins of the penicillin development program in the United States, see Hobby, *Penicillin* (n. 35), pp. 80–81, 87–92, 94; Chester S. Keefer, "Penicillin: A Wartime Achievement," in Andrus, *Advances in Military Medicine* (n. 4), vol. II, pp. 717–718; A. N. Richards, "Production of Penicillin in the United States (1941–1946)," *Nature* 201 (February 1, 1964), 441–445; W. H. Helfand, H. B. Woodruff, K. M. H. Coleman, and D. L. Cowen, "Wartime Industrial Development of Penicillin in the United States," in John Parascandola, ed., *The History of Antibiotics: A Symposium* (Madison, WI: American Institute of the History of Pharmacy, 1980), pp. 31–56. On Chester Keefer and the development of the clinical testing program, see Hobby, *Penicillin*, pp. 141–149; David P. Adams, "Wartime Bureaucracy and Penicillin Allocation: The Committee on Chemotherapeutic and Other Agents, 1942–1944," *JHM* 44 (1989), 196–217. A handful of researchers had their own supplies of the drug prior to the CMR program, and several groups continued to divert official supplies to unauthorized research. See Hobby, *Penicillin*, pp. 69–77.

37 On Keefer's career, see Robert W. Wilkins, "Chester Scott Keefer," *Transactions of the Association of American Physicians* 85 (1972), 24–26; Maxwell Finland, *The Harvard Medical Unit at Boston City Hospital* (Boston: Francis Countway Library of Medicine, 1982), pp. 189–193.

38 Keefer, "Penicillin: A Wartime Achievement," in Andrus, *Advances in Military Medicine* (n. 4), vol. II, p. 719.

of science enabled Keefer to defend the CMR's monopoly on civilian supplies of the drug against critics and queue jumpers. Government officials and drug manufacturers, fearful of the political fallout if money or privilege could buy access to the drug, similarly relied on Keefer's scientific authority to shield them from public criticism.[39]

CMR's research program focused first on the most serious infections, and those for which other drugs performed poorly.[40] For the military, syphilis was among the most serious medical problems, and existing therapies quite inadequate. The arsenical treatments favored by civilian experts took months to complete. The need for close medical supervision while these toxic drugs were being used meant that optimal therapy drained operating units and medical facilities alike. Initially, military researchers focused on accelerated arsenical treatments deemed too experimental for civilian use.[41]

Plans to evaluate the use of penicillin in syphilis did not begin until the summer of 1943 when Public Health Service researcher John F. Mahoney demonstrated that, contrary to earlier reports, the drug had a pronounced spirocheticidal effect in experimental infections.[42] Security restrictions on all penicillin research did not prevent news of Mahoney's findings from circulating rapidly among experts on venereal disease. Mahoney's report that the initial syphilitic lesions in four sailors had promptly disappeared upon treatment with penicillin heightened military interest in the drug.[43]

Penicillin would not have been the first antisyphilitic drug that failed to realize its initial promise. Given the pressing military need for a rapid and convenient syphilis treatment, army physicians began using penicillin in high dosages well in

39 On the evolution of Keefer's role as "penicillin czar," see David P. Adams, *"The Greatest Good to the Greatest Number": Penicillin Rationing on the American Home Front, 1940–1945* (New York: Peter Lang, 1991), pp. 31–39, 67–69; idem, "Wartime Bureaucracy" (n. 36). On the political concerns of OSRD and War Production Board officials, see Adams, *The Greatest Good*, pp. 71–73. These concerns intensified as the war wound down: Eleanor Poland to Dr. Fischelis, April 10, 1944, War Production Board, RG 179, Box 75, Class. No. 2219, NA; Penicillin Producers Industry Advisory Committee, *Civilian Distribution of Limited Quantities of Penicillin,* April 11, 1944, War Production Board, RG 179, Box 1691, 533.8105M, NA.

40 Chester S. Keefer, Francis G. Blake, E. K. Marshall Jr., J. S. Lockwood, and W. Barry Wood Jr., "Penicillin in the Treatment of Infections: A Report of 500 Cases," *JAMA* 122 (1943), 1217–1224.

41 Paul Padget, "Diagnosis and Treatment of the Venereal Diseases," in U.S. Army, Medical Service, *Internal Medicine in World War II,* vol. II, *Infectious Disease* (Washington, DC: Office of the Surgeon General, 1963), pp. 419–423.

42 After demonstrating its effects in rabbit syphilis, Mahoney obtained authorization to try the drug in humans. [Chester Keefer], *Memorandum on Use of Penicillin in Syphilis* [late October 1943], NRC Program Files: DIV NRC: Medical Sciences: Committee on Medicine, Subcommittee on Venereal Diseases: Correspondence, NAS. Approval for Mahoney's human trial was granted over the objections of J. E. Moore, who thought that additional animal investigations would be more productive and reliable. J. E. Moore to E. C. Andrus [CMR], July 13, 1943, OSRD/CMR, RG 227, Box 67, F Penicillin VD, NA.

43 Padget, "Diagnosis and Treatment of the Venereal Diseases" (n. 41), 419–423; William S. Middleton, "European Theater of Operations," in U.S. Army, Medical Service, *Internal Medicine in World War II,* vol. I, *Activities of Medical Consultants* (Washington, DC: Office of the Surgeon General, 1961), pp. 291–299.

advance of any carefully controlled evaluations. Recognizing the need to examine the merits of penicillin in "the spirit of impartial enquiry" that military users of the drug could not afford, army officials requested that the NRC organize a more systematic investigation of penicillin's potential in treating syphilis.[44]

By the fall of 1943, increased penicillin production made it possible to begin planning a civilian investigation of syphilis treatment, under the direction of Joseph Earle Moore, chairman of the NRC's Subcommittee on Venereal Disease.[45] The NRC's studies had two aims: to determine the optimal ways of using penicillin to treat syphilis and to evaluate its efficacy under more carefully controlled circumstances. A cooperative study, operating according to a fixed plan, would meet both objectives. It would accumulate results more quickly, and more reliably, than a series of less focused individual inquiries.[46]

Participating researchers agreed in advance to "cooperate in a planned investigation, [with] each clinic utilizing a treatment scheme indicated to it by the steering panel." They also agreed upon standardized data collection and laboratory procedures.[47] Final decisions about the research were in the hands of Chester Keefer, whose control over the civilian distribution of penicillin greatly enhanced the authority of Moore's committee.

The clinics involved represented a handful of elite investigators, selected either

---

44 The initial uses of penicillin were on the customary basis: take a few cases in extremis and see what happens. Charles Fletcher, "First Clinical Use of Penicillin," *British Medical Journal* 289 (December 22–29, 1984), 1721–1723. The need for "impartial inquiry" was noted in reference to the testing of penicillin for wound infections: U.S. Army Memo, [Report of Penicillin Conference at No. 48, General Hospital, August 24–25, 1943], OSRD/CMR, RG 227, Box 60, F Penicillin, Miscellaneous, NA. The military's evaluation of penicillin for syphilis is reported by Donald M. Pillsbury, "Penicillin Therapy of Early Syphilis in 14,000 Patients: Follow-Up Examination of 792 Patients Six or More Months after Treatment," *American Journal of Syphilology and Dermatology* 30 (March 1946), 134–135. The two figures in Pillsbury's title speak volumes about the difficulty of conducting an informative investigation of syphilis treatment within the military. On the NRC's involvement, see N.R.C.–U.S. P.H.S., *Meeting of Penicillin Investigators. 7 and 8 February 1946*, 1–2; [Chester Keefer], *Memorandum on Use of Penicillin in Syphilis* [late October 1943], NRC Program Files: DIV NRC: Medical Sciences: Committee on Medicine, Subcommittee on Venereal Diseases: Correspondence, NAS.

45 Pilot studies on humans were being explored as early as August but detailed planning of a cooperative investigation did not begin until October. [Chester Keefer], *Memorandum on Use of Penicillin in Syphilis* [late October 1943], NRC Program Files: DIV NRC: Medical Sciences: Committee on Medicine, Subcommittee on Venereal Diseases: Correspondence, NAS. Unbeknownst to Keefer, Joseph Earle Moore had proposed resurrecting the Cooperative Clinical Group in order to study penicillin in syphilis; Public Health Service officials doubted they could get a supply of the drug. J. R. Heller to Joseph Earle Moore, September 28, 1943, Public Health Service, General Classified Files (1936–1944), RG 90, Box 56, 0470 (penicillin), NA. Harry Dowling emphasizes the links between the wartime penicillin studies and the prewar Cooperative Clinical Group in his "The Emergence of the Cooperative Clinical Trial," *Transactions and Studies of the College of Physicians of Philadelphia* 43 (July 1975), 22–23.

46 OSRD/CMR, *Agenda for Penicillin Conference November 9, 1944*, OSRD/CMR, RG 227, Box 67, NA.

47 *Minutes of a Conference on Penicillin in the Treatment of Syphilis in Human Beings. October 29, 1943*, NRC Program Files: DIV NRC: Medical Sciences: Committee on Medicine, Subcommittee on Venereal Diseases: Minutes: 1940–1943, NAS.

for their expertise in syphilis or in the study of antiinfectious agents.[48] Thanks to OSRD, they did not lack for funds or manpower in pursuing their researches. But these unusually favorable circumstances found researchers no less reluctant to surrender their intellectual autonomy, even in the pursuit of agreed-upon goals. The study began by examining the value of penicillin in a range of doses up to 1.2 million units, a dosage that Mahoney had already demonstrated would work; however, no one knew if lesser amounts would do as well. Participating clinicians, who wished to cure as many patients as possible, resented the protocol's requirement to employ the lower dosages.[49] Even after dosages below 1.2 million units were abandoned, investigators objected to "merely acting as technicians, each dealing with a small phase of a large experiment."[50]

Researchers' requests to use a portion of their penicillin allocations for autonomous investigations were repeatedly rejected by senior CMR officials.[51] Not surprisingly, some individuals followed promising leads anyway, with the pursuit of scientific curiosity resulting in the neglect of patient follow-up in the cooperative study. Yet in a disease like syphilis, only data on long-term outcomes could address the question of cure.[52]

Despite the fact that they employed a prospective rather than a retrospective design, the methodological difficulties of the penicillin studies evoke those of the prewar Cooperative Clinical Group study. Nearly half the cases accumulated during the war had to be discarded, because of incomplete information or the investigators' failure to follow the protocol.[53] Loss of patients to follow-up ham-

---

48 Keefer added the clinics of infectious disease experts Francis Blake and W. Barry Wood to the study. *Twenty-First Meeting, Subcommittee on Venereal Diseases. 11 November 1943,* NRC Program Files: DIV NRC: Medical Sciences: Committee on Medicine, Subcommittee on Venereal Diseases: Minutes: 1940–1943, NAS. An undercurrent of tension between general infectious disease and disease-specific specialists runs through the wartime and postwar discussions and deserves a more careful examination than I have been able to provide.

49 The initial use of lower dosages was due both to the shortage of penicillin supplies at the outset, and to the theoretical importance of testing the drug's value in the lower ranges. See NRC, CMR, *Minutes on a Conference on Penicillin in the Treatment of Syphilis in Human Beings, 29 October 1943,* NRC Program Files: DIV NRC: Medical Sciences: Committee on Medicine, Subcommittee on Venereal Disease: Minutes: 1940–1943, NAS; and OSRD/CMR, *Agenda for Penicillin Conference November 9, 1944,* OSRD/CMR, RG 227, Box 67, NA.

50 J. E. Moore, Memorandum, May 9, 1945, OSRD/CMR Correspondence, RG 227, Box 67, F Penicillin VD, NA.

51 The NRC Subcommittee on Venereal Diseases passed these requests on to the NRC Committee on Chemotherapeutics, chaired by Chester S. Keefer, who also served as medical administrative officer for OSRD/CMR. Keefer's committee insisted that any proposed studies would have to come up through NRC and CMR for a full review. J. E. Moore to members, Penicillin Panel, Subcommittee on VD, January 24, 1945, OSRD/CMR Correspondence, RG 227, Box 56, NA; J. E. Moore, Memorandum, May 9, 1945, OSRD/CMR Correspondence, RG 227, Box 67, F Penicillin VD, NA.

52 See the remarks of Joseph Earle Moore, U.S. P.H.S., F.D.A. and N.R.C., *Penicillin Conference 26–27 March 1946* [mimeograph] (Washington, DC: n.p., n.d.), p. 159.

53 As late as 1945, Moore reported that the initial 6,000 to 8,000 cases would need to be reabstracted and reanalyzed. J. E. Moore to A. N. Richards, May 2, 1945, OSRD/CMR, RG 227, Box 67, F Penicillin VD, NA. Only 6,000 of 11,000 cases proved useful in the end. See Margaret Merrell in

pered interpretation of the remaining data.[54] Although researchers intended to compare standardized treatments across clinics, individual clinics rarely tested more than two or three of the numerous regimens being studied. Variations in race, gender, and stage of disease among the clinics further complicated investigators' efforts at interpretation, by confounding treatment with clinic effects.[55] Before NRC researchers were ready to draw even tentative conclusions from the study, the war itself was drawing to a close.

Despite their obvious problems, cooperative studies had an appeal to therapeutic reformers, which the outbreak of peace did little to reduce. If studies conducted according to a standard protocol could guide military policy, Moore and his associates saw no reason why they could not also be used to shape the therapeutic practices of civilian physicians. As military pressures abated, their attention turned to evaluating treatment schedules and modes of administering penicillin that might prove useful in postwar civilian practice.

During the war, army physicians desired a rapid and effective means of treating syphilis. The NRC's investigations focused accordingly on treatment schedules that might deliver the greatest protection in the shortest amount of time. With an end to hostilities in sight, the venereal disease specialists on the NRC committee began giving equal consideration to studies that would anticipate and guide the physician in civilian practice. Some research objectives continued to balance the aims of effectiveness and efficiency that had characterized the wartime studies. Were the various penicillin emulsions, more convenient to use, as effective as amorphous penicillin? Which dosages produced the best results with the least trouble? Other inquiries, designed to influence postwar clinical practice, brought the venereal disease specialists on Moore's committee into conflict with their superiors in the NRC.

One such conflict involved the proposal by Moore's committee to evaluate the use of bismuth in tandem with penicillin. In the traditional arsenical treatment of syphilis, physicians often alternated between injections of heavy metals like bismuth and neoarsphenamine. NRC's venereal disease specialists had no reason to believe that penicillin required such a supplement, but they were sure that physi-

"General Discussion," NRC–U.S. P.H.S., *Meeting of Penicillin Investigators. 7 and 8 February 1946*, 147. This contrasts with Lowell Reed's estimate in February 1945 that 25,000 cases would be needed to produce "statistically significant results." See report of J. E. Moore and Lowell Reed to the Committee on Chemotherapeutics, *Minutes. 9 February 1945*, NRC: Division of Medical Sciences, Committee on Chemotherapeutics and Other Agents, NAS.

54 Overall loss to follow up averaged 9.5 percent but was as high as 43.5 percent in one clinic. See J. E. Moore, "Preliminary Statement," U.S. P.H.S., *Conference of Investigators of Penicillin Therapy* [February 7–8, 1946], p. 4.

55 Other problems evocative of the Cooperating Clinic Study were the inclusion in the study of patients who had been treated prior to entry, and differences of opinion regarding the distinction between relapse and reinfection. See Paul D. Rosahn, "The Treatment of Early Syphilis with Penicillin Alone and Combined with Mapharsen and with Bismuth: Results of a Nation-Wide Study," in U.S. P.H.S., *Conference of Investigators of Penicillin Therapy* [February 7–8, 1946], and the comments of Joseph Earle Moore and Margaret Merrell in the discussion at this conference: NRC–U.S. P.H.S., *Meeting of Penicillin Investigators. 7 and 8 February 1946*, pp. 146–147.

cians would attempt such a combination, however irrational, once penicillin was available. Although opposed by the NRC's infectious disease specialists, to whom the proposed treatment made no sense, Moore's panel advocated a bismuth-penicillin study. Better knowledge, they hoped, might translate to more influence, allowing experts to guide practitioners.[56]

In January 1946, the wartime Committee on Medical Research turned responsibilities for the penicillin study over to the Public Health Service. The transfer of authority did little to alter the membership of those directing the study, or their confidence in cooperative investigations.[57] But with penicillin supplies increasing, senior investigators found it increasingly difficult to get participating researchers to stick to the study protocols. To discipline errant participants, Moore returned to the prewar tool of moral suasion:

Since money is provided for a particular purpose, it should so be employed. The individual clinics should resist pressure to abandon a given treatment method "because we have already so treated 100 patients with it," and to adopt a new one, perhaps because of the latest publication of a new penicillin fraction, of methods of administration or of absorption delaying. The Advisory Committee . . . is as anxious as individual investigators to adopt new methods but would prefer, now that military pressure has relaxed, to await definite information from special experimental centers before authorizing general application.[58]

With the war over, many medical investigators were eager to return to research of their own inspiration and under their own control. In 1947, projected cutbacks at the National Institutes of Health in funding for venereal disease research led to a phasing out of the cooperative study in favor of individual investigations, both laboratory and clinical. Those managing the study responded by eliminating clinics with poor track records in following the protocol and finding patients, while maintaining support for the Central Statistical Unit.[59] Well after the war,

---

56 J. E. Moore to Chester Keefer, November 21, 1944, OSRD (CMR), RG 227, Box 53, NA; *Minutes,* November 17, 1944, NAS-NRC Program Files: DIV NRC: Medical Sciences: Committee on Chemotherapeutics and Other Agents: Minutes, NAS. An analogous, but less controversial, proposal was to study the use of penicillin in beeswax, suggested to counteract manufacturers' promotions to private physicians. *Minutes of a Conference of the Penicillin Panel,* July 11, 1945, NAS-NRC Program Files: DIV NRC: Medical Sciences: Committee on Medicine, Subcommittee on Venereal Diseases: Bulletin: 1944–1946, NAS.

57 See Daniel M. Fox, "The Politics of the NIH Extramural Program, 1937–1950," *JHM* 42 (October 1987), 447–466. In most cases, the Public Health Service simply added two or three members to the existing NRC subcommittee overseeing the study, christened it an advisory study section to the National Institutes of Health, and continued operating as before. For a list of committee members, see J. E. Moore, "Preliminary Statement," in U.S. P.H.S., *Conference of Investigators of Penicillin Therapy* [February 7–8, 1946], p. 1.

58 Moore, "Preliminary Statement," p. 4.

59 On the extensive resistance to continuing wartime organized programs of medical research, see Harry M. Marks, *Leviathan and the Clinic: Academic Physicians and Medical Research Policy, 1945–1955,* a paper presented at the History of Science Society meeting, December 27–30, 1992, Washington, DC. For details of the tuberculosis funding, see "Financial Support for Medical Research in the Venereal Diseases," *American Journal of Syphilis, Gonorrhea and Venereal Diseases* 31 (December 1947), 664–668.

the Central Statistical Unit continued to churn out publications on the study's behalf.[60] But despite the impressive numbers of patients they enrolled, the cooperative investigators were forced to draw heavily on speculation and ad hoc interpretations of the data when defending specific findings against the conclusions of other researchers.[61] For the study's statisticians, the most important result had been learned much earlier:

It is less important to get very large numbers of patients on a particular schedule and then not pay much attention to following them, than it is to get a smaller number who are followed through. There is a balance between the two problems of getting large numbers and devoting enough energy to following them up, so that conclusions are not based primarily on pure assumptions.[62]

The need for more planning and better follow through was an experiential lesson, not easily taught in the textbooks. Many more researchers would have to share the frustrations of the penicillin investigators before the message took hold. Meanwhile, for a new generation of therapeutic reformers, the systematic approach pioneered in the NRC's studies of penicillin served as testimony to the virtues of cooperative research:

The first step in the evaluation of a chemotherapeutic agent is the discovery that X drug is "good" in the treatment of Y disease. In the past, once that step has been made, there has been a great tendency for the responsible leaders of the medical profession to lose interest in the subsequent all important but infinitely less dramatic subsequent steps. These include attempts to decide: *how* "good" is X drug? in what forms is it of little value? does one administer it by the pound or by the ton? daily, weekly or for 18 month periods?; under what circumstances is the treatment definitely worse than the disease from the standpoint of toxicity? from the standpoint of naturally acquired resistance? or from the standpoint of the health of the general public?[63]

60 Margaret Merrell, "Estimates of Relapse and Reinfection Rates in Early Syphilis Treated with Penicillin," *American Journal of Syphilis, Gonorrhea and Venereal Disease* 35 (November 1951), 532–543.
61 Frank W. Reynolds, "Penicillin in Early Syphilis: An Analysis of the Discrepancies between the Results of Arnold et al. and Those of the Central Statistical Unit," in U.S. Public Health Service, *Recent Advances in the Study of Venereal Diseases: A Symposium, April 8–9, 1948* (Washington, DC: Venereal Disease Education Institute, 1948), pp. 113–121. In comparing the Cooperative Study with the superior results obtained by John Mahoney and his colleagues, Reynolds notes that the superior "cure" rates obtained by the latter group may have been due to the Cooperative Study's greater diligence in following patients, which lowered their overall success rate.
62 Margaret Merrell in "General Discussion," N.R.C.–U.S. P.H.S. *Meeting of Penicillin Investigators. 7 and 8 February 1946*, pp. 147–148. Another lesson, even harder won, was the need to simplify the number of questions being asked. See Margaret Merrell, "Report from Central Statistical Unit on Comparative Failure Rates for Early Syphilis Treated with Penicillin," in *A Symposium on Current Progress in the Study of Venereal Diseases*, held under the auspices of the Syphilis Study Section, Division of Research Grants and Fellowships, NIH, April 7–8, 1949 (Washington, DC: Public Health Service, 1949), p. 40.
63 [Walsh McDermott] to Doctors Palmer, Bogen, Barnwell, Hinshaw, Willis, and Long [March 27, 1947], *Suggestion for the Report from the Panel on Dose Regimens to the Tuberculosis Study Section*, Esmond Long papers, Box 15, NLM (hereafter cited as Long papers).

The cooperative studies of penicillin demonstrated that it was possible to collapse radically the interval between introducing a new drug and obtaining the knowledge that would enable the practitioner to use it intelligently:

> Ehrlich made the X-drug-Y-disease step almost forty years ago and yet there is pathetically little information available today on the proper use of the organic arsenicals in the treatment of syphilis.
>
> Mahoney made the X-Y step for penicillin in syphilis less than four years ago and by means of the cooperative approach a vast amount of information on the subsequent steps has already been accumulated.[64]

It comes as no surprise that the specialists who guided the NRC's studies sought to maintain their influence on medical research after the war. During World War II specialists had consolidated their hold on *all* areas of medicine.[65] But that the tradition of cooperative therapeutic studies should survive with them was by no means a foregone conclusion. Even under the most favorable circumstances – and for getting scientists to cooperate, national emergencies were the most favorable circumstances – obtaining the sustained cooperation of clinical investigators had been difficult to engineer.

At the end of the war, medical researchers faced the question of whether to continue working under a common yoke or be free to pursue their intellectual curiosity without restraint. In medicine, as elsewhere in the scientific community, opinions about the merits of organized, purposeful research were mixed.[66] Therapeutic reformers would require more than their scientific ideals to continue the tradition of cooperative research after the war. They would need influential allies from outside medicine and a credible justification for withholding drugs from the rest of the medical community while they were studied. They would find both in the newest wonder drug: streptomycin.

A TALE OF TWO STUDIES

The introduction of streptomycin toward the close of the war provided reformers a ready-made opportunity to continue the tradition of cooperative investigation. First isolated by microbiologist Selman Waksman in 1943, streptomycin initially received little attention from either the military or civilian authorities. Lacking

---

64 Ibid.

65 Paul R. Beeson and Russell C. Maulitz, "The Inner History of Internal Medicine," in Russell C. Maulitz and Diana E. Long, eds., *Grand Rounds: One Hundred Years of Internal Medicine* (Philadelphia: University of Pennsylvania Press, 1987), pp. 27–29; Daniel M. Fox, *Health Policies, Health Politics: The British and American Experience, 1911–1965* (Princeton: Princeton University Press, 1986), pp. 115–123.

66 On debates about the control and direction of postwar science policy generally, see J. Merton England, *A Patron for Pure Science: The National Science Foundation's Formative Years, 1945–1957* (Washington, DC: National Science Foundation, 1982); Daniel J. Kevles, "The National Science Foundation and the Debate over Postwar Research Policy, 1942–1945," *Isis* 68 (1977), 5–26. For medicine, see Marks, *Leviathan and the Clinic* (n. 59).

federal encouragement, companies pursued only limited and exploratory research on the drug.[67] But in September 1945, the announcement by two researchers at the Mayo Clinic (H. Corwin Hinshaw and William Feldman) that streptomycin showed promise in treating advanced cases of tuberculosis generated widespread civilian demand for the drug.[68] With the army, private industry, and government planners soon "besieged by panic requests for the drug," all three turned to Chester Keefer and the NRC to "establish an integrated clinical research program" in which Keefer would once again take charge of allocating the drug to researchers who would be able to determine its most beneficial uses.[69]

Preliminary research had identified tuberculosis as one of the conditions for which streptomycin showed therapeutic promise. For more aggressive forms of the disease, such as "miliary tuberculosis," the drug demonstrated dramatic effects. For the initial stages, its advantages over conventional therapies were far from clear-cut. Researchers concluded that additional studies were needed to specify the precise benefits (and hazards) of treating tuberculosis with streptomycin.[70]

67 Selman A. Waksman, *My Life with the Microbes* (New York: Simon and Schuster, 1954), pp. 214–215, 230–231; Penicillin Producers Industry Advisory Committee, April 20, 1945, RG 179, Box 1697, F 533.8105M, NA; Geoffrey Rake to Chester S. Keefer, March 29, 1945; and Lewis H. Weed to Rake, March 23, 1945, NRC: Div Med Sci: CMR: Subcommittee on Chemotherapeutics, 1945–1948: Streptomycin, NAS. By the summer of 1945, the army was interested in an organized research program modeled on the penicillin studies. CMR officials, hoping to wind down their research activities, were not. See Chester S. Keefer to Brigadier Gen F. W. Rankin, July 5, 1945, RG 227, Box 88, "streptomycin," NA.

68 On the early preclinical and clinical testing of streptomycin, see H. C. Hinshaw and W. H. Feldman, "Streptomycin in Treatment of Clinical Tuberculosis: A Preliminary Report," *Proceedings of the Staff Meetings of the Mayo Clinic* 20 (September 5, 1945), 313–317; William H. Feldman, "The Chemotherapy of Tuberculosis – Including the Use of Streptomycin: The Harben Lectures," *Journal of the Royal Institute of Public Health and Hygiene* 9 (1946), 348–362; H. Corwin Hinshaw, "Historical Notes on Earliest Use of Streptomycin in Clinical Tuberculosis," *American Review of Tuberculosis* 70 (1954), 9–14; idem, "Tuberculosis Chemotherapy: Reminiscences of Early Clinical Trials," *Scandinavian Journal of Respiratory Disease* 50 (1969), 197–203. For additional details, see Julius H. Comroe Jr., "Pay Dirt: The Story of Streptomycin: Part II. Feldman and Hinshaw; Lehmann," *American Review of Respiratory Disease* 117 (April 1978), 957–963.

69 The lead role in organizing this program was taken by Lawrence Brown of the Civilian Production Administration, which had taken over rationing and distribution of industrial goods from the War Production Board. Drug companies, concerned about maintaining control over their own research programs on streptomycin, were somewhat reluctant about participating in an NRC research program. They hoped instead that the federal government would simply purchase all the streptomycin the companies did not need, and give Chester Keefer the unpleasant job of saying no to those who did not get the drug. The final administrative arrangements for the NRC-CPA program preserved the autonomous corporate research programs on the drug. On the CPA initiative, see Lawrence Brown to Brigadier Gen. James S. Simmons, January 18, 1946, Bureau of the Budget, RG 51, Series 39.14A, Box 17, NA; NRC, Committee on Chemotherapeutics and Other Agents, *Minutes,* February 19, 1946, NAS-NRC Div Med Sci: Comm on Chemotherpeutics: Minutes, NAS; Brown to Lewis H. Weed, February 1, 1946, NRC: Div Med Sci: CMR: Subcommittee on Chemotherapeutics, 1945–1948: Streptomycin, NAS. On the industry position, see Streptomycin Producers Industry Advisory Committee, January 15, 1946, RG 179, 533.8405, Box 1699, NA; Civilian Production Administration, Chemical Division, Drugs Section, *Initial Report on Operations. July 1 1945 to March 31, 1946* (June 5, 1946), RG 179, Chemicals: Drugs, Box 73, NA.

70 By January 1946, streptomycin appeared "as a potentially useful adjunct to approved and time-tested therapeutic procedures in tuberculosis, but by no means a substitute for them." H. Corwin

In the spring of 1946, NRC officials began meeting with representatives of the Veterans Administration (VA), Army, Navy, and the Public Health Service (PHS) to discuss plans for a collaborative investigation of streptomycin.[71] Almost all the individuals involved had extensive personal knowledge of the NRC's wartime penicillin studies.[72] The continuity of personnel assured a continuity of methods and purpose between the two investigations: a cooperative study, by accumulating more patients and handling them in a uniform manner, promised to provide results more quickly and more reliably than any independent, albeit coordinated, series of researches.[73] Moreover, proponents argued, such a study would prevent the present "profligate misuse" of the scarce drug by "uninformed physicians" who had little idea of when the drug might be effective.[74]

Hinshaw et al., "Report of the Committee on Therapy [American Trudeau Society, January 11–12, 1946]," *American Review of Tuberculosis* 54 (October–November 1946), 442; H. Corwin Hinshaw and William H. Feldman, "Streptomycin in Treatment of Clinical and Experimental Tuberculosis," *Ann NY Acad Sci* 48 (September 27, 1946), 177–182; H. McLeod Riggins and H. Corwin Hinshaw, "American Trudeau Society: The Streptomycin-Tuberculosis Research Project," *American Review of Tuberculosis* 56 (August 1947), 168–173.

71 As the CMR official in charge of allocating streptomycin supplies, Chester Keefer was in a position to indicate the best research opportunities for the drug; as an NRC official, Keefer was involved in planning the cooperative study. See Civilian Production Administration, Chemical Division, Drug Section, *Initial Report on Operations. July 1, 1945 to March 31, 1946*, RG 179, Box 73, NA; Streptomycin Industry Advisory Committee, Civilian Production Administration, *Meeting. January 15, 1946*, RG 179, 533.8405, NA; Civilian Production Administration, *Memo*, February 13, 1946, RG 179, 533.845, NA; and Ernest M. Allen to R. E. Dyer, February 20, 1946, RG 443, NIH, Office of the Director, Box 142, NA; Chester Keefer to Esmond Long, March 9, 1946, Box 15, Long papers. For an earlier account of the VA and PHS trials, which emphasizes the contentious issue of "control groups" in the two studies, see Dowling, "Emergence of the Cooperative Clinical Trial" (n. 45), 23–25.

72 The VA's Arthur Walker took charge of the streptomycin investigation after completing a history of the penicillin studies for OSRD. Esmond Long, who spent the war as a consultant on tuberculosis to the U.S. Army, joined the study as the NRC's representative, at the request of Lewis Weed, head of NRC's Division of Medical Sciences. Both Walsh McDermott and Chester Keefer brought their experience with the NRC's penicillin studies to the task of analyzing streptomycin. Carroll E. Palmer taught statistics for six years at the Johns Hopkins School of Hygiene alongside Dr. Margaret Merrell, the statistician for the penicillin studies. Only John Barnwell, newly appointed head of the VA's Tuberculosis Division, had no obvious personal connection to the wartime studies. William B. Tucker, "The Evolution of the Cooperative Studies in the Chemotherapy of Tuberculosis of the Veterans Administration and Armed Forces of the U.S.A.," *Advances in Tuberculosis Research* 10 (1960), 3–4; Veterans Administration, *Minutes of the Third Streptomycin Conference. May 1, 2 & 3, 1947* (St. Louis: Veterans Administration, 1949), 7; George W. Comstock, *Ripples in a Pond: How the Work of One Scientist Can Influence Public Health around the World*, unpublished lecture, April 6, 1982, Continuing Education Course in Preventive Medicine, School of Hygiene and Public Health, Johns Hopkins University. I am grateful to Dr. Comstock for calling this lecture to my attention, and for providing me with a copy. Contrast Dowling "Emergence" (n. 45), 23, which emphasizes only Arthur Walker's role.

73 *Projected Plan for a Joint Study of TB. April 25, 1946*, Box 15, Long papers.

74 Surgeon General [Parran] to Watson B. Miller [Federal Security Administrator], January 25, 1946. The "efficiency" argument was key in appeals to senior administration officials and Congress on behalf of the proposed centralized allocation for research. See also Surgeon General [Parran] to William D. Hassett [Secretary to the President], January 21, 1946; Surgeon General to Honorable Angier L. Goodwin, January 29, 1946. All NIH, General Records, 1930–1948, RG 443, Box 27, F 0470 (Streptomycin), NA.

As originally planned, the proposed streptomycin study was intended as a joint venture between the VA, the army, navy, and the PHS. Lack of funding prevented the PHS from immediately joining a major research initiative.[75] With 9,000 tuberculosis patients in its hospitals, and more on the way, the VA could not afford to wait: in June 1946, the first of its studies began.[76]

Research in the bureaucracy

The VA may have seemed like the ideal organization to conduct a controlled investigation of streptomycin treatment – a centralized bureaucracy, newly invigorated by an infusion of medical and scientific talent.[77] The reality was somewhat different. Study organizers in Washington kept an eye on the veterans' lobbies, whose strength in many congressional districts gave local concerns substantial weight with the VA's central bureaucracy. The very idea that the VA was conducting experiments had to be approached gingerly: "We don't like to use the word 'experiments' in the Veterans Administration; 'investigation' or 'observations,' I believe is the approved term for such a study in the VA hospitals."[78]

The VA's delicacy posed difficulties for what was initially planned as a controlled experiment.[79] In principle, the arguments for including a control group were well understood. Clinical researchers had long been aware that spontaneous recoveries confounded the interpretation of treatment results. The experiences of the war-

---

75 In June 1946, the Public Health Service refrained from adding streptomycin to its research program due to "conditions prevailing in Congress at that time." Discussions of a study, within the PHS and by the Bureau of the Budget, continued, however. National Health Advisory Council, *Minutes. December 6–7, 1946*, vol. 1, p. 51, NIH, Office of the Director, Minutes, National Advisory Health Council, 1945–1960, RG 443, Box 2, NA.

76 Tucker, "Evolution of Cooperative Studies" (n. 72), 6. While the VA study was getting started, joint discussions with the PHS continued. Even after beginning its own study, PHS representatives, along with various NRC figures, continued to advise the VA on its own investigation. The overlap in membership between the VA's Streptomycin Committee, the Tuberculosis Study Section of NIH, and the Committee on Research of the American Trudeau Society makes it difficult to determine at times which study is being discussed, especially in the spring and summer of 1946 when the VA study was just getting underway. The continuing involvement of the NRC only further complicates the problem. The key players with multiple hats were John Barnwell, who served as head of the VA's TB Division and on the NIH's tuberculosis study section; Esmond Long, a key figure in the American Trudeau Society, who served as the NRC's representative to the VA study, and later helped design the PHS investigation; and Carroll E. Palmer, who headed the PHS's tuberculosis division and consulted frequently to the VA study. Other ubiquitous players include H. Corwin Hinshaw, J. Burns Amberson, Chester Keefer, and Walsh McDermott.

77 Paul R. Hawley, "Medical Problems of the Veterans Administration," *JAMA* 129 (October 13, 1945), 521–522; Paul R. Hawley, "New Opportunities for Physicians in the Veterans Administration," *JAMA* 130 (February 16, 1946), 403–405.

78 [John Barnwell] in Veterans Administration, *Minutes of the First Streptomycin Conference. December 12, 13 & 14, 1946* (Chicago: Veterans Administration, 1949), 29. See also U.S. Army, U.S. Navy, Veterans Administration, U.S. Public Health Service, National Research Council, and National Tuberculosis Association, *Streptomycin Conference. May 10, 1946*, Box 15, Long papers.

79 Streptomycin Committee, "The Effect of Streptomycin upon Pulmonary Tuberculosis in Man – Preliminary Report of a Cooperative Study of 223 Cases by the Army, Navy and Veterans Administration," *Veterans Administration Technical Bulletin* TB 10-37 (September 24, 1947), 4.

time penicillin investigators had only reinforced prewar concerns about studies that lacked a group of untreated control patients. Without "simultaneously run" controls, statisticians had found it difficult to distinguish between the effects of penicillin and the numerous other factors that might have affected treatment results: patient selection, adjunct therapies, and the complex natural history of syphilis itself.[80]

The course of tuberculosis was similarly erratic: relapses and spontaneous recoveries were common enough events to confound treatment assessments. In the absence of an untreated control group, crediting improvements to streptomycin, or any novel treatment, was problematic.[81] But for the VA investigators to withhold treatment from one group of patients while providing it to others required additional justification:

In general, and in particular with a disease as various and unpredictable as pulmonary tuberculosis, there can be no doubt as to the theoretical desirability of untreated controls, selected by alternation or randomization. In the laboratory, this is axiomatic. In the clinic, however, such a series seems justifiable to us on only one of two grounds: (1) a genuine ignorance or doubt that the drug in question has any therapeutic value; or (2) a shortage of supply which, by making it *impossible* to treat all cases, makes it fair to treat alternate cases.[82]

The use of a control group was better science, but the VA investigators proved unwilling to abandon existing treatments purely in the name of science. Within a few months of starting the study, investigators fearful that the study hospitals held too few eligible patients dropped their plans for a control group. Sacrificing half their patients to a control group would impede the VA's ability to provide quick answers about the merits of streptomycin. What began as a pragmatic decision soon became a matter of policy. Fearful that withholding treatment would produce "undesirable repercussions" from "certain groups in this country," the researchers' commitment to untreated controls flagged.[83] Despite the arguments of outside consultants that a control group was necessary, the study proceeded without such a safeguard.[84]

80 See the remarks of Margaret Merrell, N.R.C.–U.S. P.H.S., *Meeting of Penicillin Investigators. 7 and 8 February 1946*, pp. 147–148. For earlier discussions of the problems of chance and spontaneous recoveries, see Frederick T. Jung, "Centripetal Drift: A Fallacy in the Evaluation of Therapeutic Results," *Science* 87 (May 20, 1938), 461–462; Donald Mainland, "Problems of Chance in Clinical Work," *British Medical Journal* ii (August 1, 1936), 221–224.

81 Streptomycin Committee, "The Effect of Streptomycin" (n. 79), 4.

82 Arthur M. Walker and John Barnwell, "Clinical Evaluation of Chemotherapeutic Drugs in Tuberculosis," *Ann NY Acad Sci* 52 (December 14, 1949), 746.

83 See Streptomycin Committee, "The Effect of Streptomycin upon Pulmonary Tuberculosis" (n. 79), 4; Veterans Administration, *Minutes of the Fourth Streptomycin Conference. October 9, 10, 11, & 12, 1947* (St. Louis: Veterans Administration, 1947), 61.

84 The most insistent of these critics was Carroll Palmer, PHS representative to the planning group. See VA, *Minutes of the First Streptomycin Conference* (n. 78), 5–6; VA, *Minutes of the Third Streptomycin Conference* (n. 72), 155–156. See also NRC, Subcommittee on Tuberculosis, *Minutes*, May 2, 1947. Palmer was supported in his views by both VA and NAS statisticians, who were increasingly skeptical of the VA's ability to produce reliable conclusions. See Gilbert W. Beebe, Memo for Lewis Weed, *Organization of Research in Use of Streptomycin in TB*, June 11, 1947. Both documents in

The lack of an untreated control group forced the VA researchers to rely on ad hoc comparisons of study patients with the results of conventional therapy obtained in the recent past on comparable patients.[85] The difficulties of interpreting such comparisons soon became evident.[86] The study was further compromised by the investigators' decision, in October 1947, to abandon a two-month baseline period of observations on patients before beginning treatment.[87] But despite its methodological shortcomings, the VA study remained the largest, if not the only, program investigating streptomycin treatment: "Absolutely the whole profession is going to have to depend on the Veterans Administration to tell us what we are going to be able to learn about streptomycin. There is no other organization which is likely to be able to learn about streptomycin on such a wide scale."[88]

To the community of tuberculosis researchers, the value of the VA study depended upon the organization's capacity to treat large numbers of patients according to a standard protocol. VA investigators were hopeful that they would lose fewer observations of treatment results, as VA patients had to return for periodic exams if they wished to collect their disability checks.[89]

To deliver on these promises, VA investigators had to secure effective compliance with the aims and conditions of therapeutic research:

The integrity of this whole thing depends upon regarding it as an investigative job. It is not indifference to the welfare of the patient in my mind but there is something much more important than the welfare of any particular patient – we are trying to find out something which will be of use to a great many thousand patients, in the future, or not of use.[90]

In maintaining the scientific integrity of their study, organization and ideology were the VA's principal assets. In the long run, neither proved adequate. Initially, the "Streptomycin Committee" in charge of the research made all decisions about

NRC: Division of Medical Sciences: Committee on Medicine: Subcommittee on TB: General, NAS. See also the call for "more adequately controlled" studies from the American Trudeau Society: "Annual Report of the Committee on Therapy and the Subcommittee on Streptomycin," *JAMA* 135 (November 8, 1947), 642. As new regimens came under consideration, the issue of controls recurred, with the same themes being sounded. See the discussion on a control group for thoracoplasty: *Minutes of the Third Streptomycin Conference* (n. 72), 33–34.

85 VA, *Minutes of the First Streptomycin Conference. December 12, 13 & 14, 1947* (n. 78), 5.

86 In an effort to prevent knowledge of treatment from influencing assessments of outcome, "blind" evaluations of x-ray results were obtained from observers who did not know whether they were scoring cases that had received streptomycin. Statisticians reviewing these results reported that interobserver agreement about the degree of improvement was no better than might have been expected by chance. See VA, *Minutes of the Third Streptomycin Conference* (n. 72), 147–165, esp. 150–152; Streptomycin Committee, "Effect of Streptomycin upon Pulmonary Tuberculosis" (n. 79), 6.

87 VA, *Minutes of the Fourth Streptomycin Conference October 9, 10, 11 & 12, 1947* (n. 83), 67.

88 The importance of the VA program only increased as other projects encountered funding difficulties. [H. Corwin Hinshaw], in Veterans Administration, *Minutes of the Second Streptomycin Conference. January 23 & 24, 1947* (Chicago: Veterans Administration, 1949), 87, 50–51; see also [Esmond Long], Veterans Administration, *Minutes of the Fifth Streptomycin Conference. April 15, 16, 17 & 18, 1948* (Chicago: Veterans Administration, 1948), 149.

89 Walker and Barnwell, "Clinical Evaluation of Chemotherapeutic Drugs in Tuberculosis" (n. 82), 742–743.

90 [Arthur M. Walker], in VA, *Minutes of the Second Streptomycin Conference* (n. 88), 59.

which VA institutions and patients were eligible to participate.[91] Backed by the authority of the VA's medical director, the Streptomycin Committee initially was able to restrict use of streptomycin to the elite group of VA hospitals and physicians "most competent" to assess the drug. So long as little streptomycin was available, centralized allocation according to the guidelines of the research protocol seemed to work – almost too well in the view of some companies, which criticized the hospitals "for adhering too strictly to the conditions for which the drug is definitely indicated."[92] But as supplies of the drug improved, regulating the use of streptomycin within the VA became increasingly difficult.[93]

As with penicillin, publicity concerning streptomycin created a demand for the drug among both patients and physicians. Of the two groups, VA researchers considered patients and their families easier to manage: "What we tell the relatives is this – that this is an experimental drug, that its efficacy has not been proven and that we feel sure they would not want their own husband, father or brother being experimented upon because we have heard so many times, complaints about people being experimented upon."[94]

The demands of VA physicians and hospitals for streptomycin proved more difficult to control. To the leadership, allowing more hospitals into the study seemed the only alternative to abandoning the research entirely. If streptomycin had to be made more available, then increasing the number of VA hospitals in the study seemed the most prudent course.[95] But as the study grew larger and more complex, continuing centralized selection and monitoring of patients seemed less feasible. The alternative was to delegate control of the study to coordinators in the VA's regional offices, but with the regions in charge, "each and every individual in our offices who has political power will attempt to break down the investigative program into one of purely therapy."[96]

---

91 On the organization of the study, see ibid., 66–67, 72–74, and, more generally, Tucker, "Evolution of Cooperative Studies" (n. 72), 8–15.

92 Streptomycin Producers Industry Advisory Committee, November 15, 1946, Civilian Production Administration, RG 179, Box 1699, F 533.8405, NA.

93 VA, *Minutes of the Second Streptomycin Conference* (n. 88), 5–6, 67, 69, 84–85. Discussions of the implications of increasing streptomycin supply began almost as soon as the study started. See A. M. Walker to John B. Barnwell, Esmond Long, and George Owen, June 17, 1946, Box 15, Long papers. In November 1946, less than six months into the study, the VA decided to make streptomycin available generally available for all non-TB uses, while keeping the Streptomycin Committee in charge of allocations for TB cases. Paul Hawley to Esmond Long, November 25, 1946, Box 15, Long papers.

94 Patients who persevered were successfully discouraged by a detailed enumeration of hazards on the consent form they were asked to sign. [Delmar Goode], in VA, *Minutes of the Second Streptomycin Conference* (n. 88), 88.

95 By December 1946, the principal investigators believed that restricting the study (and use of the drug) to the original units was no longer a viable strategy. Arthur M. Walker to John B. Barnwell, Esmond Long, H. Corwin Hinshaw, et al., December 3, 1946; and also see A. M. Walker to John B. Barnwell, Esmond Long, and George Owen, June 17, 1946, Box 15, Long papers. For the arguments, pro and con, on expanding the study, see VA, *Minutes of the Second Streptomycin Conference* (n. 88), esp. 65–74.

96 [F. G. Bell], in VA, *Minutes of the Second Streptomycin Conference* (n. 88), 72.

Researchers' fears about the consequences of abandoning centralized control proved well founded. With an increasing number of VA institutions enrolled in the study, the directors' ability to ensure compliance with the protocol diminished.[97] As reports from other, smaller, studies became available, the impulse to explore new directions suggested by these findings grew stronger.[98] University-based VA affiliates posed a particular problem: "Streptomycin is a new toy with a lot of our attending men and in one of our hospitals I think our Dean's Committee has been wanting to use it. We are not particularly sure about the type of cases in which they are using it."[99]

Once the study's leaders decentralized decisions about patient enrollment, moral suasion provided their principal means for ensuring that participating investigators followed the research protocol: "It is strongly urged that each unit remember that this is an experiment. Whenever any question of interpretation arises in the selection of cases or in the post-treatment management, the investigator should adopt that course which will supply the most valid evidence."[100] Apart from appeals to the scientific conscience of researchers, threats that the Bureau of the Budget would defund the study "if it [streptomycin] becomes too widely disbursed" were the leadership's only remaining recourse for persuading errant investigators.[101]

To nonmedical observers, the VA study looked like their idea of research: focused, purposeful investigation in a large bureaucracy.[102] The watchword of the VA was organization, but the organizational means available to the VA study ultimately proved inadequate to the task. To the medical community, the VA's investigation of streptomycin demonstrated the limits of organization alone in producing convincing findings. Another avenue to producing reliable cooperative studies had to be found.

---

97 In general, there were two distinct kinds of protocol violation: one involved continuing the study at sites without the correct laboratory facilities to monitor reactions to the drug; the other involved selecting patients who did not fit the protocol's rules of eligibility, or varying the treatment regimen in some fashion. The latter type of deviation caused difficulties in interpreting results. VA, *Minutes of the Third Streptomycin Conference* (n. 72), 63, 67, 69, 152–153, 157.

98 See the discussion in VA, *Minutes of the Fifth Streptomycin Conference* (n. 88), 147–150.

99 [H. L. Mantz], in VA, *Minutes of the Third Streptomycin Conference* (n. 72), 66, and discussion, 57–58.

100 Investigators were granted permission to use the drug on ineligible patients at their discretion, so long as they did not include those patients in their reports on the study. Streptomycin Committee to Study Units, December 20, 1946, Box 15, Long papers.

101 [John Barnwell], in VA, *Minutes of the Third Streptomycin Conference* (n. 72), 51. In 1949, cutbacks in the size of the study enabled the directors to request that units that did not feel comfortable following the protocol elect to leave "active" status in the study; despite these initiatives, protocol deviations still continued. Veterans Administration, *Minutes of the Seventh Streptomycin Conference. April 21, 22, 23 & 24, 1949* (Washington, DC: Veterans Administration, 1949), 335–336.

102 On contemporary promotions of the industrial model of medical research, see Richard Harrison Shryock, *American Medical Research* (New York: Commonwealth Fund, 1947), p. 104; Marks, *Leviathan and the Clinic* (n. 59).

Politics in the service of science

While the VA study was getting underway, the Public Health Service was planning its own researches into streptomycin. Mindful of the penicillin experiences, PHS advisors anticipated some of the difficulties physicians would face in following the research protocols:

It was the experience in the penicillin-syphilis investigation that the directing committee were subjected to almost constant temptation to add this or that therapeutic regimen to the general program. The tuberculosis investigators may anticipate similar temptations and must attempt to exert the most rigid self-control. . . . Innumerable physicians throughout the country will be treating small series of patients with this or that regimen and will be publishing their results. This will constitute a pressure in the form of competition which is most difficult to resist. We must be prepared, however, to accept the risk that some one of these unsponsored programs may discover something which we have not yet had an opportunity to study.[103]

To keep participating physicians in line, the planners called for a strictly defined protocol, with explicit rules about eligibility and treatment schedules. Physicians would be expected to continue treating patients on a given regimen, until authorized by a steering committee to discontinue treatment.[104]

Public Health Service officials contemplated an organized program of cooperative research, complementary to the ongoing VA investigation. Individual tuberculosis researchers, however, wanted the PHS to sponsor a free-ranging program of research, not purely confined to evaluating streptomycin treatment in humans. The announcement of cutbacks in congressional appropriations for streptomycin research from $1.25 million to $500,000 forced tuberculosis researchers to accept a change in

philosophy from free research to a target[ed] study directed at the specific question of the merit of streptomycin in tuberculosis therapy. . . . The essence of this portion of the program, as distinguished from the various proposals of the Study Section, is that a group of special experts in the field of clinical tuberculosis, in different institutions, in different parts of the country, agree to cooperate in a large scale, rigidly controlled project, which is operated in such a way as to insure the collection of uniform observations that may be combined or pooled to furnish statistically significant evidence in the treatment of certain well defined types of pulmonary tuberculosis.[105]

---

103 [Walsh McDermott] to Doctors Palmer, Bogen, Barnwell, Hinshaw, Willis, and Long, *Suggestions for the Report from the Panel on Dose Regimens to the Tuberculosis Study Section* [March 27, 1947], Box 15, Long papers.

104 Ibid. Even at this date, incorporation with the VA study was not yet ruled out. Two of the "advisors," Bogen and Barnwell, were deeply engaged in the VA study, while the others (especially McDermott and Long) were actively involved in discussions of the VA's interim results and future plans.

105 National Health Advisory Council, *Minutes. June 6–7, 1947,* vol. 1, 168, NIH, Office of the Director, Minutes, National Advisory Health Council, 1945–1960, RG 443, Box 2, NA; testi-

The Bureau of the Budget approved funding for the PHS study on condition that the research would "be carefully coordinated with similar work by other government agencies . . . and be closely controlled in extent and direction by the Study Section, the [National Health Advisory] Council and appropriate specialists in the Public Health Service." In the midst of a contentious struggle over Truman's plans for national health insurance, the Bureau of the Budget's principal concern was that appropriations for medical treatment not be slipped in under the guise of research. There is no evidence that Bureau of the Budget officials had any particular interest in the details of the experimental design. Their intervention nonetheless provided PHS officials with an opportunity to engage the contentious issue of experimental controls.[106]

Carroll Palmer, in charge of Public Health Service "field studies" on tuberculosis, had been an outspoken critic of the VA's decision to abandon the use of a control group. A former member of the Biostatistics Department at Johns Hopkins, where he taught with Margaret Merrell in the 1930s, Palmer was convinced of the need for controlled studies in tuberculosis research.[107] Unsuccessful in his initial efforts to have the VA and PHS studies managed by a single statistical office, Palmer subsequently used the threat of funding cutbacks to convince the remaining PHS researchers that their study, unlike the ongoing VA investigation, contain a preselected control group of patients who did not receive streptomycin: "The cases chosen by the Panel shall, by proper random device, to avoid all possibility of bias, be divided by the Central Unit into cases for treatment and cases for control."[108]

Like the VA investigators, PHS researchers anticipated difficulties from physicians asked to withhold streptomycin from one group of patients while treating others with the drug:

mony of R. E. Dyer, U.S. Congress, House of Representatives, Committee on Appropriations, *Hearings. Department of Labor-Federal Security Appropriation Bill for 1948. February–March 1946,* part II, 491, 80th Congress, 1st Session.

106 National Health Advisory Council, *Minutes. June 6–7, 1947,* vol. 1, pp. 167–168, NIH, Office of the Director, Minutes, National Advisory Health Council, 1945–1960, RG 443, Box 2, NA. The Bureau of the Budget's own records shed little light on the matter, but are consistent with this interpretation. See Mr. C. Martin to Director, January 5, 1948, Bureau of the Budget Estimates Division, RG 51, Series 39.14a, Federal Security Agency, 1939–1952, Box 12, NA. On the political struggles over health insurance at this time, see Monte M. Poen, *Harry S. Truman vs. the Medical Lobby: The Genesis of Medicare* (Columbia: University of Missouri Press, 1979), pp. 93–116.

107 On Palmer's career, see George W. Comstock, "In Memoriam: Carroll Edwards Palmer, 1903–1972," *American Journal of Epidemiology* 95 (April 1972), 305–307; idem, *Ripples in A Pond* (n. 72). On Palmer's advocacy of controls, see also Esmond Long, "The Award of the Trudeau Medal for 1972," *American Review of Respiratory Disease* 106 (1972), 627.

108 *Minutes. Meeting of the Tuberculosis Study Section Steering Committee and Special Consultants,* May 24–25, 1947, Box 16, Long papers. See also Gilbert W. Beebe, Memo for Lewis Weed, *Organization of Research in Use of Streptomycin in TB,* June 11, 1947; and *Minutes, Subcommittee on Tuberculosis,* May 2, 1947, NRC: Division of Medical Sciences: Committee on Medicine: Subcommittee on TB: Conferences on Streptomycin in TB, NAS. George Comstock implies that Palmer had an "in" at the Bureau of the Budget, Emory Ferebee, who helped him in persuading the PHS to conduct a randomized controlled trial. See *Ripples in a Pond* (n. 72), p. 12.

It seems very likely that the men responsible for various phases of this project may encounter criticism from people who are already convinced of the value of streptomycin, or who for some other reason do not consider necessary a program providing for withholding the drug from one group of patients. Since we have agreed to go ahead with such a program, it is important to protect the individual investigators from possible serious consequences of this criticism.[109]

Advocates of a control group wanted backing from the medical authorities on the study's steering committee, in the form of a statement justifying the withholding of streptomycin. The limited amounts of streptomycin available, coupled with uncertainty about the drug's precise value, could serve as an initial justification. Skeptics doubted that any such statement would serve its purpose: to stiffen the backbone of investigators faced with a patient whose conditions was deteriorating.[110] The proposed compromise was "that physicians do not communicate to patients the fact that they are being considered for inclusion in this series. Hence patients who are in the control group are not to realize that they have been denied streptomycin."[111]

The majority of investigators participating in the PHS study proved willing to go along with the idea of a control group.[112] Unresolved was the question of handling control patients whose disease worsened substantially during the study. Should they receive the drug, and under what circumstances? Palmer and his PHS associate, Dr. Shirley Ferebee, proposed that investigators submit such cases to an appeals board, which would decide if an exemption was warranted. Provided the exemption criteria were sufficiently narrow, and specified in advance, only a few patients would be lost and the research design need not be compromised.[113] Their proposal only altered the terms of the debate. According to one dissenting study section member, it all boiled down to a question of clinical integrity:

As a matter of fact I do not believe it is possible to give a definition [of life-threatening conditions] which would cover all the possibilities. Fundamentally, it rests on the judgement

109 Carroll E. Palmer to Esmond R. Long, October 21, 1947, Box 15, Long papers.
110 Ibid.; H. C. Hinshaw to Palmer, October 29, 1947; Walsh McDermott to Palmer, November 3, 1947, Box 15, Long papers. Hinshaw's and McDermott's letters make it clear that both were uncomfortable with signing a statement denying that streptomycin had *any* value, but whereas Hinshaw proposed a modified statement justifying a control group, McDermott thought that the best approach was saying nothing at all on the subject.
111 H. C. Hinshaw to Carroll E. Palmer, *Proposed Statement of Investigations . . .* , October 29, 1947, Box 15, Long papers. George Comstock implies that at one point Carroll Palmer had proposed giving a placebo injection to the control group, a suggestion that was abandoned in the compromise. See Comstock, *Ripples in a Pond* (n. 72), p. 12.
112 It appears, however, that both control patients and those receiving streptomycin were permitted to have other traditional treatments such as "collapse therapy'; when the control group is referred to as "untreated," it is the use of streptomycin which is meant. In the event, 79.2 percent of the streptomycin patients and only 73 percent of the controls received *no* surgical intervention. Esmond R. Long and Shirley H. Ferebee, "A Controlled Investigation of Streptomycin Treatment in Tuberculosis," *Public Health Reports* 65 (November 3, 1950), 1424.
113 Tuberculosis Study Section, Steering Committee, *Minutes. November 22, 1947,* 6, Box 16, Long papers; Shirley H. Ferebee to Esmond Long, December 2, 1947, Box 15, Long papers.

of the physician who is treating the case and who knows the patient best. He is in a far better position than anyone else to make the decision. If he is capable of undertaking a clinical investigation of therapy, he is certainly capable of assuming the responsibility for such judgement.[114]

To advocates of experimental controls, this approach, if allowed free rein, "would completely invalidate the control study" and "jeopardize the entire program of the Study Section."[115]

The PHS study of streptomycin was smaller and less complex than the VA investigations, enabling PHS officials to exercise an unusual degree of influence over the conduct of the research. Senior investigators reviewed all decisions to admit patients to the study; the central statistical unit assigned eligible patients to treatment or control groups. But organization alone could not forestall the desire of investigators to raise questions not contemplated in the original research plans.

Nearly eighteen months into the study, the Evaluation Policy Committee proposed that "an adequate evaluation [of outcome] must take into account everything that can be known about a patient," including data that only the treating physician could provide.[116] The VA study had begun to demonstrate problems with the traditional reliance on roentgenographical measures of outcome.[117] Holding an improvised case conference on each patient, clinicians argued, would

---

114 J. Burns Amberson to Esmond R. Long, December 18, 1947, Box 15, Long papers. The continued obstructions placed by Amberson in the face of maintaining effective controls are all the more striking as in 1931 he had conducted what appears to be the first U.S. clinical study employing an untreated control group where the assignment of treatment or no treatment was left to chance. J. Burns Amberson, B. T. McMahon, and Max Pinner, "A Clinical Trial of Sanocrysin in Pulmonary Tuberculosis," *American Review of Tuberculosis* 24 (1931), 401–435.

115 H. McLeod Riggins to Esmond Long, November 14, 1947; and Riggins to H. Stuart Willis, November 10, 1947, Box 15, Long papers. The subsequent decision to create an appeals board did not, however, permanently resolve the underlying issue: questions about the scope and operating procedures of the appeals process continued to recur. See Tuberculosis Study Section, *Report of Informal Meeting. June 17, 1948,* Box 16, Long papers. This discussion implies that some physicians were referring cases which could not possibly meet the appeals criteria, perhaps in the hopes of having the appeals board take responsibility for withholding the drug. The document also raises questions about the investigators' understanding of the concept of blind allocation to treatment and controls: at several points it is suggested that the panel reviewing patient eligibility would be better off knowing whether the patients are intended for control or treatment.

116 Shirley H. Ferebee to J. Burns Amberson, October 20, 1948, Box 15, Long papers.

117 William B. Tucker, "Evaluation of Streptomycin Regimens in the Treatment of Tuberculosis: An Account of the Study of the Veterans Administration, Army and Navy, July 1946 to April 1946," *American Review of Tuberculosis* 60 (1949), 745–746; Lawrence B. Hobson and Walsh McDermott, "Criteria for the Clinical Evaluation of Antituberculosis Agents," *Ann NY Acad Sci* 52 (December 14, 1949), 782–787. The initial VA discussions (prior to 1949) emphasize the problem of interobserver agreement in interpreting x-rays, and means to improve it. Hobson and McDermott's discussion implies a more fundamental problem: x-rays are simply not good prognostic indicators in early pulmonary tuberculosis. Observer variation simply aggravates the lack of sensitivity inherent in the method, which cannot detect at an early stage of disease the tissue changes that are predictive of subsequent course.

"lend greater accuracy to interpretations of questionable features and in the long run give greater significance to the interpretation of results."[118]

To the statisticians in the PHS study, there were enough difficulties producing trustworthy measurements for data they had agreed to collect, without trying to introduce clinical material that was neither standardized nor uniformly available: "It would be a tragic mistake to distort the original pattern of the study now to try to make it yield information it was not designed to produce, because in so doing, the kind of answers it can give will lose their validity."[119] The statisticians' inclination was to distrust measures that could not be reliably reproduced. In this, as in other respects, the future of clinical research was theirs.[120]

Both the PHS and VA cooperative investigations remained in operation for well over a decade, evaluating newer drugs in the treatment and prevention of tuberculosis, and serving as models (and training grounds) for physicians interested in therapeutic research.[121] The primary interest of the VA and PHS studies, however, lies neither in their scientific accomplishments nor in their subsequent historical influence, but in what they can tell us about the changing purposes and means of therapeutic investigation.

"GOOD" SCIENCE AND ORGANIZED RESEARCH

The initial impetus for cooperative studies came from clinical investigators in the 1920s and 1930s, eager to improve on what they regarded as the scientific limitations of individualistic therapeutic research. During World War II, clinical researchers turned again to cooperative studies, now emphasizing their capacity to get reliable answers about the merits of novel therapies quickly and efficiently. Greatly aided by the wartime centralization of research funding and policy, academic physicians represented on the National Research Council organized cooperative studies of the new wonder drug, penicillin, itself a product of a novel coordinated approach to industrial research and production.

Whether the penicillin investigations deserved this confidence remains an open question. The NRC's findings concerning the drug's use in treating syphilis, published from one to three years after the war was won, can hardly be described as timely. Nonetheless, during the war cooperative research came to represent the

---

118 J. Burns Amberson to Esmond R. Long, November 3, 1948, Box 15, Long papers.

119 Shirley H. Ferebee to J. Burns Amberson, October 20, 1948, Box 15, Long papers.

120 Emil Bogen, a VA clinician, had an interesting response to the statisticians' plaint that experienced clinicians cannot agree even in judging x-rays. He replied, in effect: they can if you throw out the bad films. Veterans Administration, *Minutes of the Eighth Streptomycin Conference. November 10, 11, 12, & 13, 1949* (Washington, DC: Veterans Administration, 1949), 279.

121 On the subsequent activities of the VA and PHS enterprises, see the discussions by Harry Dowling, "Emergence" (n. 45), 20–29; Shirley Ferebee Woolpert, "Acceptance of the Trudeau Medal for 1972," *American Review of Respiratory Disease* 106 (1972), 629–630; and that of William Tucker, "Evolution of Cooperative Studies" (n. 72).

ideal blending of science with efficiency: to the talents of individual researchers, cooperative studies added the leaven of organization. Both within and beyond the medical community, the development and clinical investigation of penicillin served as an eloquent testimony to the virtues of cooperative research.[122]

The streptomycin studies conducted by the VA and PHS represent the principal attempt to carry on the tradition of cooperative studies immediately after the war. Once again, an innovative drug was in short supply and, once again, cooperative studies were proposed as a way of producing the most knowledge in the most efficient manner. The VA and PHS studies, without question, involved experienced investigators, knowledgeable about the vagaries of tuberculosis and the mechanisms of drug action and resistance. Yet what distinguished these studies from other research on streptomycin was not the involvement of specialists, but their apparent willingness in this instance to subordinate individual judgment to a common purpose.

If decisions about the future of the VA and PHS studies had been left solely up to the scientific community, it is an open question whether they would have been supported, or if they would have taken the precise form they did. But to those footing the bill, the streptomycin studies represented *organized,* purposeful research: a means of quickly finding answers to practical questions about the therapeutic use of streptomycin. What gave cooperative studies like these a competitive advantage, in the quasi-public debates over the direction and funding of postwar medical research, was not their association with better science but their reputation for efficiency.

In 1946, streptomycin was scarce; in 1947, Congress made money for tuberculosis research scarcer. Both circumstances made it easier for the advocates of cooperative studies in the Veterans Administration and the Public Health Service. Organizers of both studies benefited from the initial desires of drug manufacturers to have someone stand between them and a public demanding a drug the producers could not yet supply in commercial quantities. PHS advocates for untreated controls benefited again from Congress's decision to cut funding for tuberculosis research in half. But like the shortages of streptomycin, the resulting consensus on the aims and means of cooperative studies was ephemeral.[123] VA physicians could not be so easily persuaded to treat their patients as experimental subjects, nor clinical investigators to give up their intellectual autonomy.

The VA and PHS studies of streptomycin relied heavily on the tools of organization – standardization, centralized planning, and monitoring – to achieve their scientific goals. The irony of these studies is that, in tandem, they demonstrated the inadequacy of good organization alone to produce good science. To the

---

122 The wartime work with penicillin, along with that on radar, were the two examples with which Vannevar Bush, head of OSRD, introduced his report to President Roosevelt on postwar science policy, *Science, The Endless Frontier* (Washington, DC: Government Printing Office, 1945), p. 5.

123 On the fragile social consensus produced by the politics of scarcity, see Harry M. Marks, "Cortisone, 1949: A Year in the Political Life of a Drug," *BHM* (Fall 1992), 419–439.

generation of clinical investigators trained before the war, the participation of specialists in joint projects of therapeutic evaluation was in itself a partial guarantee of a study's scientific merit. The VA investigations of streptomycin demonstrated that specialists, no less than anyone else, were capable of self-deception, selecting the most or least promising cases for treatment, depending on their particular prejudices.[124] Both studies testified favorably on behalf of streptomycin, but it was the PHS studies, properly randomized, which received credit for demonstrating the new drug's benefits in treating tuberculosis.[125] To contemporaries, the lessons were clear: cooperation and expertise, planning and standardization, were necessary but not sufficient to ensure a successful investigation.

Long after the technical details of the procedures they employed were obsolete, the PHS's studies of streptomycin served as an example of scientific progress in therapeutics. Along with centrally controlled randomization, their use of objectively measured indicators of progress and blinded assessments of therapeutic outcomes constituted adherence to a program of methodological reform in the postwar era. The rationale contemporaries offered for such innovations was that they served to limit the exercise of subjective judgment: rather than pitting the clinical acumen of individual physicians against each other, evaluations conducted according to the new methodological canons would provide an objective measure of therapeutic progress. What went unmentioned was that these procedures also reduced the clinician's ability to deviate spontaneously from an agreed-upon plan of research, *whatever* the reason.

The scientific accomplishments of the PHS study were credited to its superior methodology. But the methodological advances adopted by the PHS served organizational purposes as well. By taking decisions about treatment assignment and

---

124 [Morris C. Thomas], *VA Minutes of the Fifth Streptomycin Conference* (n. 88), 15; William Stead, "A Suggested Change in the Method of Randomization of Patients in Therapeutic Trials," in Veterans Administration, *Transactions of the 16th Conference on the Chemotherapy of Tuberculosis. February, 1957* (Washington, DC: Veterans Administration, 1957), 117–119. Manipulation of treatment assignment by physicians who "randomized" on the basis of patients' chart numbers was widely suspected in another VA study, of anticoagulants, conducted in the 1950s. See Louis Lasagna, "The Controlled Clinical Trial: Theory and Practice," *JCD* 1 (April 1955), 357–358.

125 The PHS shared credit for demonstrating the value of streptomycin with the British Medical Research Council, whose trials also used randomized controls. See Dowling, "Emergence" (n. 45), 24. The subsequent VA decision to "finally" adopt randomization was influenced by disagreements between the three cooperative groups (VA, PHS, and MRC) concerning the relative value of isoniazid versus streptomycin plus PAS (para-amino-salicylic acid). William B. Tucker, "A Controlled Study of the Variables in the Chemotherapy of Pulmonary Tuberculosis: An Account and Critique of the Investigation by the Cooperative Group of the Veterans Administration, Army and Navy, 1946–1953," in Veterans Administration, *Transactions of the 12th Conference on the Chemotherapy of Tuberculosis. February 1953* (Washington, DC: Veterans Administration, 1953), 31–32; Tucker, "Evolution of Cooperative Studies" (n. 72), 28.

It is difficult to reconcile Tucker's claim in 1960 that "repeated checks" found only "minor deviations" from randomization (30) with Stead's observation as late as 1957 that statistically significant differences existed among the treatment arms in severity of disease. What is clear is that even "internal" critics of the VA study such as Stead and Tucker continued to believe in the VA findings: the adoption of centralized randomization was to convince others. Stead, "A Suggested Change in the Method of Randomization" (n. 124), 119.

outcome evaluation out of clinicians' hands, the PHS provided researchers with a mechanism that reduced the investigator's opportunity to change his mind in midstream about the methods and purposes of a study. None of these innovations could eliminate the need for *someone* to enforce the details of the experimental protocol. But putting the central statistical office in charge of this task relieved participating clinicians of the duties of policing themselves. How and why statisticians came to play the policeman's role is the subject of Chapter 5.

PART II

Of methods and institutions, or
The triumph of statistics

Almost every phase of the practice of medicine necessitates at least the rudimentary application of statistical ideas.[1]

Statistics and statistical analyses are ubiquitous in contemporary medical science. Statistical methods appear in reports of laboratory and clinical experiments as well as in epidemiological assessments of disease and medical treatment. Since 1970, the Food and Drug Administration (FDA) has required drug firms to obtain evidence of the safety and "effectiveness" of new drugs "consisting of adequate and well-controlled investigations" incorporating "appropriate statistical methods," a standard most therapeutic reformers would extend to surgical and nondrug therapeutic innovations.[2] The leading clinical journals routinely employ biostatistical consultants; literacy in statistics is a prerequisite of medical graduation; and few academic medical centers are without a biostatistical unit, if not a full fledged department.[3] By all apparent indicators, the second half of the twentieth century represents the "statistical era" of clinical medicine.

1 Harold F. Dorn, "Some Applications of Biometry in the Collection and Evaluation of Medical Data," *JCD* 1 (1955), 638.
2 The standard of "well-controlled investigations" was set in law by the "Drug Amendments of 1962," section 102, 2, Public Law 87-781, October 10, 1962. The FDA did not define the standards for such "well-controlled" studies until 1970, when it indicated that such studies must (ideally) incorporate a contemporaneous control group assigned at random, and "permit quantitative evaluation" of treatment effects using "appropriate statistical methods." *Federal Register* 35 (May 8, 1970), 7250–7253. A series of legal challenges to the FDA's authority under the new statute to review the efficacy of pre-1962 drugs delayed implementation of these regulations. An adequate historical account of the implementation of the "efficacy" standard at FDA after 1962 remains to be written. For a useful and reliable account of the legislative and judicial history, see "Drug Efficacy and the 1962 Drug Amendments," *Georgetown Law Journal* 60 (1971), 185–224.
3 On the scope of biostatistical reviewing, see Stephen L. George, "Statistics in Medical Journals: A Survey of Current Policies and Proposals for Editors," *Medical and Pediatric Oncology* 13 (1985), 109–112; Douglas G. Altman, "Statistics in Medical Journals: Developments in the 1980s," *Statistics in Medicine* 10 (1991), 1897–1913. On biostatistics in the exams prepared by the National Board of Medical Examiners, see Beth Dawson-Saunders, Paul K. Jones, and Steven J. Verhulst, *The History of the Subsection on Teaching of Statistics in the Health Sciences.* I am grateful to Dr. Dawson-Saunders for making a copy of this unpublished paper available to me.

The notion of using statistical analysis in medicine is an old one, dating back virtually to the origins of modern probability theory. Despite a few celebrated advocates and examples, the use of statistical analysis in medical research did not take hold in either the eighteenth or the nineteenth centuries. In the early twentieth century, a handful of researchers introduced statistical methods and concepts into physiological, biochemical, and clinical research. For the most part, these remained isolated examples, scarcely known, much less imitated.[4] As late as 1950, few would have imagined the central place statistics now holds in medicine.

As historians of statistics have emphasized, the triumph of statistics after 1950 was not limited to medicine. In the 1930s and 1940s, the statisticians R. A. Fisher, Jerzy Neyman, and Egon Pearson developed a series of novel statistical methods for assessing experimental data and judging scientific conclusions. Along with their counterparts in medicine, researchers in genetics, psychology, economics, and physics turned to these "inference experts" with their newly developed ideas of how to gain secure, objective knowledge of nature and society with the aid of statistical methods and concepts.[5]

The turn to statistical concepts and methods after World War II was undeniably widespread. Yet the historian interested in the development of statistics within a particular domain such as medicine faces a series of problems in interpreting these intellectual changes. What did medical researchers know (or care) about developments in statistical theory (or in the social sciences)? For what practical and scientific problems were statistical analysis and expertise deemed suitable (or unsuitable) in medicine? Were the uses of statistical techniques and concepts uniform across the disciplines, or were particular techniques introduced and favored in medicine, economics, or psychology? In what ways were the respon-

---

4 On the use of probability theory in eighteenth-century debates over smallpox, see Lorraine Daston, *Classical Probability in the Enlightenment* (Princeton: Princeton University Press, 1988), pp. 82–91; on quantification more generally in these debates, see Andrea Rusnock, *The Quantification of Things Human: Medicine and Political Arithmetic in Enlightenment England and France* (Ph.D. thesis, Princeton University, 1990). For medical statistics in the nineteenth century, see the discussion in Chapter 2. For examples of statistical analysis in early twentieth-century biochemistry and physiology, see H. L. Rietz and H. H. Mitchell, "On the Metabolism Experiment as a Statistical Problem," *Journal of Biological Chemistry* 8 (1910–1911), 297–326; Halbert L. Dunn, "Application of Statistical Methods in Physiology," *Physiological Reviews* 9 (1929), 275–398. The earliest use of statistical analysis in the leading journal of clinical investigation was Isaac Starr, Leon Collins, and Francis Clark Wood, "Studies of the Basal Work and Output of the Heart in Clinical Conditions," *Journal of Clinical Investigation* 12 (1933), 13–43. For further discussion of statistics in clinical research prior to 1945, see Chapter 5.
5 Gerd Gigerenzer, Zeno Swijtink, Theodore Porter, Lorraine Daston, John Beatty, and Lorenz Krüger, *The Empire of Chance: How Probability Changed Science and Everyday Life* (Cambridge: Cambridge University Press, 1989); Theodore M. Porter, "Statistics and the Politics of Objectivity," *Revue de synthèse*, 4th ser., 1 (January–March 1993), 87–101. Gigerenzer et al. (pp. 90–106) provide a succinct discussion of the methodological and philosophical differences between Fisher's theories of statistical inference and those of Neyman and Pearson. On statistics in economics, see also Mary S. Morgan, "Statistics without Probability and Haavelmo's Revolution in Econometrics," in Lorenz Krüger, Gerd Gigerenzer, and Mary S. Morgan, eds., *The Probabilistic Revolution* (Cambridge: MIT Press, 1987), vol. 2, pp. 171–200; Neil de Marchi and Christopher Gilbert, eds., *History and Methodology of Econometrics* (Oxford: Clarendon Press, 1989).

sibilities and authority of the medical statistician similar to those of workers in other settings?

The temptation is great for the historian to assume that if statistical concepts were influential across a wide variety of domains, then this "influence" flowed from some central source, whether that be a common set of theoretical ideas, a general cultural need for "objective" techniques of analysis, or a social force common to multiple settings after World War II – e.g., bureaucratization or the professionalization of expertise.[6] As historians long ago noted, the notion of intellectual "influence" is extremely nebulous and often substitutes for a more substantive analysis of change in intellectual concepts, scientific practices, cultural authority, or social institutions.[7]

Existing historical accounts of statistics in the post–World War II era rely heavily on the published writings of a handful of leading theoreticians. Ideally, one would like to examine the working lives of individuals – both prominent and obscure – from a variety of institutions, and be able to track their intellectual and professional activities both on and off the public stage.[8] Given the spotty nature of the archival record for post-World War II science, and the still limited interest in the history of statistics, we are unlikely to have such accounts soon.[9]

The historian interested in the history of statistical practice as well as statistical

6 The analysis of mid-twentieth-century statistics by Gigerenzer et al., *The Empire of Chance* (n. 5), seems at times to skate dangerously close to methodological thin ice, without ever explicitly employing the notion of intellectual "influence." Yet in not providing a detailed analysis of the institutional settings in which statisticians worked or of the intellectual resistances they encountered in agriculture, biology, or industry, they inadvertently give the impression of the inevitable triumph of statisticians' intellectual influence. The same authors present a more nuanced account in other work: see the articles by Gigerenzer and Danziger on statistical traditions in psychology in Krüger et al., *The Probabilistic Revolution* (n. 5), vol. 2, pp. 11–72. Despite the authors' claims, however, there is very little analysis of "institutionalization" here. For two influential historiographical discussions of statistics, see Ian Hacking, "How Should We Do the History of Statistics," *Ideology & Consciousness* 8 (Spring 1981), 15–26; Porter, "Statistics and the Politics of Objectivity" (n. 5).

7 See the discussions in Quentin Skinner, "Meaning and Understanding in the History of Ideas" [1969], in James Tully, ed., *Meaning and Context: Quentin Skinner and His Critics* (Princeton: Princeton University Press, 1988), pp. 29–67; Michel Foucault, *The Order of Things: An Archaeology of the Human Sciences* (New York: Pantheon Books, 1970), pp. xi–xiv, 125–128. For an exemplary historical analysis of intellectural influence and borrowed authority, see JoAnne Brown, *The Definition of a Profession: The Authority of Metaphor in the History of Intelligence Testing, 1890–1930* (Princeton: Princeton University Press, 1992). See also Joel D. Howell's discussion about the difficulties of analyzing technological innovation from programmatic statements or isolated examples in *Technology in the Hospital: Transforming Patient Care in the Early Twentieth Century* (Baltimore: Johns Hopkins University Press, 1995), esp. pp. 12–21.

8 The model for this sort of study remains Robert E. Kohler's *From Medical Chemistry to Biochemistry: The Making of a Biomedical Discipline* (Cambridge: Cambridge University Press, 1982). See also the studies collected in Gerald L. Geison, ed., *Physiology in the American Context, 1850–1940* (Bethesda, MD: American Physiological Society, 1987).

9 See my Note on Sources. Even the standard tool of the intellectual historian, the published correspondence of major figures, is largely absent from this field. Just recently, selections of R. A. Fisher's correspondence have become available: J. H. Bennett, ed., *Statistical Inference and Analysis: Selected Correspondence of R. A. Fisher* (Oxford: Clarendon Press, 1990). We lack comparable published editions for any of the other major figures of twentieth-century statistics: Jerzy Neyman, Abraham Wald, Egon Pearson, M. S. Bartlett, L. J. Savage.

theory, and in institutions as well as ideas, can nonetheless proceed by examining contemporary representations of statistical ideas, techniques, and personnel. When statisticians entered a field, whom did they address, and with what kinds of arguments? Who were their allies, and how were they enlisted? Which tasks did statisticians undertake and which did they leave to others? Such questions lead easily to an analysis of resistances. What were the alternatives to statistical methods and what were the consequences of adopting them? Who remained indifferent to the appeals of statisticians and their allies, and who entered into active opposition? How did indifference and opposition affect the working statistician or the representation of statistical concepts and methods?

In the next four chapters, I explore these questions for the medical domain by examining the history of the randomized clinical trial (RCT). Within the world of academic medicine, the RCT is widely esteemed for its contribution to the validity and scientific purity of therapeutic experiments: "no other method for studying the merits of clinical treatment regimens can approach the precision of estimating effects and the strength of inference permitted by sound RCTs."[10]

An extension of the statistician R. A. Fisher's ideas about experimental design, the RCT was introduced into medicine following World War II with the U.S. Public Health Service's and the British Medical Research Council's trials of streptomycin for tuberculosis.[11] Since that time, therapeutic reformers have invested controlled randomized experiments with the faith they once had in the integrity and skill of experienced researchers, in the productivity and scientific rigor of cooperative studies, and in the ability of gate-keeping institutions such as the AMA's Council on Pharmacy and Chemistry to transform medical knowledge and practice.

Unlike the dinosaurs, cooperative studies did not die a sudden, unexplained death in the 1950s. Veterans Administration (VA) researchers turned from organized programs for studying tuberculosis to cooperative studies of psychopharmacology and hypertension treatments. Officials at the National Cancer Institute independently established regional centers for assessing new cancer chemotherapies.[12] Similarly, the organizations reformers created to pass judgment on the

---

10 John C. Bailar III, "Introduction," in Stanley H. Shapiro and Thomas A. Louis, eds., *Clinical Trials: Issues and Approaches* (New York: Marcel Dekker, 1983), p. 1. For introductions to the literature on randomized controlled trials, see Thomas Louis, Frederick Mosteller, and Butnam McPeek, "Timely Topics in Statistical Methods for Clinical Trials," *Annual Review of Biophysics and Engineering* 11 (1982), 81–104; Sonja M. McKinley, "Experimentation in Human Populations," *Milbank Memorial Fund Quarterly. Health and Society* 59 (1981), 308–323; and Stanley H. Shapiro and Thomas Louis, eds., *Clinical Trials: Issues and Approaches* (New York: Marcel Dekker, 1983); Curtis L. Meinert, *Clinical Trials: Design, Conduct and Analysis* (New York: Oxford University Press, 1986).

11 See Chapter 4.

12 On the VA, see William G. Henderson, "Some Operational Aspects of the Veterans Administration Cooperative Studies Program from 1972 to 1979," *Controlled Clinical Trials* 1 (1980), 209–226; Testimony of Joseph H. McNinch, in House of Representatives, Committee on Government Operations, *Hearings on Drug Safety. April–June 1964*, 360–364, 88th Congress, 2nd session. On clinical trials at the NCI, see Edmund A. Gehan and Marvin A. Schneiderman, "Empirical and Methodological Developments in Clinical Trials at the National Cancer Institute," *Statistics in*

quality of therapeutic studies did not suddenly vanish after World War II. The National Research Council contemplated and the AMA's Council on Pharmacy and Chemistry initiated a national brokerage agency to locate qualified researchers for drug firms with new products in need of clinical evaluation.[13] Yet academic physicians no longer emphasized these cooperative institutional endeavors in their discussions of therapeutic reform. Rather, reformers counted on improvements in the methodology of clinical research, and especially the randomized controlled trial, to regulate physicians' enthusiasm for innovative treatments.

This transfer of authority from institutions to methods is a central theme of the following four chapters. As described in Chapter 5, in the 1950s methodological reformers attempted to persuade medical researchers to adopt the unfamiliar procedures of the RCT, in which patients are randomly assigned to treatment and control groups, while physicians "blinded" to these assignments assess their progress following a prearranged schedule of examinations and tests. Reformers claimed that such objective measures would provide a more reliable, less biased assessment of therapeutic value, and thereby moderate practitioners' uncritical use of novel therapies. By the end of the decade, many researchers accepted the RCT in principle as the ideal instrument for producing "scientific" therapeutic knowledge, a consensus acknowledged by the FDA, which soon adopted the RCT as the standard of proof for judging new therapies.

By 1968, National Heart Institute director Donald Fredrickson, could speak wryly of clinical researchers working under the "benevolent tyranny of statisticians." Based on remarks like Fredrickson's, it would be possible to tell a triumphal story of methodological reform and statistical dominance. Such is the story told by medical critics of the statistical enterprise, and by some historians of statistics.[14] Yet the successes of the RCT as the arbiter of therapeutic merit in theory and in law must be weighed against the continuing obstacles methodological reformers faced in practice. As reformers themselves have emphasized, the use of RCTs lags in some medical fields, ostensibly well-designed studies suffer from numerous methodological flaws, and the average medical practitioner remains blissfully ignorant of the statistical concepts that underwrite the design and interpretation of

Medicine 9 (1990), 871–880; Sidney J. Cutler and Howard B. Latourette, "A National Cooperative Program for the Evaluation of End Results in Cancer," *Journal of the National Cancer Institute* 22 (1959), 633–646; Barth Hoogstraten, ed., *Cancer Research: Impact of the Cooperative Groups* (New York: Masson Publishers, 1980). A good historical study of the NCI clinical trials program is sorely needed.

13 On the NRC and AMA enterprises, see Chapter 5.

14 Donald S. Fredrickson, "The Field Trial: Some Thoughts on the Indispensable Ideal," *Bull NY Acad Med* 44 (August 1968), 989. Fredrickson's ironic comments about excessive statistical authority were taken more seriously by critics of the statistical enterprise. See Alvan R. Feinstein, "Clinical Biostatistics: VI. Statistical Malpractice – and the Responsibility of a Consultant," *Clinical Pharmacology and Therapeutics* 11 (1970), 898–914. Historians have subsequently taken up this line of interpretation. See Porter, "Statistics and the Politics of Objectivity" (n. 5), 98–99; J. Rosser Matthews, *Quantification and the Quest for Medical Certainty* (Princeton: Princeton University Press, 1995), esp. pp. 139–149.

clinical trials.[15] Such examples speak to the partial and incomplete character of the statistical revolution in clinical medicine.

In Chapters 6 and 7, I examine the difficulties methodological reformers encountered in two clinical domains: heart disease and diabetes. In Chapter 6, I describe how a group of prestigious clinical researchers were drawn to the controlled clinical trial to demonstrate their conviction that a low-fat diet would reduce heart attacks, only to find that they could not convince other researchers to fund the large study needed. In Chapter 7, I analyze the controversy that erupted when investigators from a federally funded RCT concluded that patients receiving a widely used drug for treating diabetes were dying of heart disease at an unexpectedly high rate. Chapter 8 concludes the book with an analysis of the contests for authority over drug evaluation between consumer activists and therapeutic reformers in the 1980s.

A reader of my manuscript cautioned that by selecting these controversial examples of the Diet-Heart study and the University Group Diabetes Program, I might give readers the impression that the RCT was a failure, and the program for methodological reform a paper tiger. Given the prominence of statisticians and statistical methods in contemporary medical research, that would be a serious mistake. Yet there remains a gap between the world of methodological dicta and the social realities of clinical research, a gap best explored by examining the remarks and actions of those who must conduct, interpret, and apply clinical studies. I would not quarrel with anyone who pointed out that many RCTs are more easily mounted or more enthusiastically received than the two I have focused on in these chapters. Nonetheless, even the simplest RCT is the product of a negotiated social order, replete with decisions – some contested, some not – and with unexamined assumptions.[16] Ordinarily, such contests are part of the worka-

---

15 On variable standards of clinical research, see Suzanne W. Fletcher, Robert H. Fletcher, and M. Andrew Greganti, "Clinical Research Trends in General Medical Journals, 1946–1976," in Edward B. Roberts, Robert I. Levy, Stan N. Finkelstein, Jay Moskowitz, and Edward J. Sondik, eds., *Biomedical Innovation* (Cambridge: MIT Press, 1981), pp. 284–300; Roger D. MacArthur and George Gee Jackson, "An Evaluation of the Use of Statistical Methodology in the Journal of Infectious Diseases," *Journal of Infectious Diseases* 149 (1984), 349–354; James P. Kahan, C. R. Neu, Glenn T. Hammons, and Bruce J. Hillman, *The Decision to Initiate Clinical Trials of Current Medical Practices* R-3289-NCHSR (Santa Monica, CA: Rand Corporation, 1985); E. Juhl, E. Christensen and N. Tygstrup, "The Epidemiology of the Gastrointestinal Randomized Clinical Trial," *NEJM* 296 (January 6, 1977), 20–22. On statistical competence among medical researchers and physicians, see Don M. Berwick, Harvey V. Fineberg, and Milton C. Weinstein, "When Doctors Meet Numbers," *American Journal of Medicine* 71 (1981), 991–998; Douglas G. Altman and J. Martin Bland, "Improving Doctors Understanding of Statistics," *Journal of the Royal Statistical Society,* ser. A, 154 (1991), 223–248; Jonas H. Ellenberg, "Biostatistical Collaboration in Medical Research," *Biometrics* 46 (March 1990), 1–32.

16 I prefer Anselm Strauss's notion of a "negotiated social order" to the more fashionable terminology of "social construction." See Anselm Strauss, Leonard Schatzman, Danuta Ehrlich, Rue Bucher, and Melvin Sabshin, "The Hospital and Its Negotiated Order," in Eliot Freidson, ed., *The Hospital in Modern Society* (New York: Free Press, 1967), pp. 147–169; Anselm Strauss, *Negotiations: Varieties, Contexts, Processes, and Social Order* (San Francisco: Jossey-Bass Publishers, 1978), pp. 1–26, 234–262. For other studies that take a social view of RCTs, see Marcia Lynn Meldrum, *Departures from the*

day world of clinical investigators, undeserving of comment. Only the more celebrated, more elaborate studies leave a paper trail permitting the outsider a look into the social world of clinical research.

The historian's convenience alone provides a poor justification for concentrating on a series of cases that reformers might regard as a biased sample. Such cases also provide an unusual vantage point for exploring the relation between judgment and authority. The statisticians who entered medicine did so to provide physicians with a set of intellectual tools for judging the strengths and weight of evidence. Yet statisticians offered at best limited guidance for situations in which the statistician's judgment and that of the clinician's did not coincide.[17] Working in institutions where physicians held much of the power, what kind of influence could statisticians expect to have on research practices and therapeutic beliefs in situations where their judgments were contested?

The dilemma of methodological reformers in the 1960s, 1970s, and 1980s recapitulates that of their predecessors analyzed in Chapters 1 and 2: how much authority can "science" have in medicine when both the knowledge that underwrites that science and the circumstances for producing it are not widely shared? To what degree does progress in therapeutic reform depend on physicians understanding the concepts and methods of statistics?

Contests for intellectual authority over the evaluation of medical research did not conveniently end in the 1970s. In recent decades, consumer activists have joined a previously intraprofessional debate, challenging the authority of medical researchers to unilaterally determine policies for evaluating new drugs. These new struggles over the role of science and politics in therapeutic reform make it even more necessary to examine the justifications offered by methodological reformers on behalf of the randomized clinical trial, a task I take up in the concluding chapter.

Design: The Randomized Clinical Trial in Historical Context, 1946–1970 (Ph.D. thesis, State University of New York at Stony Brook, 1994); Ilana Löwy, *Between Bench and Bedside: Science, Healing and Interleukin 2 in a Cancer Ward* (Cambridge: Harvard University Press, 1996); Steven Gary Epstein, *Impure Science: AIDS, Activism and the Politics of Knowledge* (Ph.D. thesis, University of California at Berkeley, 1993).

17 Statistically minded readers may wonder at this point about the roles of Bayesian and likelihood analysis, intended for just such situations. They are discussed briefly in Chapters 5 and 8.

5

Managing chance: Statistics and therapeutic experiments, 1950–1960

To a certain extent we are all necessarily statisticians, whether doctors or not.[1]

In the decades prior to World War II, a handful of leading investigators had argued for the importance of statistical methods and knowledge in clinical research, arguing that the phenomena of disease were so variable as to require the aid of statistics. Statistical analysis in clinical medicine nonetheless remained the rare exception, not the rule, through the 1940s. The first authors to use statistical analysis in the *Journal of Clinical Investigation* found it necessary to explain such basic technical terms as the standard deviation and the correlation coefficient to their 1933 medical readers.[2]

Although statisticians were occasionally employed to prepare tables and analyze data, statistical methods took second place to organizational reforms – standardization and cooperative studies – in improving the quality of therapeutic research. The fact that the "computers" employed in cooperative studies were often women may have facilitated their continued relegation to a subordinate role.[3]

As late as 1950, most physicians still thought of statistics as a public health domain largely concerned with records of death and sickness.[4] Although most medical schools taught something about statistics, few budding physicians found

---

1 Edwin B. Wilson, "Statistics and the Doctor," *BMSJ* 189 (November 23, 1923), 804.
2 The article in question was Issac Starr, Leon Collins, and Francis Clark Wood, "Studies of the Basal Work and Output of the Heart in Clinical Conditions," *Journal of Clinical Investigation* 12 (1933), 13–43.
3 On the early history of statistical methods in clinical research, see the discussion in Chapters 2 and 4. On women and statistical work before 1950, see Margaret W. Rossiter, *Women Scientists in America: Struggles and Strategies to 1940* (Baltimore: Johns Hopkins University Press, 1982), pp. 231–232; idem, *Women Scientists in America: Before Affirmative Action 1940–1972* (Baltimore: Johns Hopkins University Press, 1995), p. 13. Among women statisticians involved in clinical research were the Public Health Service's Lida J. Usilton, the FDA's Lila Knudson, the American Heart Association's Dorothy Fahs Beck, Johns Hopkins University professor Margaret Merrell, and Alfred Cohn's collaborator Claire J. Lingg in their epidemiological study, *The Burden of Diseases in the United States* (New York: Oxford University Press, 1950).
4 Donald Mainland, "Statistics in Medical Research," *Methods in Medical Research* 6 (1954), 123–124; Frank L. Roberts, "Teaching of Statistical Analysis in Medical Schools," *Journal of the Association of American Medical Colleges* 16 (1941), 46–48. Graduating physicians were expected to be able to define

the instruction pertinent.[5] In laboratory disciplines that had long ago embraced quantification, researchers still regarded a merely statistical study as intellectually inferior to a carefully planned out program of experimental investigation.[6] Clinical researchers relied little on statistics and, in the opinion of statisticians, understood even less.[7]

Statisticians, correspondingly, saw little opportunity in biological research and less in clinical medicine. As a discipline, statistics was dominated by economic researchers.[8] "Biometry," as many statisticians with biological interests termed their field, was concerned largely with problems of laboratory research in agronomy and biology.[9] The statistical aspects of clinical research, consisting of the

terms such as "specific death rate" or "infant mortality rate," and on occasion might be asked to analyze the diagnostic value of serological testing for syphilis or tuberculin testing for tuberculosis, questions that might call for statistical knowledge. See National Board of Medical Examiners, *Bulletin No. 8. Examination Questions. Parts I and II, 1943–1948* (n.p., n.d.), pp. 51, 59, 77, 165. See also the autobiographical account of Louis Dublin, which captures the centrality of vital statistics to pre–World War II generations of statisticians: Louis I. Dublin, "The Statistician and Institutional Policy," *AJPH* 54 (June 1964), 875–879.

5 In 1942, only 29 percent of all medical schools taught statistics. By 1952, 82 percent of all medical schools provided some teaching in biostatistics. Roberts, "Teaching of Statistical Analysis" (n. 4), 46; "Preventive Medicine in Medical Schools: Report of the Colorado Springs Conference, November 1952," *Journal of Medical Education* 28 (October 1953), part II, p. 44. On student complaints regarding the relevance of prewar quantitative training, see Charles Doan, "Research and Medical Education," *Journal of the Association of American Medical Colleges* 22 (1947), 12. At least one school with biostatistical expertise (Johns Hopkins) had, by 1950, developed courses that aimed at teaching a medical student "to read the medical literature more intelligently and critically" and "to realize when he needs further advice from a biometrician." W. G. Cochran, "Discussion," *Biometrics* 6 (1950), 96. For a pioneering prewar educational effort in statistics, see John Wyckoff, "The Statistical Method As an Adjunct to the Teaching of Medicine in the Clinic," *Journal of the Association of American Medical Colleges* 5 (1930), 210–215.

6 On the resistance of laboratory-trained workers to statistics, see Donald Mainland, "Some Undesirable Effects of Laboratory Tradition," *Methods in Medical Research* 6 (1954), 172; A. A. Miles, "Problems in the Measurement of Immunity and of the Potency of Immunizing Agents," *Federation Proceedings* 13 (February 1954), 799–807; Lloyd C. Miller, "Official Standards for Immunology: A Challenge to Biometry," *Federation Proceedings* 13 (February 1954), 797–799. On the quantitative (but nonstatistical) tradition in physiology, see Frederic L. Holmes, "The Intake–Output Method of Quantification in Physiology," *Historical Studies in the Physical and Biological Sciences* 17 (1987), 235–270; see also Halbert L. Dunn, "Application of Statistical Methods in Physiology," *Physiological Reviews* 9 (1929), 276.

7 On prevailing attitudes to statistics in clinical research, see Evarts A. Graham to Samuel C. Harvey, September 8, 1943, Office of Scientific Research and Development/Committee on Medical Research, RG 227, Box 28, NA; Ortho B. Ross Jr., "Use of Controls in Medical Research," *JAMA* 145 (January 13, 1951), 72–75; Walter R. Houston, *The Art of Treatment* (New York: Macmillan, 1936), pp. 20–21. For the statistician's view, see Chester Bliss to H. C. Meakins, October 3, 1955, Box 32, Chester I. Bliss papers, Manuscripts and Archives, Yale University Library.

8 Economists and business researchers comprised 46 percent of all American Statistical Association members in 1946, as compared with the less than 3 percent who were engaged in biological research and public health. Abner Hurwitz and Floyd C. Mann, "The Membership of the American Statistical Association: An Analysis," *Journal of the American Statistical Association* 41 (June 1946), 158.

9 William G. Cochran, "The Present Status of Biometry," *Biometrics* 6 (March 1950), 75–78; Lila F. Knudson to Harold F. Dorn, February 16, 1950, 045.9, Box 36, Accession 88-63A-292, Food and Drug Administration records, W-NRC. See also the emphases on public health and bioassay in National Research Council, Committee on Applied Mathematical Statistics, *Personnel and Training Problems Created by the Recent Growth of Applied Statistics in the United States*, NRC Report 128 [1947

application of known principles to new experimental situations, seemed neither remarkable nor exciting.[10]

Given the mutual indifference of statisticians and medical researchers, how do we explain the extraordinary social success and intellectual influence of statistics in contemporary medicine? The answer may well differ for each medical domain to which statistical methods were applied: the laboratory, the epidemiologic study of disease, and the clinic.[11]

In the case of clinical research, statisticians succeeded by forging an alliance with therapeutic reformers. Academic physicians in the 1950s, faced with a seemingly endless stream of innovative drugs, found in statisticians' ideas about controlled experimentation a dependable means for distinguishing products with therapeutic merit from those which merely had good copywriters. For many physicians, the statisticians' randomized controlled trial came to represent both symbol and substance of the statistical method in medicine.

Reformers' emphasis on statistical analysis and the randomized clinical trial posed a challenge to traditional notions of medical research and the sources of medical authority. Statisticians aided reformers by presenting their innovative ideas about experimentation to the broader medical community as if they represented little more than the conventional wisdom of conscientious and intelligent investigators. The result was an incomplete revolution, one in which the most physicians were acquainted neither with the intellectual power that lay behind the procedures advocated by statisticians nor with the limitations of statistical methods.

The geneticist and statistician R. A. Fisher is generally credited with orienting the theory of experimental design within the conceptual framework of statistical inference. I begin the chapter by examining Fisher's ideas about the uses and purposes of randomization in experiments. Fisher's views and arguments about experimental controls are contrasted with pre–World War II ideas about controls in therapeutic research, as well as with the arguments and concepts presented by postwar advocates of randomized experiments in medicine. In subsequent sections, I examine the allegiance of statisticians to the cause of therapeutic reform, and the changing relation between statistician and clinician implicit in postwar ideals of

or 1948], p. 5. On the prewar history of biometric research in biology, see Sharon E. Kingland, *Modeling Nature: Episodes in the History of Population Biology* (Chicago: University of Chicago Press, 1985), esp. pp. 50–126.

10 Nathan Mantel, "A Personal Perspective on Statistical Techniques for Quasi-Experiments," in D. B. Owen, ed., *On the History of Statistics and Probability* (New York: Marcel Dekker, 1976), pp. 124–125; W. G. Cochran, "Designing Clinical Trials," in Francis M. Forster, ed., *The Evaluation of Drug Therapy* (Madison: University of Wisconsin Press, 1961), p. 71.

11 On the development of epidemiology, see Daniel M. Fox, "Health Policy and the Politics of Research in the United States," *Journal of Health Politics, Policy and Law* 15 (Fall 1990), 481–499. I know of no comparably useful historical studies of statistics in the medical sciences. See also Richard G. Cornell, "Biostatistics Instruction: A Historical Perspective," in *Proceedings of the ASA: Sesquicentennial Invited Paper Sessions* (1988–1989), 317–318 on the important role of the Centers for Disease Control in the statistical development of epidemiology. On the prewar tradition of vital statistics, see Dublin, "The Statistician and Institutional Policy" (n. 4), 875–879.

therapeutic experimentation. The concluding section explores the unresolved conflicts between statisticians and physicians in their views of medical treatment and therapeutic research.

THE MANAGEMENT OF CHANCE: THREE PERSPECTIVES ON EXPERIMENTAL CONTROLS

Many people believe [statistical methods] eliminate chance when in fact they merely give us an idea as to the probability of the results being due to chance.[12]

Chance is always considered to be guilty or responsible for the differences until its innocence *has been proved* by the results of technical tests of significance. (emphasis added)[13]

Most medical students will recall their first introduction to the fallacy of hasty conclusions. Consider, their teachers advised, the comforting illusion engendered when the initial patients treated with a new drug respond dramatically to the innovation. Do not be deceived, statisticians warn: chance alone could easily produce a run of spontaneous recoveries. Only a proper attention to experimental design and the procedures of statistical analysis can protect the unwary.

However salutary the lesson, statisticians were hardly the first to call attention to such chance effects, nor the first to advocate the use of experimental controls to guard against them. To understand statisticians' contribution to the theory and practice of experimental design, it is necessary to consider the views and practices of their predecessors.

In the initial decades of the twentieth century, experienced researchers repeatedly counseled the inexperienced physician about the role of chance in creating the illusion of effective treatment. The use of experimental controls was one means to protect oneself against this illusion, as were care in the selection of cases and efforts to study treatment outcomes in large numbers of patients.[14]

A purely statistical knowledge, such as might be gained by the comparative review of large series of cases was, however, regarded as inferior.[15] Even statisticians, caught in the grip of a determinism in which all causes were ultimately knowable, confessed to the inadequacies of the knowledge gained through statistics: "Let the experimenter who is driven to use statistical methods not forget this,

---

12 Cornell Conference, "How to Evaluate a New Drug," *American Journal of Medicine* 17 (November 1954), 727.
13 D. D. Reid, "Statistics in Clinical Research," *Ann NY Acad Sci* 52 (March 10, 1950), 933.
14 Donald Mainland, "Problems of Chance in Clinical Work," *British Medical Journal* 2 (August 1, 1936), 221–224; Frederic T. Jung, "Centripetal Drift: A Fallacy in the Evaluation of Therapeutic Results," *Science* 87 (May 20, 1938), 461–462.
15 See, for example, the arguments of W. D. Sutliffe in "Adequate Tests of Curative Therapy in Man," *Ann Int Med* 10 (July 1936), 89–96. Sutliffe, an advocate and practitioner of controls, nonetheless accepted most of Claude Bernard's criticisms of statistical approaches to therapeutics and experimentation.

that the very fact that he is compelled to use statistical methods is a reflection on his experimental work. It shows that he has failed to attain the very object of experiment and exclude disturbing causes."[16]

Clinical researchers aspired to the conditions of the laboratory experiment, where ideally the factors that affected outcomes were both known and manipulable. Yet even the best clinical study could only approximate this ideal: "Clinical observations can be made just as accurate as laboratory observations; but in the human subject, observation cannot be as readily controlled, the conditions cannot be so easily kept uniform or varied – in one word, the problems cannot be analyzed, as they can be in the animal."[17]

Unable to stabilize the conditions of therapeutic research, clinical investigators in the first half of the twentieth century sought to master uncertainty by accumulating experience. Experience alone brought detailed knowledge of the vagaries of specific disease, knowledge that might then be applied in devising proper experimental controls. Within this context, a "well-controlled" experiment might refer to one in which a carefully selected comparison group was employed to "control for" the effects of disease severity and spontaneous recovery, but it might equally refer to a study in which the perturbing factors of diet, comorbidity, and the like had been minimized to the greatest extent possible.[18] In both instances, the use of "controls" depended on the experimenter's ability to recognize those circumstances that might affect the results of treatment. The value of a study depended on the prior state of knowledge concerning disease and treatment. The more that was known, the better the experiment which could be designed. The quality of research also depended, as we have seen in previous chapters, on one's

---

16 G. Udny Yule, *The Function of Statistical Method in Scientific Investigation*, Medical Research Council, Industrial Fatigue Research Board, Report No. 28 (London: His Majesty's Stationary Office, 1924), p. 5. See also Edwin Wilson's discussion of the superiority of physical controls (uniform breeding) over statistical controls in feeding experiments: Edwin Bidwell Wilson, "The Statistical Significance of Experimental Data," *Science* 58 (August 10, 1923), 99. As Ian Hacking notes, the introduction of statistical methods and data in the late nineteenth century often reinforced, rather than undermined, deterministic thinking about natural phenomena. See his *The Taming of Chance* (Cambridge: Cambridge University Press, 1990).

17 Torald Sollman, "Experimental Therapeutics," *JAMA* 58 (January 27, 1912), 243. Obviously, this comparison relies on an idealization of actual laboratory work. Statisticians convinced that variability was, if not inherent in biological research, far more common than most laboratory investigators realized, argued for the use of statistics in those domains as well. See Dunn, "Application of Statistical Methods in Physiology" (n. 6), 278, 298; Wilson, "Statistics and the Doctor" (n. 1), 805.

18 The 1931 study by J. Burns Amberson and his colleagues, previously cited by myself and others as an early example of controls chosen at random, is typical of contemporary thinking on the subject. The experimenters took twenty-four carefully selected tuberculous patients and divided them into twelve pairs, with the cases "individually matched, one with another" on the basis of the experimenters' clinical assessments. Group A was then assigned to receive a drug treatment; Group B to serve as controls "by a [single] flip of the coin." Such a procedure has little in common with the statistical theory underlying randomization, however much an advance it may have seemed on the standard experimental procedures of the day. See J. Burns Amberson, B. T. McMahon, and Max Pinner, "A Clinical Trial of Sanocrysin in Pulmonary Tuberculosis," *American Review of Tuberculosis* 24 (1931), 403–404.

confidence in the experimenter. The more experienced and skilled the particular observer, the more reliable the findings.

Before World War II only a handful of investigators saw any need to rely on statistical analysis to assess the effects of random variations on therapeutic outcomes.[19] For the most part, chance was regarded as an enemy of knowledge rather than an ally, working its most powerful effects when the researcher was ignorant of "true" causes: no researcher could afford to overlook these effects but each researcher hoped to reduce them to a minimum. Experimental controls, in this context, gave researchers a technique for managing chance. In contrast, R. A. Fisher's ideas about randomized experiments called for researchers not merely to acknowledge but to embrace chance: in the face of a sometimes perverse nature, the prudent investigator would give up trying to approximate certainty and concentrate on finding a means to measure the inevitable uncertainty that remained.

Along with Egon Pearson and Jerzy Neyman, the British geneticist R. A. Fisher was responsible for developing the statistical theory of modern experimental design. Much of the literature about Fisher is written by statisticians, eager to arbitrate the methodological and philosophical differences between Fisher and other statistical theorists concerning the nature of statistical inference and probability statements.[20] While the debate over Fisher's legacy does demonstrate how difficult he could be to understand and how easy to misconstrue, despite the apparently simple nature of his ideas, it has little relevance to the issues discussed here.[21]

Fisher's involvement with experimentation began in 1919, when he was appointed statistician to the agricultural experiment station at Rothamsted. As might be expected, Fisher's initial interest was in plants, not patients. He was conducting experiments comparing the yields of different varieties of grain and was looking

19 For early advocacy of statistical analysis in clinical research, see A. Graeme Mitchell, "Critical Interpretation of Clinical Observations," *JAMA* 105 (July 27, 1935), 241–244; Roger I. Lee, "Some Desirable Supplements to the Present Trends in Medical Investigation," *Ann Int Med* 12 (1938), 692–698; Horace E. Campbell, "The Statistical Method: A Vital Tool in Clinical Medicine," *Surgery* 9 (June 1941), 825–831.

20 Among the more useful assessments by Fisher's contemporaries, students, and successors are Harold Hotelling, "The Impact of R. A. Fisher on Statistics," and F. Yates, "The Influence of *Statistical Methods for Research* on the Development of the Science of Statistics," both in *Journal of the American Statistical Association* 46 (March 1951), 35–46 and 19–34; and Leonard J. Savage, "On Rereading R. A. Fisher," *Annals of Statistics* 4 (1976), 441–500.

21 On Fisher's career and ideas, see the biography by his daughter, Joan Fisher Box, *R. A. Fisher: The Life of a Scientist* (New York: John Wiley and Sons, 1978). One intriguing argument about the early, pre-Fisherian, history of experimental randomization which should be consulted, however, is Ian Hacking, "Telepathy: Origins of Randomization in the Design of Experiments," *Isis* 79 (September 1988), 427–451. In a speculative coda to this article, Hacking suggests that Fisher's ideas about randomization may have developed in response to early twentieth-century efforts to debunk claims made for telepathy. Gerd Gigenrenzer et al. provide a useful overview of the Fisher-Neyman debates: see Gerd Gigerenzer, Zeno Swijtink, Theodore Porter, Lorraine Daston, John Beatty, and Lorenz Krüger, *The Empire of Chance: How Probability Changed Science and Everyday Life* (Cambridge: Cambridge University Press, 1989), pp. 90–109.

for a way to solve two problems simultaneously: first, to maximize the information gained from a single experiment and, second, to maximize the likelihood that a given experimental result could be relied on. Suppose, Fisher asked, an experimenter finds a 10 percent difference in yields between two grain varieties planted in different fields. How can one tell if the difference in yields is due to a real difference between the grains, or to differences in the soil, temperature, moisture, and light in the two fields?

One way is to rely on the experimenter's past experience that a difference of such magnitude is never due solely to variations in plot conditions. This approach, Fisher objected, leaves us in the expert's hands, dependent solely on his experience and authority. For Fisher, who sought "principles of scientific inference" that "any thinking man" could understand and apply, reliance on such "an authoritarian method of judgement" was unacceptable.[22] A second option is to replicate the experiment several times, an alternative Fisher rejected as uneconomical. It could take as long as five hundred years, he calculated, to demonstrate that this particular finding was due to chance only once in twenty times.[23]

Instead, Fisher proposed that the experimental plots be divided into narrow strips, and that the grains be assigned to their place in the field by use of a chance mechanism. The practice of subdividing a field into narrow strips was already common in agricultural experimentation. Fisher's contribution was to provide a rationale for the practice within the framework of statistical inference. By subdividing a single field, Fisher noted, the number of observations gained from a single experiment is vastly increased, and the effects of variations in soil and atmospheric conditions on experimental error are greatly reduced.[24] For Fisher these were laudable but not crucial consequences of the proposed experimental procedure.

The essential advantage for Fisher was only gained by the use of a chance mechanism (randomization) to assign treatments, which ensures the validity of the inference that the experimental difference in yields reflects a true difference in grain productivity. Where no chance mechanism is employed to allocate treatments in an experiment, what Fisher termed the experimental "estimate of error" is invalid.[25] The "physical act of randomization," Fisher wrote, "is necessary for the validity of [using] any test of significance."[26]

Couched in terms of evaluating new crops and fertilizers, Fisher's arguments

22 R. A. Fisher, *The Design of Experiments* (London: Oliver and Boyd, 1935), p. 2. See also pp. 69–70.

23 R. A. Fisher, "The Arrangement of Field Experiments" [1926], in R. A. Fisher, *Collected Papers* (Adelaide: University of Adelaide Press, 1972), vol. 2, p. 86.

24 Ibid.; Fisher, *Design* (n. 22), pp. 66–68. On the tradition of agricultural experimentation, Joan Fisher Box, "R. A. Fisher and the Design of Experiments, 1922–1926," *American Statistician* 34 (1980), 1–7; W. G. Cochran, "Early Development of Techniques in Comparative Experimentation," in Owen, *On the History of Statistics and Probability* (n. 10), pp. 3–25.

25 Fisher, "The Arrangement of Field Experiments" (n. 23), pp. 87–88; idem, *Design* (n. 22), pp. 46–49.

26 Fisher, *Design* (n. 22), p. 51. Fisher argued that any single experiment produces only an estimate of the real error (or difference between treatments), and that for this estimate to reflect the true

nonetheless provided a conceptual basis for the use of statistical methods in all forms of experimentation. Ultimately, Fisher's work would prove relevant to an expansive range of practical and theoretical problems in the experimental sciences.[27] But in the years immediately following publication of his views regarding experimental design, Fisher and his followers had sufficient difficulty in convincing agricultural experimenters to apply the methods and theories developed with regard to grains to studies in animal breeding and care.[28] For much of the 1930s, only a small group of agricultural and biological researchers were familiar with Fisher's work. Despite a steady stream of pilgrims to Fisher's experimental farm at Rothamsted, the visibility and import of Fisher's ideas for medical research remained minuscule.[29] Regardless of their intellectual power and ultimate influence, Fisher's ideas about randomization would deserve little more than a footnote here, were it not for the illuminating contrast they provide with the way in which the virtues of randomization were initially articulated to medical audiences.[30]

"error," it is necessary that causes of variation which do not influence the true "error" should not be allowed to influence the estimate, while making it equally certain that any causes which do affect the real difference must equally affect the estimate (pp. 46–47). For Fisher, the use of a chance mechanism to assign treatment determines "whether this particular ingredient of error [location in the field] shall appear in our average with a positive or negative sign. Since each particular error has thus an equal and independent chance of being positive or negative, the error of our average will necessarily be distributed in a sampling distribution, centered at zero, which will be symmetrical in the sense that to each possible positive error there corresponds an equal negative error, which, as our procedure guarantees, will in fact occur with equal probability" (p. 48).

27 For accounts of the initial lag among statisticians in accepting Fisher's ideas, see Hotelling, "The Impact of R. A. Fisher on Statistics" (n. 20), 45–46 and Yates, "Sir Ronald Fisher and the Design of Experiments" (n. 20), 316. Not the least of the controversies over Fisher's methods was the dispute with his friend and colleague, W. S. Gosset, of "Student's t-test" fame, over the virtues of randomized versus systematic designs. See Cochran, "Early Development of Techniques" (n. 24), pp. 21–23; and E. S. Pearson, " 'Student' as Statistician," in E. S. Pearson and M. G. Kendall, eds., *Studies in the History of Statistics and Probability* (London: Griffin, 1970), pp. 360–364. For a more assertive reading of Fisher's (and Neyman's) influence, see Gigerenzer et al., *The Empire of Chance* (n. 21), pp. 117–120 (which nonetheless takes World War II to be the key turning point in the fortunes of the "inference experts").

28 As summarized by John Wishart, the technical objections to randomized experimentation with animals sound remarkably similar to the reservations of medical and biological researchers who subsequently emphasized the variability of individual subjects. And, like medical researchers, the instinct of agricultural researchers was to look for, and seek to control, the biological factors that accounted for variable outcomes. See John Wishart, "Statistical Treatment of Animal Experimentation," *Journal of the Royal Statistical Society* 6 (1939) Supplement no. 1, 1–12. See also Yates, "Sir Ronald Fisher and the Design of Experiments" (n. 20), 314. A full history of the reception of Fisher's ideas in agricultural experimentation would be most welcome.

29 On the pilgrimages to study with Fisher, see Box, *R. A. Fisher: The Life of a Scientist* (n. 21); and W. J. Youden, "The Fisherian Revolution in Methods of Experimentation," *Journal of the American Statistical Association* 41 (March 1951), 49–50. Unfortunately, neither Box nor Youden offers anything near a complete list of the individuals who came to study and work with Fisher, although Youden mentions the existence of such a list for the period 1934–1944. Beginning in 1931, and intermittently after that, Fisher reversed the flow by coming to the United States to lecture at various statistical centers, most notably the University of Iowa.

30 Donald Mainland suggests that some of the problem is due to Fisher himself, Fisher's influence coming initially through his book on *Statistical Methods* rather than the more sophisticated *Design of Experiments*. See Mainland, "The Use and Misuse of Statistics in Medical Publications," *Clinical Pharmacology and Therapeutics* 1 (July–August 1960), 412–413.

For Fisher, the paramount virtue of randomization was that it enabled the statistics to work: with randomization, you knew how to interpret an experimental finding; without it you were lost. An important but secondary advantage of randomized experiments was that they limited the sources of *objective* bias, by which Fisher meant the factors which might favor one outcome over another, without the investigator's realizing it. But for Fisher, it was not the randomization *per se* that reduced the effects of bias, so much as the multiple replications of the experimental comparison that occur in randomized agricultural experiments.[31] Both devices nonetheless had a common purpose: aiding the experimenter to orient himself in what Fisher apparently regarded as forays against a capricious, if not malevolent, nature.

According to his biographer, Fisher viewed experimentation as a form of gambling with a somewhat perverse devil:

> To play this game with the greatest chance of success, the experimenter cannot afford to exclude the possibility of any possible arrangement of soil fertilities, and his best strategy is to equalize the chance that any treatment shall fall on any plot by determining it by chance himself. Then if all the plots with a particular treatment have higher yields, it may still be due to the devil's arrangement, but then and only then will the experimenter know how often his chance arrangement will coincide with the devil's.[32]

In contrast to Fisher, randomization's medical advocates emphasized the credulity of man over the perversities of nature. To medical researchers, randomization's greatest asset was to neutralize the investigator's beliefs about the value of novel therapies: "This principal of the elimination of personal bias is fundamental in all experiments but it is of particular importance in clinical research."[33] To physicians engaged in therapeutic experimentation, randomization appeared to offer a mechanism that, by limiting the investigator's role in the selection and assignment of patients, would augment the medical community's confidence in the therapeutic claims being made.

For many physicians in the United States, the writings of another British statistician, A. Bradford Hill, provided their initial introduction to the methods and purposes of the clinical trial. As the architect of the Medical Research Council's (1948) study of streptomycin, Hill's success in getting British physicians to adopt the principles of controlled experimentation was admired and envied by American statisticians.[34] By 1945, statisticians in this country needed no introduc-

---

31 See Fisher, *Design of Experiments* (n. 22), pp. 68–71, 78–79.
32 Box, "R. A. Fisher and the Design of Experiments" (n. 24), p. 3. For a reading of Fisher's statement that erroneously makes the "devil" to be the doctor's subjectivity, see Stephen Senn, "Fisher's Game with the Devil," *Statistics in Medicine* 13 (1994), 217–225. Senn's reading says more about fifty subsequent years of medical discussions of randomization than about Fisher. The remainder of Senn's analysis regarding the purposes of randomization (226–229) is nonetheless orthodox Fisher.
33 D. D. Reid, "Statistics in Clinical Research" (n. 13), 932.
34 Hill had advocated the use of "alternating" treatment assignments in a small prewar study of serum treatments for pneumonia, and first used randomization in a study of pertussis vaccines begun

tion to the newer ideas about controlled experimentation. Nonetheless, Hill's work and writings served as an example through which reformers hoped to persuade domestic medical audiences of the proper approach to therapeutic evaluation: the randomized clinical trial (RCT).[35] And in certain crucial respects, the principal claims of Hill and his American interpreters regarding randomization had little to do with Fisher's ideas about the logical basis of statistical inference.

The arguments of Hill and his admirers resembled the traditional skepticism of therapeutic reformers: human disease is highly variable, making individual case reports inadequate for assessing the merits of new treatments; clinicians have a limited ability to determine the factors (other than treatment) that might affect the outcome of therapy, making control groups a necessary adjunct to therapeutic studies; and so on.[36]

To medicine's scientific elite, these were familiar and plausible arguments. But the reservations of earlier generations regarding the clinician's capacity to assess new therapies critically now applied with equal force to the researchers themselves. To Fisher's concept of objective bias, advocates of randomized therapeutic experiments added the notion of *subjective* bias, the hopes of the experimenter that a new treatment might work. The most compelling reason for randomization in medicine, according to its advocates, was to regulate the effects of the investigator's therapeutic preferences on the conduct of experimentation. The use of randomization ensured "that neither our personal idiosyncrasies, consciously or consciously applied, nor our lack of judgement have entered into the construction of the two (or more) treatment groups and thus biased them in any way."[37]

Traditionally, investigators using controls sought to carefully match the characteristics of patients in the control group with those receiving the experimental treatment. The difficulty with the traditional selection of controls by experts, Hill

---

during World War II. The 1948 study of tuberculosis has nonetheless received the credit for introducing randomization to therapeutic studies. For a full discussion of the evolution of Hill's ideas and research practices, see Peter Armitage, "Bradford Hill and the Randomized Controlled Trial," *Pharmaceutical Medicine* 6 (1992), 23–67. For additional biographical background on Hill, see the various essays gathered in *Statistics in Medicine* 1 (1982), especially that by Sir Harold Himsworth, "Bradford Hill and Statistics in Medicine," 301–303. For analyses that place Hill's work in historical context, see the forthcoming dissertations by Desiree Cox-Maximov, *The Making of the Clinical Trial in Britain, 1900–1950: A Cultural History* (Cambridge University), and Alan Yoshioka, *British Clinical Trials of Streptomycin: 1946–1951* (Imperial College).

35 For citations of Hill's work with the MRC, see E. K. Marshall and Margaret Merrell, "Clinical Therapeutic Trial of a New Drug," *Bulletin of the Johns Hopkins Hospital* 85 (1949), 228–229; D. D. Reid, "Statistics in Clinical Research" (n. 13), 932; Donald Mainland, "Statistics in Medical Research" (n. 4), 152. For a (retrospective) account of Hill's influence on E. K. Marshall, and, through Marshall, on a generation of researchers at the National Cancer Institute, see Edmund A. Gehan and Marvin A. Schneiderman, "Empirical and Methodological Developments in Clinical Trials at the National Cancer Institute," *Statistics in Medicine* 9 (1990), 872–873.

36 A. Bradford Hill, "The Clinical Trial," *British Medical Bulletin* 7 (1951), 279; idem, "Assessment of Therapeutic Trials," *Transactions of the Medical Society of London* 68 (1953), 129–131, 136; Marshall and Merrell, "Clinical Therapeutic Trial of a New Drug" (n. 35), 224.

37 Hill, "Assessment of Therapeutic Trials" (n. 36), 132.

argued, is that one could never be sure that the groups were truly comparable or that factors other than treatment had not affected the results.[38] Even trained investigators have prejudices which may operate "unconsciously," if not consciously, to undermine the comparability of treatment groups. Efforts to correct for such preferences simply result in "reverse" biases which undermine the integrity of the study.[39] "The best way to avoid such bias is to assign cases by some technique which eliminates the possibility of prejudice."[40]

As statisticians acknowledged, randomization could not, in fact, guarantee that experimental groups were comparable. Although statistically trained authors were at pains to insist on the need to check the comparability of the experimental groups after randomization, it was not difficult for the unmethodical and less informed reader to overlook such caveats, arriving at the conclusion that randomization took care of the problem. The occasional remarks by Hill and others that randomization led to equalization of the groups "in the long run" no doubt contributed to this perception.[41] When used in tandem with other recommended methodological reforms, such as "blinded" assessment of outcomes, reformers promised that randomization would free a researcher from the accusation that his beliefs had affected a study's execution. The researcher who followed correct procedure could reassure not only himself but his colleagues that the results could be trusted. By freeing the investigator from the charge of bias as well as the act, randomization ensured that even "the sternest critic is unable to say eventually when we dash into print that quite likely the groups were biased through our predilections or through our stupidity. The random method removes all responsibility from the observer."[42]

The naiveté of such statements would discomfort subsequent generations of statisticians.[43] Behind such imprecise exaggeration lay a desire to impress research-

38 Hill, "The Clinical Trial" (n. 36), 278–279.
39 A. Bradford Hill, *Principles of Medical Statistics,* 3rd ed. (London: Lancet, 1945), p. 8; idem, "The Clinical Trial" (n. 36), 280; idem, "Assessment of Therapeutic Trials" (n. 36), 132. See also Mainland, "Statistics in Medical Research" (n. 4), 155. "Blinding" or concealing the identity of experimental and control subjects was also advocated as a counter to "unconscious bias." See Torald Sollman, "Fundamentals of Medical Research," in Austin Smith, ed., *Medical Research: A Symposium* (Philadelphia: J. B. Lippincott, 1946), p. 24. Sollman had introduced blinded tests to U.S. pharmacological researchers in the 1910s: see A. W. Hewlett, "Clinical Effects of 'Natural' and 'Synthetic' Sodium Salicylate," *JAMA* 61 (August 2, 1913), 319–320.
40 Louis Lasagna, "The Controlled Clinical Trial: Theory and Practice," *JCD* 1 (April 1955), 357. On the myriad ways in which "bias" creeps into clinical research, see also Hugo Muench, "Biostatistics – and Why!," *Postgraduate Medicine* 13 (April 1953), 336–337.
41 See A. B. Hill, "Principles of Medical Statistics: I. The Aims of the Statistical Method," *Lancet* i (January 2, 1937), 42; Brian MacMahon, "Statistical Methods in Medicine," *NEJM* 253 (October 13, 1955), 648. For caveats, see Hill, "The Clinical Trial" (n. 36), 281–282; idem, "The Assessment of Therapeutic Trials" (n. 36), 132; Marshall and Merrell, "Clinical Therapeutic Trial of a New Drug" (n. 35), 225; Reid, "Statistics in Clinical Research" (n. 13), 932.
42 Hill, "Assessment of Therapeutic Trials" (n. 36), 132.
43 Jerome Cornfield, "Recent Methodological Contributions to Clinical Trials," *American Journal of Epidemiology* 104 (1976), 408–421; Frederick Mosteller, personal communication. For an interesting example of medical naiveté on this point, see Mantel, "A Personal Perspective" (n. 10), 109.

ers with the critical contribution that statistical methods and reasoning might make to therapeutic experimentation. Even reformers sympathetic to statistical methods cautioned against the "professional statisticians' " propensity to make "a simple common sense problem unduly complex by the use of too much mathematics and a little-understood terminology."[44] The message was not lost on Bradford Hill: "My skill, if any, was, I believe, in offering the clinician something simple that he could understand. . . . If one had started with something abstruse, the answer would have been 'Go to Hell' – and we would still be there."[45]

Early advocates of randomized controlled trials were engaged in a campaign to persuade as well as to explain. In such a campaign, there was neither need nor opportunity to explain R. A. Fisher's complex and subtle ideas about the need for randomization. Where Fisher had sought to give the experimenter a measure of the uncertainty that characterized his results, later statisticians offered randomization to medical researchers as a technique for bolstering confidence in their experimental findings.[46] An earlier generation's trust in the judgment of experienced researchers was to be replaced by a reliance on experimental method: "The use of properly designed clinical trials permits us to move from an authoritative frame of reference to a scientific one."[47]

Therapeutic reformers had always spoken in the name of science. Yet it was sometimes difficult to know just whom "science" had authorized to speak on its behalf. Previously, reformers had relied on organizations such as the AMA's Council on Pharmacy and Chemistry for the sifting and winnowing of therapeutic claims. Following World War II, several groups, inspired by examples of cooperation between industry and academia, attempted to create centralized, professionally controlled committees to evaluate innovative drugs. The National Research Council's Division of Medical Science and the National Academy of Sciences each briefly contemplated such undertakings.[48] The AMA's Council on Pharmacy and Chemistry organized a Therapeutic Trials Committee, which for nine years offered to organize clinical studies for interested manufacturers. In each case,

---

44 American Medical Association, Therapeutic Trials Committee, *Minutes*, May 19, 1948, T48, James Harold Austin papers, College of Physicians of Philadelphia.

45 Harold M. Schoolman, "The Clinician and Statistician," *Statistics in Medicine* 1 (1982), 315.

46 It is interesting to note that Fisher's argument on behalf of randomization does not appear in any of A. Bradford Hill's most oft-cited papers. Individuals who had studied with Fisher, or who followed the logic of his arguments in the *Design of Experiments* acknowledged the importance of randomization in providing "a basis for valid inference." Yet few took the trouble to explain to medical audiences what this might mean. However, for a view that strongly emphasizes the role of statistics as obtaining a measure of uncertainty rather than eliminating it, see Gilbert W. Beebe, "Statistics and Clinical Investigation," Department of Medicine and Surgery, Veterans Administration, *Medical Bulletin*, MB-2, December 13, 1957. I am grateful to Dr. Beebe for providing me with a copy of this article.

47 James J. Nickson and Arvin S. Glicksman, "Clinical Trials in Radiation Therapy: An Application of Statistical Methods to Clinical Research," *American Journal of Roentgenology* 96 (July 1966), 236.

48 The National Academy of Sciences briefly offered its services as an impartial broker of therapeutic claims for cortisone. See Harry M. Marks, "Cortisone, 1949: A Year in the Political Life of a Drug," *BHM* 66 (Fall 1992), 419–439. The National Research Council's Division of Medical

organizational efforts foundered in the face of drug company indifference to reformers' objectives and professional disagreements about whose expertise was needed.[49] Experts, it seemed, could always disagree. But who could quarrel about adopting a reliable, efficient, and transparent procedure for improving therapeutic experiments?

THE GIFT RELATIONSHIP: STATISTICIANS AND CLINICIANS

Once the clinician has grasped the simple techniques that have been brought to his aid, the statistician has no further part to play. Along with the old soldier he can fade away, contentedly if, sometimes, wistfully.[50]

It is currently fashionable in some circles to consider the clinician member of the team as some sort of minor excrescence, "a fifth cousin about to be removed."[51]

Before the late 1940s, the statisticians involved in clinical research played an ancillary and subordinate role to their physician colleagues. Statisticians generally served as collectors and computers of data, called in to provide technical services in analyzing quantitative results. Like the pathologist, the statistician was consulted only after the damage was done – as one wag put it, to determine "what the experiment died of."[52] Yet by the mid-1960s, no clinical researcher embarking on a major therapeutic experiment would think of planning such a study without the active collaboration of one or more professional statisticians, a curious outcome for a group whose stated purpose was "professional suicide."[53] The circumstances that led to such results bear further examination.

Sciences considered but then rejected a proposal to organize therapeutic studies once the war was over. See NRC, *Minutes of Annual Meeting,* June 1, 1944, DIV NRC: MED: Meetings: Annual: 1944, NAS; *Minutes of Meeting of Executive Committee,* June 28, 1944, DIV NRC: MED: Executive COM: Meetings: Minutes: 1944, NAS.

49 Although the AMA's Therapeutic Trials Committee did broker some clinical evaluations, it was by and large unsuccessful in its ambitions to become the central agency in new drug evaluation. On the history of the TTC, see Council on Pharmacy and Chemistry, "The Therapeutic Trials Committee," *JAMA* 131 (June 15, 1946), 596–597. For some of the committee's difficulties with manufacturers, see Walton Van Winkle Jr., "Activities of the Therapeutic Trials Committee," Veterans Administration, *Minutes of the 8th Streptomycin Conference. November, 1948* (Veterans Administration, 1949), 320; and Therapeutic Trials Committee, *Bulletin* (1946), 63, 100–101; "Report of a Committee of the Council to Consider the Status of the Therapeutic Trials Committee," *Bulletin* (1950), 2–6; *Bulletin* (1950), 132–133; Committee on Research, *Bulletin* (1953), 104–105, American Medical Association Archives, Chicago. See also Issac Starr, *Memorandum,* March 1960; and Issac Starr to Harold D. Katz, May 10, 1960, both in Committee on Policy, Council on Drugs, A. McGehee Harvey papers, RG 121GG5, Chesney Archives.

50 A. Bradford Hill, "Reflections on the Controlled Trial," *Annals of Rheumatic Diseases* 25 (1966), 113.

51 Lasagna, "The Controlled Clinical Trial" (n. 40), 354.

52 R. A. Fisher, quoted in C. Radhakrishna Rao, "R. A. Fisher: the Founder of Modern Statistics," *Statistical Science* 7 (1992), 44. See also Lasagna, "The Controlled Clinical Trial" (n. 40), 356.

53 Hill, "Reflections on the Controlled Trial" (n. 50), 113.

To the modern sociologist of science, on the lookout for Hobbesian forays in discipline building and professional self-aggrandizement, the behavior of medical statisticians may seem self-defeating. Rather than emphasize the esoteric aspects of their technical craft, statisticians disparaged the importance of "statistical arithmetic"; rather than lay claim to unique theoretical insights, they insisted that "modern statistics does not claim to be something intrinsically different from the principles and methods of experimenters in general"; rather than recording each minor assist to members of the research community, they accepted credit in the literature only for contributions "above and beyond the ordinary call of duty."[54]

Statisticians' insistence that the planning of clinical trials was more "a matter of hard work and attention to detail" than an application of "esoteric intellectual principles" was hardly insincere. Their initial counsels to clinical investigators *were* little more than "common sense talk" with few pretensions to theoretical originality.[55] Although not the product of a self-conscious strategy to accumulate influence, the conduct of statisticians could not have been better calculated to do so. In emphasizing the need to raise the standards of therapeutic experimentation, statisticians created a natural alliance with reformers who sought to improve the practice of medicine, and thereby created an opportunity for themselves to contribute to the cause of reform.

The 1950s were the decade of the "wonder drugs" when antibiotics, steroids, and other therapeutic novelties flowed from manufacturers' laboratories and plants in a seemingly endless stream. As in the past, reformers sought to regulate the exaggerated therapeutic claims put forth through commercial channels, but it now seemed that newer methods, more efficient and reliable, were needed to manage the stream of drugs and drug promotions. The flourishing production of new remedies required that the doctor abandon the time-consuming process of "weighing imponderables" and slowly "coming to a decision."[56] Statisticians emphasized that traditional procedures for discriminating among the relative mer-

---

54 See Mainland, "Statistics in Medical Research" (n. 4), 122; idem, "The Use and Misuse of Statistics" (n. 30); and Reid, "Statistics in Clinical Research" (n. 13), 934. In assisting experimenters, statisticians initially saw themselves as carrying out the logical implications of a developed theory; the idea that some of their contributions might in fact be of scientific interest, and hence publishable, only gradually emerged. See Mantel, "A Personal Perspective" (n. 10), 124–125; idem, "Jerome Cornfield and Statistical Applications to Laboratory Research: A Personal Reminiscence," *Biometrics* 38 (1982), Supplement, 18.

55 Cochran, "Designing Clinical Trials" (n. 10), p. 71; see also Cochran's letter to William G. Madow, December 6, 1961, characterizing the existing literature as "common sense talk with precautions about the [?] sources of bias." W. G. Cochran papers, Box 5, Harvard University Archives. Muench, "Biostatistics" (n. 40), 338, poses a similar attitude.

56 L. J. Witts, "Introduction," in L. J. Witts, ed., *Medical Surveys and Clinical Trials: Some Methods and Applications of Group Research in Medicine* (London: Oxford University Press, 1959), p. 3. See also Lasagna, "The Controlled Clinical Trial: Theory and Practice" (n. 40), 353; Cornell Conference, "How to Evaluate a New Drug" (n. 12), 722; J. Solon Mordell and C. K. Himmelsbach, "An Objective Approach to New Drug Therapy," *Public Health Reports* 68 (January 1953), 47. For discussions of undue commercial influence, see Chauncey D. Leake, "Current Pharmacology: General Principles in Practical Clinical Applications," *JAMA* 138 (November 6, 1948), 732; Mindel C. Sheps, "The Clinical Value of Drugs: Sources of Evidence," *AJPH* 51 (May 1961), 647–653.

its of "undoubtedly effective drugs" were inefficient as well as unreliable: "For instance, I do not think the relative values of aureomycin, chloramphenicol and penicillin in clinical pneumonias could have been determined without a fairly large-scale and statistically designed trial."[57] Moreover, the enthusiasm physicians formerly expressed for remedies of questionable value was of even greater concern in the case of newer, more powerful drugs coming on the market.[58] What better time to get "away from the old type clinical testing which has misled so many people; and has caused doctors to prescribe drugs which are no good and has caused the poor sufferer to mortgage his home."[59]

The potential of "properly designed" trials to curb physicians' enthusiasm for novel treatments did not go unnoticed.[60] "Modern methods of experimental design" offered a means to avoid the "needless suffering of animals and human beings [which] occurs when an investigation is so conducted that any conclusion that can be drawn from it must inevitably be equivocal."[61]

From the reformers' perspective, equivocation about the merits of new treatments was as undesirable as unwarranted enthusiasm. Their aim was not to prevent progress but to provide a reliable basis for distinguishing it from puffery:

The doctor of today is under constant bombardment with claims as to the efficacy of drugs, new and old. It is difficult, if not impossible, to read a journal, attend a medical meeting, or open the morning mail without encountering a new report on the success or failure of some medication. The clinician who would avoid nihilistic rejection or trusting acceptance of all such claims, or capricious decisions as to their merits, is well advised to adopt a yardstick, a set of criteria, that will improve his chances of making sound evaluations.[62]

57 Hill, "Assessment of Therapeutic Trials" (n. 36), 136.
58 See James Whorton, " 'Antibiotic Abandon': The Resurgence of Therapeutic Rationalism," in John Parascandola, ed., *The History of Antibiotics: A Symposium* (Madison, WI: American Institute of the History of Pharmacy, 1980), pp. 125–136. My only quarrel with Whorton's excellent discussion of the elite's critical reaction to antibiotics is the tacit implication that between Osler and the antibiotic era, therapeutic rationalism was in suspended animation. On the general postwar confidence in medical innovation, see William A. Silverman, *Retrolental Fibroplasia: A Modern Parable* (New York: Grune and Stratton, 1980), pp. 69–89. On concerns over medical "enthusiasm" in the British case, see David Cantor, "Cortisone and the Politics of Drama, 1949–1955," in John V. Pickstone, ed., *Medical Innovations in Historical Perspective* (Basingstoke: Macmillan, 1992), pp. 165–184.
59 Walter Bauer, Therapeutic Trial Committee, Subcommittee on Steroids and Cancer, *Minutes* (June 9, 1952), 9, AMA Archives.
60 Hill, *Principles of Medical Statistics* (n. 39), p. 171; E. M. Glaser, "Volunteers, Controls, Placebos and Questionnaires in Clinical Trials," in Witts, *Medical Surveys and Clinical Trials* (n. 56), p. 111. On the links between therapeutic efficacy and the management of clinical practice, see the prescient discussion of François Dagonet, *La raison et les remèdes* (Paris: Presses Universitaires de France, 1964), pp. 60–61.
61 Donald Mainland, "The Planning of Investigations," *Methods of Research in Medicine* 6 (1954), 138.
62 Lasagna, "The Controlled Clinical Trial" (n. 40), 353. For a similar argument, see Sheps, "The Clinical Value of Drugs" (n. 56), 650–652. Sheps's account is unusual for its emphasis on the need to have hospitals and "organized medical groups" support such evaluations, by participating in such studies and by creating institutional policies based on such evaluations (653). Sheps is also unusually frank about the propensity of drug firms to use clinical trials to "serve promotional [rather than scientific] ends."

The techniques of modern statistical experimentation offered just such a yardstick: a well-designed trial should offer clinicians "as decisive an answer" to questions of therapeutic merit as "can be foreseen or as the statistical approach can ever give."[63]

In allying themselves with reformers, statisticians eschewed therapeutic nihilism. In this respect, statisticians conformed to the traditional ideal of the medical researcher who combined "imaginative enthusiasm" with "critical judgment."[64] The RCT's function, accordingly, was to be "as informative and as convincing as possible."[65] To convince, a clinical study not only needed to offer guarantees of impartiality, but to be as simple and as transparent as possible. A trustworthy answer to a simply put question, statisticians argued, was preferred to a contestable reply to a more complex inquiry.[66] The key to a successful investigation was planning, necessary not only to determine which questions were to be asked but to decide if they were worth asking: "Proper planning does not guarantee a successful experiment, but it makes success more likely; and attempts to draw up a plan are equally valuable if they reveal that a proposed investigation would be futile."[67]

As much as any methodological innovations, what distinguished the "modern" clinical trial was the participation of statisticians in its planning. The investigator was advised to "consider your statistical colleague rather as an architect, to be consulted *before* the work is started, so that" the experiment can produce "the maximum amount of accurate information."[68]

In improving the quality of therapeutic experimentation, it was not the statistician's technical contributions – his repertoire of experimental designs or his ability to calculate the necessary sample size and choose the appropriate statistical tests – that mattered so much as his gift for "ferreting out weaknesses in experiment[al]

63 A. Bradford Hill, *The Philosophy of the Clinical Trial: National Institute of Health Annual Lectures – 1953* (Washington, DC: Public Health Service, 1953), p. 28.
64 A. McGehee Harvey, "The Individual in Medical Research and the Role of the University Center in His Training," *Journal of Clinical Investigation* 35 (1956), 684. On therapeutic nihilism, see Hill, "The Clinical Trial" (n. 36), 282.
65 A. Bradford Hill, "Aims and Ethics," *Conference on Controlled Clinical Trials – Vienna, 1959* (Oxford: Blackwell Scientific Publishers, 1960), p. 4.
66 Hill, "The Clinical Trial" (n. 36), 279; Marvin Schneiderman, "Controlled Clinical Trials: Monday's Countdown for Tuesday's Launching," *Journal of New Drugs* 1 (November–December, 1961), 251.
67 A group of investigators who could not agree on the kinds of patients to be enrolled, the appropriate schedule of treatment, and the means for measuring improvements probably were "not ready" to undertake a trial. See Cochran, "Designing Clinical Trials" (n. 10), 71.
68 Reid, "Statistics in Clinical Research" (n. 13), 931. On the importance of having the statistical contribution made while the study is being planned, see also Donald Mainland, "Statistics in Clinical Research: Some General Principles," *Ann NY Acad Sci* 52 (March 10, 1950), 923; idem, "The Planning of Investigations," *Methods of Medical Research* 6 (1954), 138–145; Lasagna, "The Controlled Clinical Trial" (n. 40), 356; Dorothy Wiehl, "Statistical Appraisal of Nutritional Data," *Federation Proceedings* 9 (June 1950), 564–565; Paul M. Densen, "Long-Time Follow Up in Morbidity Studies: The Definition of the Group to Be Followed," *Human Biology* 22 (December 1950), 237; Beebe, "Statistics and Clinical Investigation" (n. 46), 2, 14–15; Muench, "Biostatistics" (n. 40), 334–335.

design, risks of bias, and undesirable variability."[69] "Clinicians," Harvard's Walter Bauer announced to a group of medical colleagues, "frequently do some very loose thinking." They need a biostatistician on hand "who could trip us, each one of us time and again in these sessions about the looseness of our methods."[70]

As statisticians were quick to acknowledge, they had no particular monopoly on such "statistical tact," which was as much a matter of temperament as of training. But if professional education provided "no guarantees" of such aptitudes, the individuals drawn to statistics were more likely to possess that affinity for obsessive doubt, which in their view made for good experiments.[71] And if neither nature or nurture engendered a taste for the "policeman's duties" in statisticians, circumstances did. Detecting (and repairing) problems in the design and conduct of experiments required time, and the statisticians had more such time (if never enough) than the busy clinicians with whom they worked. Moreover it helped, as Donald Mainland pointed out, that two "experienced" statisticians could be had for the price of one "suitable" clinician.[72]

The role of house skeptic was an uncomfortable one, which statisticians sought, unsuccessfully, to abdicate.[73] In the short run, their place in medical schools depended on their ability to help, not hinder, the experimenter's progress.[74] If it often fell to the statistician to remind the investigator "too readily persuaded by his data . . . just how significant or insignificant" the results were, statisticians also elected to "concentrate on what has been accomplished positively," thereby allaying the reservations of young investigators about the merits of their contributions and assisting them in getting products out the door.[75] In the long run, however, the success of their program for experimental reform depended on the "investigator himself" mastering "the principles of statistical reasoning."[76]

69 Donald Mainland, "The Clinical Trial: Difficulties and Suggestions," *JCD* 11 (May 1960), 493.
70 Therapeutic Trials Committee, Subcommittee on Steroids and Cancer, *Minutes* (June 9, 1952), 12–13, AMA Archives.
71 The notion of statistical tact, "which is rather more than simple good sense," is Major Greenwood's, cited by Bradford Hill: "some are born with it; the rest of us have to acquire it." "Statistics in Medicine," Manchester Statistical Society, *Transactions* (1946–1947), 4–5. On the affinity of statisticians for their duties see Mainland, "The Clinical Trial: Difficulties and Suggestions" (n. 69), 492–495.
72 Mainland, "The Clinical Trial: Difficulties and Suggestions" (n. 69), 492.
73 On the reluctance of statisticians to assume the preeminent role in managing clinical trials, see J. Yerushalmy, "The Planning of a Clinical Trial – Introduction," in Forster, *Evaluation of Drug Therapy* (n. 55), 60.
74 Donald Mainland, "We Wish to Hire a Medical Statistician. Have You Any Advice to Offer?," *JAMA* 193 (July 26, 1965), 290–291. Mainland's article, a paper composed in 1958 but rejected for publication then, is largely about the difficulties medical school statisticians will face in *refusing help* to colleagues in the face of demands that they serve as methodological fireman, offering consultations by the bushload. Mainland's point is that the quality of advice, and hence of the resulting research, depends on the statistician's opportunity to immerse himself in the experimenter's problem to a greater extent than circumstances generally allowed.
75 Mantel, "A Personal Perspective" (n. 10), 120.
76 Reid, "Statistics in Clinical Research" (n. 13), 929.

Statisticians expected that clinically trained investigators would ultimately take responsibility for routine therapeutic investigation, as understanding of the relevant statistical principles became more commonplace.[77] The most effective statistical education was propaganda by the deed, requiring the active collaboration of statisticians and clinicians in identifying and solving the problems of therapeutic experimentation.[78] After a few "intimate collaboration[s]," the qualified medical investigator might obtain enough "insight into the methods of applying the general principles" of statistics to enable him to work on his own, limiting future consults to particular technical questions or instances where more abstruse methodological issues came into play.[79]

The most successful statisticians were those with gifts for persuasion as well as polemic, those who learned to speak the clinician's language well and to present complicated statistical ideas as if they were little more than common sense.[80] Above all, the work required statisticians willing to learn about the "special features of medical problems," by immersing themselves in medical institutions as an earlier generation of applied statisticians had gone "into laboratories, fields, greenhouses and kitchens, among machinery and chemical vats."[81] Walter Bauer warned medical colleagues contemplating a study that they needed "a statistician who is not only biologically and clinically oriented but also biologically and clinically interested. Because this committee without such a statistician wouldn't get to first base."[82] Not all statisticians qualified for the work: some were too "rigid," others were too "abstruse," and yet others seemed to think "that no one should work with statistics but statisticians."[83]

In the early 1950s, most available statisticians had acquired their expertise in nonmedical fields, such as economics, or were autodidacts like Donald Mainland, a physician who had gone after statistical training on his own. Reformers aware of the need for "biostatistical expertise" in judging research proposals encouraged

---

77 Ibid., 929; Mainland, "The Rise of Experimental Statistics and the Problems of a Medical Statistician," *Yale Journal of Biology and Medicine* 27 (September 1954), 8–9; Hill, "Statistics in Medicine" (n. 71), 3–5; Muench, "Biostatistics" (n. 40), 338. Contrast Gilbert Beebe's view that this represented an "ideal unattainable" in most cases. See Beebe, "Statistics and Clinical Investigation" (n. 46), 2.

78 Mainland, "Statistics in Clinical Research" (n. 68), 929; and "Statistics in Medical Research" (n. 4), 124–125.

79 Mainland, "Statistics in Medical Research" (n. 4), 125.

80 See the remarks of Fred Ederer on Jerome Cornfield and of Sir Harold Himsworth on Bradford Hill: Fred Ederer, "Jerome Cornfield's Contributions to the Conduct of Clinical Trials," *Biometrics* 39 (March 1982), Supplement, 25–26; Himsworth, "Bradford Hill and Statistics in Medicine" (n. 34), 302–303.

81 Donald Mainland, "Safety in Numbers," *Circulation* 16 (November 1957), 788.

82 Therapeutic Trials Committee, Subcommittee on Steroids and Cancer, *Minutes* (1952), 19, AMA Archives.

83 Ibid.; Therapeutic Trials Committee, *Bulletin* (1947), 266; *Bulletin* (1948), 132, AMA Archives. The latter two remarks were made during a discussion of statistical consultants invited to prepare a series of articles explaining statistics to physicians. For a similar point of view, expressed by a medical statistician, see Mainland, "We Wish to Hire a Medical Statistician" (n. 74), 291.

the National Institutes of Health to fund training programs in biostatistics, but NIH efforts succeeded in the mid-1950s only after several false starts.[84]

The supply of "suitably trained" statisticians, moreover, could provide only a fraction "of the guidance that is needed." To investigators unable to undertake a suitable apprenticeship, statisticians could only offer the admittedly second-best prescription of "a limited number of simple techniques of design and analysis, which should be rigidly adhered to."[85] The articles and then books on "modern" methods of therapeutic investigation that began to appear in the 1950s were part of this missionary effort.[86]

Yet the desire to inculcate the philosophy, and not merely the techniques, of statistics among physicians could not be fulfilled by the writing of books and the organizing of symposia. Reformers found methodological progress in clinical research unbearably slow. Even worse than the fact that few clinical investigators employed statistical methods was the fact that even fewer used them correctly.[87] Despite reformers' protests that "the chanting of a few mathematical formulas or Greek symbols over the corpse of an ill-planned experiment will [not] restore the breath of life," researchers used statistics in a ritualistic and uncomprehending way.[88] Yet reformers themselves bore some of the responsibility for these misuses of statistics.

84 The early NIH statisticans recruited by Harold Dorn, for example, had a background in economic statistics. See Mantel, "A Personal Perspective" (n. 10), 123. On Mainland's self-tutoring, see Mainland, "The Rise Of Experimental Statistics" (n. 77), 1–2. In 1951, NIH established a biometrical review committee to evaluate "population" studies proposed by university researchers. In 1953, Lowell Reed's proposal for a program to train biostatisticians was approved by the National Advisory Health Council (NAHC) but two years later Thomas Dublin saw to the creation of an Advisory Committee on Epidemiology and Biometry for much the same purpose. See NAHC, *Minutes*, October 19, 1951; NAHC, *Minutes*, February 20–21, 1953; NAHC, *Minutes*, October 27–28, 1955, NIH, Office of the Director, Minutes of the National Advisory Council, RG 443, Boxes 3 and 4, NA. For a retrospective history of the program, see James Shannon to John W. Tukey, December 9, 1960, NIH, Office of the Director, Central Files (research), OD, NIH.

85 Mainland, "Statistics in Medical Research" (n. 4), 125.

86 One of the major efforts along this line was a regular series from Donald Mainland, in which statistical principles were explained through specific research examples. Beginning in 1959, Mainland's essays – available through request – were subsidized by the National Institute of General Medical Sciences; the Veterans Administration took up support in the late 1960s. Now hard to find, Mainland's essays have been collected and reprinted in several series: Donald Mainland, *Notes from a Laboratory of Medical Statistics*, 2 vols. (Ann Arbor, MI: Medical Biometry Press, 1979); idem, *Mainland's Notes on Biometry in Medical Research* (Ann Arbor, MI: Medical Biometry Press, 1978); idem, *Mainland's Statistical Ward Rounds* (Ann Arbor, MI: Medical Biometry Press, 1978). Mainland's talents were exceptional: as the American Medical Association already had found out, it was difficult to find a suitable statistician to write a few short articles on medical research.

87 Robin Badgley, "An Assessment of Research Methods Reported in 103 Scientific Articles from Two Canadian Medical Journals," *Canadian Medical Association Journal* 103 (July 29, 1961), 246–250; Stanley Schor, "Statistical Evaluation of Medical Journal Manuscripts," *JAMA* 195 (March 28, 1966), 145–150; Harold M. Schoolman, "Medical Research: A Profession Peopled by Amateurs," *Clinical Research* 14 (January 1966), 9–10.

88 Lasagna, "The Controlled Clinical Trial" (n. 40), 356. For contemporary jeremiads on the ritualistic use of statistics, see Mainland, "The Use and Misuse of Statistics" (n. 30), 411–422; Mainland "Safety in Numbers" (n. 81).

In offering up statistical methods as a means for attaining greater certainty and objectivity in therapeutic experiments, reformers had missed an opportunity to enlighten physicians about the fragility of all claims to produce authoritative knowledge, even those of the statistician. Reformers did not want to be reminded that "statisticians disagree with each other in evaluating evidence."[89] Still less did they wish to have the reasons for these disagreements explained. Practical men, medical researchers were looking for statisticians who would teach them how "to repair a gasoline engine" without instructing them on "thermodynamics."[90] Yet the limitations of the statistical enterprise were often embedded in the arcana of statistical theory which reformers sought to avoid.

ETHICS AND EPISTEMOLOGY: THE SHADOW WARS

The true question for the jury is not, "Do hospital or other physicians try experiments?" for, strictly speaking, every administration of a remedy is an experiment – but, "Do they study diligently the claims of all new and old methods, and do they know how to select those which offer the best chance of proving useful?"[91]

To judge from the published writings of medical statisticians in the 1950s, the road to responsible therapeutic investigation was paved over the objections of clinicians, which had to be dismantled before RCTs could become a routine practice. Whatever reservations physicians held privately about the statistical enterprise, however, few voiced their doubts publicly.[92] For the most part, historical records document a shadow war, in which therapeutic reformers marshaled arguments to persuade a largely silent medical community of the necessity of randomized clinical trials. Though reformers' arguments cannot tell us what physicians "really thought" about RCTs, they can reveal how much was at stake in reformers' efforts to reorganize the research enterprise.

To many clinicians, the basic procedures of the randomized controlled trial were unfamiliar. Allowing a roll of the dice to determine a patient's treatment, withholding innovative therapies from one group of patients, keeping treating physicians in the dark about what medications their patients were receiving –

89 AMA, Therapeutic Trials Committee, *Bulletin* (July 19, 1948), 164, AMA Archives. For a related argument, regarding the role statistics texts in psychology played in suppressing awareness of theoretical differences between Fisher and Jerzy Neyman, see Gerd Gigerenzer, "Probabilistic Thinking and the Fight against Subjectivity," in Lorenz Krüger, Gerd Gigenrenzer, and Mary S. Morgan, *The Probabilistic Revolution* (Cambridge: MIT Press, 1980), vol. 2, pp. 19–22; Gigenrenzer et al., *The Empire of Chance* (n. 21), pp. 207–211.

90 AMA, Therapeutic Trials Committee, *Bulletin* (September 16, 1947), 291, AMA Archives.

91 O. W. Holmes, "Experiments in Medicine," *BMSJ* 30 (April 3, 1844), 202.

92 One measure of physician resistance is the propensity to subvert random treatment assignments in clinical trials. See Kenneth F. Schultz, "Subverting Randomization in Controlled Trials," *JAMA* 274 (November 8, 1995), 1456–1458. For evidence of physician qualms over participating in RCTs during the 1950s, see Silverman, *Retrolental Fibroplasia* (n. 58), pp. 37–41, 152–153.

these were all innovative and somewhat disturbing practices.[93] Just how innovative can be seen by reformers' efforts to naturalize these practices, presenting them as a simple extension, albeit an improvement, on traditional clinical skills:

After all, clinical observation becomes in the last analysis an attempt at statistical study and it is of value only when it has been put on that basis. For example, I may say that I have a patient with actinomycosis who had a striking cure as a result of the use of potassium iodide. You may say, however, that you have tried the alleged remedy in six cases with no results at all. In this case, it would be the fact that you had six negative results which would influence both you and me in concluding that potassium iodide is of little, if any, value in the treatment of actinomycosis.[94]

The only difference, Bradford Hill argued, between the statistician and the "careful clinician" who refuses to generalize about the merits of a new therapy until he has tried it on a half-dozen patients is that the latter "might sometimes fare better if he straightaway walked boldly up the path and without any ado opened the gate to a designed and controlled clinical trial."[95] Michael Shimkin, a researcher at the National Cancer Institute, put the case more strongly. The clinician experiments "continually" on his patients with each new treatment; one simply learns more from the "deliberate experimentation" of the statistically informed investigator.[96]

Despite their insistence that "modern statistics does not claim to be something intrinsically different from the principles and methods of experimenters in general," reformers in the 1950s were asking medical researchers for more than the careful observation expected in traditional clinical research. Enlisting one's patients in a randomized controlled trial called for physicians to acknowledge how little they really knew, not only about treatment but about disease. The statistician's insistence on randomization represented a not too subtle reminder of the limitations of medical knowledge: "It is impossible to identify all the elements that affect the outcome and therefore we require some process that will bring about similarity in our groups without attempting to categorize all the important factors and match the groups on these."[97] Reformers had good reason to insist on medical

---

93 The practice of "blinding," or keeping physicians ignorant of which patients were receiving placebo and which were getting the experimental treatment, was publicly criticized. See Robert C. Batterman and Arthur J. Grossman, "Effectiveness of Salicylamide As an Analgesic and Antirheumatic Agent: Evaluation of the Double Blindfold Technique for Studying Analgesic Drugs," *JAMA* 159 (December 24, 1955), 1619–1622; H. Haas, H. Fink, and G. Hartfelder, "The Placebo Problem," *Psychopharmacology Service Bulletin* 1 (1962), 12–13. The later article, while it reflects German debates on this issue, was translated for American consumption by researchers at the National Institute of Mental Health.

94 Evarts A. Graham to Samuel C. Harvey, September 8, 1943, CMR/OSRD, RG 227, Box 28, NA.

95 Hill, "Assessment of Therapeutic Trials" (n. 36), 131.

96 Michael B. Shimkin, "Problem of Experimentation of Human Beings. I. The Research Worker's Point of View," *Science* 117 (February 27, 1953), 205. See also Donald Mainland, "The Modern Method of Clinical Trial," *Methods in Medical Research* 6 (1954), 157.

97 Marshall and Merrell, "Clinical Therapeutic Trial of a New Drug" (n. 35), 224.

ignorance, apart from their conviction that many physicians knew far less than they claimed to about the vagaries of human disease.[98] Advocates of randomized clinical trials insisted that the best test of a new therapy was to try it on a group of patients while withholding it from another group. Such rationing was hard to justify, unless the physician came to doubt his own "knowledge" about a therapy's promise:

It is the physician's duty to do his best for his patients, and if he believes that there is some evidence in favor of a certain treatment, he will feel bound to use it. If, however, he is acquainted with the requirements for valid proof, he will often see that what looked like evidence is not evidence at all, and he will feel free to experiment.[99]

Creating doubt about the basis for physicians' beliefs was a necessary part of the statisticians' job. Once it was claimed that a new therapy worked, it became increasingly difficult to deny that treatment to other patients, even for the sake of testing the claim. Trials should be begun, statisticians argued, before physicians come to believe in a new treatment or they will not begin at all.[100]

Historians have puzzled over the relative absence of ethical discussions over medical research in the first twenty years after World War II.[101] In part, they have been looking in the wrong place. Reformers' remarks about the medical knowledge that underwrote physicians' therapeutic practices were highly ethically charged. The ethics in question was the traditional ethics of therapeutic reformers, who tried to persuade physicians that their beliefs about therapy were unjustified. It was, reformers asserted, the physician's responsibility to be guided by medical knowledge, not by drug company misinformation or the uninformed desires of patients.[102] The physician who did not rely on evidence from controlled clinical trials was behaving unethically: "In treating patients with unproved remedies we are, whether we like it or not, experimenting on human beings, and a good

98 Walter Modell, "The Protean Control of Clinical Pharmacology," *Clinical Pharmacology and Therapeutics* 4 (1963), 378; Schoolman, "Medical Research: A Profession Peopled by Amateurs" (n. 87), 9–10.

99 Mainland, "Statistics in Clinical Research" (n. 68), 927.

100 For the statistician's insistence on the need to conduct well-controlled trials *before* the credibility of new therapies was established on the basis of inferior evidence, see Marshall and Merrell, "Clinical Therapeutic Trial of a New Drug" (n. 35), 230; and Hill, "The Clinical Trial" (n. 36), 279. Concern about other studies foreclosing the opportunity to do a "strictly controlled clinical trial" of cortisone and ACTH in treating rheumatic fever prompted the organization of an international study of these drugs. Rheumatic Fever Working Party [MRC] and American Council on Rheumatic Fever and Congenital Heart Disease, "The Treatment of Acute Rheumatic Fever in Children: A Cooperative Clinical Trial of ACTH, Cortisone and Aspirin," *Circulation* 11 (March 1955), 343–371.

101 See David J. Rothman, *Strangers at the Bedside: A History of How Law and Bioethics Transformed Medical Decision Making* (New York: Basic Books, 1991), esp. pp. 47–69. Rothman, moreover, overlooks the many references to research ethics in discussions of clinical trials. See Mainland, "The Modern Method of Clinical Trial" (n. 96), 152, 157; Lasagna, "The Controlled Clinical Trial" (n. 40), 355.

102 Harry F. Dowling, "Twixt the Cup and the Lip," *JAMA* 165 (October 12, 1957), 658–661.

experiment well reported may be more ethical and entail less shirking of duty than a poor one."[103]

To members of the research community, claims for the application of controlled experimentation to new treatments were most compelling when contrasted with uncontrolled testing by individual clinicians: "Deliberate experimentation on a group of cases with adequate controls is merely an efficient and convenient means of collecting and interpreting data that would otherwise be dispersed and inaccessible."[104] Yet not all researchers were persuaded that the statistician's contribution to experimental design and analysis improved on traditional research practices. Morris Fishbein, editor of the *Journal of the American Medical Association*, worried about statisticians' "failure . . . to recognize the value of papers which do not meet statistical standards. One case reported from a qualified clinic is worth more than 300 cases reported from an unqualified clinic."[105] Torald Sollman, the veteran leader of the AMA's Council on Pharmacy and Chemistry, observed: "Medical research has made many if not most of its discoveries without any mathematical statistical analysis in the strict sense. This seems to indicate that such analysis is not essential in some types of research; and when it is not needed, it is a handicap, as all unnecessary complications impede direct progress."[106] The question was, Which complications were unnecessary, the statistician's or the clinical investigator's? More important, who would decide?

DILEMMAS OF AUTHORITY: RANDOMIZED EXPERIMENTS IN THEORY AND PRACTICE

A method is a dangerous thing unless its underlying philosophy is understood, and none more dangerous than the statistical. . . . In a mathematical or strictly logical discipline the care is one of technique; but in a natural science and in statistics the care must extend not only over the technique but to the matter of judgment, as is necessarily the case in coming to conclusions upon any problem of real life where the complications are great.[107]

Although the protocol is surely the chief instrument for insuring the soundness of a therapeutic trial, other considerations enter when one looks at such an investigation as a social enterprise.[108]

103 Bradford Hill, quoted in Donald Mainland, "The Modern Method of Clinical Trial" (n. 96), 157.
104 Michael Shimkin, "Problem of Experimentation of Human Beings" (n. 96), 205. See also the discussion of the proposal from the National Cancer Institute's John R. Heller that the AMA's Therapeutic Trials Committee take a role in reducing the proliferation of "clinical testing" by unqualified researchers. AMA, Therapeutic Trials Committee, *Bulletin* (April 3, 1948), 166–168, AMA Archives.
105 AMA, Therapeutic Trials Committee, *Bulletin* (January 1, 1949), 7, AMA Archives.
106 AMA, Therapeutic Trials Committee, *Bulletin* (July 19, 1948), 133, AMA Archives. Sollman nonetheless endorsed the proposal under discussion to get a statistical consultant for the *Journal of the American Medical Association*.
107 Wilson, "Statistical Significance of Experimental Data" (n. 16), 94.
108 Beebe, "Statistics and Clinical Investigation" (n. 46), 12.

Therapeutic reformers in the 1950s promoted the controlled clinical trial as a standard of scientific excellence in therapeutic research. Yet, as with any purely methodological standard, reformers failed to specify how randomized experiments would be judged in the absence of any authoritative body to perform the judging. Previous generations of reformers had relied on professional organizations such as the AMA's Council on Pharmacy and Chemistry to represent the profession's expertise, but by the mid-1950s academic researchers no longer regarded the AMA council as a standard bearer of scientific therapeutic reform.[109] Drug companies, reformers complained, operated with singular abandon in using clinical trials for "promotional ends." Yet in bypassing organizations such as the council, methodological reformers left it up to the individual physician's "critical eye" to discern when the terms "controlled," "random," and "blind" were merely being applied as "complimentary adjective[s]" and when they demonstrated adherence to the new standards of scientific excellence.[110]

Similar issues of authority affected researchers planning therapeutic experiments. In most settings, clinical and laboratory researchers had the last word on the conduct of such studies. To statisticians, it seemed that medical researchers were unhappy with the limited scientific ambitions of the controlled clinical trial: "There seems little Nobel about a clinical trial. If you complicate it with some biochemistry, a little epidemiology, and so forth, perhaps it will seem more worth doing."[111] Clinical investigators sought to augment the scientific yield of clinical trials by collecting data on various physiological, biochemical, and clinical parameters of disease. Such data, while often incidental to the study's principal aim of determining therapeutic benefit, satisfied researchers interested in adding to the store of knowledge about the biology and natural history of disease. To methodological reformers intent on promoting studies with fewer objectives and simpler protocols, even the most noteworthy clinical trials of the 1950s represented compromises with their experimental ideals. The multiyear study of anticoagulants in the prevention of coronary thrombosis, sponsored by the American Heart Association and the National Institutes of Health, provides an extreme example of the genre, with its 656 pages of text and dozens of tables providing data about the natural history of coronary thrombosis.[112] Similarly, the 1954 trials of the Salk polio vaccine, largest and best known of postwar "therapeutic" experiments,

---

109 For criticisms of the council, see Harry F. Dowling, *Medicines for Man: The Development, Regulation and Use of Prescription Drugs* (New York: Alfred A. Knopf, 1970), pp. 159–162, 166–177.
110 Sheps, "Clinical Value of Drugs" (n. 56), 649–651; Louis Lasagna and Paul Meier, "Clinical Evaluation of Drugs," *Annual Review of Medicine* 9 (1958), 347. Similarly, the legal fiction prior to 1962 that the FDA dealt only with the safety and not the efficacy of new drugs left it up to individual firms to reform their standards of clinical investigations. See Louis Lasagna, "Gripesmanship: A Positive Approach," *JCD* 10 (December 1959), 464–465.
111 To the researcher so tempted, the statistician's advice was "Don't! Resist the temptation! Keep it simple!" See Schneiderman, "Controlled Clinical Trials" (n. 66), 251. See also Mainland, "The Clinical Trial – Some Difficulties and Suggestions" (n. 61), 486–487.
112 American Heart Association, Committee on Anticoagulants, *Myocardial Infarction: Its Clinical Manifestations and Treatments with Anticoagulants* (New York: American Heart Association, 1954).

reflect the interests of virologists in collecting massive amounts of data on antibody formation within the vaccinated and control populations. The polio investigators were quite fortunate that there were no obvious points of contradiction between the immunological and the clinical evidence, and that the vaccine seemed effective regardless of whether clinical or laboratory-confirmed diagnoses were taken as a measure of outcome.[113]

As statisticians were often reminded, clinical investigation was ultimately a medical domain. When conflicts arose between physicians and statisticians over the competing aims of a clinical trial, it was the physician researcher who would decide which questions would be asked.[114] Although cognizant of the power relations in medical institutions, statisticians rarely analyzed the therapeutic trial as "a social enterprise," preferring instead the cleaner, less contested language of scientific method.[115]

According to reformers, randomized experiments offered physicians a "scientific" frame of reference for judging new therapies. Yet statisticians at best provided limited guidance in defining the rules by which experimental results should be interpreted. Statisticians generally agreed that any given experiment had both substantive scientific aspects and formal statistical aspects. In interpreting experimental results, it was the scientist's job to speak to the substantive aspects of the research; the statistician's to examine critically the quantitative aspects.[116] But statisticians had very little to say about where (or how) to draw the boundary between the two. Such border problems proved particularly acute in medicine, where the statistician's role extended to policing the conclusions that clinical investigators attempted to draw from their studies.

However much research physicians might agree in theory about the ability of randomized controls to improve the reliability of therapeutic knowledge, in practice the experienced clinician often claimed to know more about the factors that made one group of patients respond to experimental treatment and another not.[117]

---

113 Thomas Francis Jr., "An Evaluation of the 1954 Poliomyelitis Vaccine Trials – Summary Report" *AJPH* 45 (1955), 26–32. But see the critical discussion by K. A. Brownlee, "Statistics of the 1954 Polio Vaccine Trials," *Journal of the American Statistical Association* 50 (December 1955), 1005–1013, esp. 1010–1013. A full analysis of the debates in virology and public health communities regarding the effectiveness of the Salk vaccine would be welcome.

114 Robert P. Gage, "Statistics and Medicine: The Need for Close Co-operation between the Physician and the Statistician in Medical Statistics," *Proceedings of the Staff Meetings of the Mayo Clinic* 21 (March 20, 1946), 130; Paul M. Densen, "Long-Time Follow-Up in Morbidity Studies: The Definition of the Group to Be Followed," *Human Biology* 22 (December 1950), 237.

115 For a rare exception to the genre, see Beebe, "Statistics and Clinical Investigation" (n. 46), which explicitly treats the therapeutic trial as a "social enterprise" that needs to be carefully managed if success is to be achieved.

116 George W. Snedecor, "The Statistical Part of the Scientific Method," *Ann NY Acad Sci* 52 (March 10, 1950), 792–799.

117 The British biologist Lancelot Hogben made this a central issue in his critique of randomized experiments in medicine. See Lancelot Hogben, "The Assessment of Remedies," *Medical Press* (October 13, 1954), 331–338. For a favorable American mention of Hogben's concern (and proposed solutions), see Lasagna and Meier, "Clinical Evaluation of Drugs" (n. 110), 349–350.

The clinician who noticed that a subgroup of study patients responded differently to treatment was tempted to find a reason for the difference somewhere in the data. To statisticians, such findings, "however striking," were mere "impressions." They cautioned medical researchers against "drawing any *conclusions* from an experiment *except those for which it has been designed*."[118]

The clinician's impulse to reinterpret experimental data was most easily accommodated in the small, short-term trials of acute episodes of disease. Where small amounts of money or time would suffice to conduct a study, the physician with different assumptions about the patients who would best benefit from treatment or the dosages that would produce the best results could conceivably follow the statistician's advice to conduct another controlled experiment. In instances where the outcomes of treatment were unambiguous, and academic physicians had well-established interests in determining the relative merits of specific drugs, the counsels of methodological reformers increasingly took hold. The incorporation of statistical methods in these domains accordingly enhanced, rather than subtracted from, the authority of academic physicians to direct therapeutic practice.[119]

In the treatment of chronic diseases, where controversies over the merits of particular therapies ran deepest, the promise of improvements in experimental method to adjudicate differences of opinion about clinical and scientific questions was harder to realize. Here the strategy of collecting more and more data in the course of a study ran the risk of producing more, not less, controversy, as physicians attached different interpretations to voluminous data reported.[120] And the obvious methodological solution to scientific disputes – conduct another, better study – was hardly a routine option in circumstances where hundreds of patients and years of follow-up might be needed to complete an experiment.

While acknowledging that the study of chronic disease might pose greater logistical and organizational difficulties than short-term studies of acute disease, statisticians had no reason to think that the biological complexity of chronic disease posed more fundamental challenges to the program of methodological reforms. Here, if anywhere in medicine, the statisticians' injunctions – randomize and simplify – were meant to apply. Yet biological complexity and clinical individ-

118 Mainland, "Planning of Investigations" (n. 61), 141, 145; Beebe, "Statistics and Clinical Investigation" (n. 46), 14.

119 Drug companies' support for improvements in the methods of clinical evaluation assisted in these developments. See Hart E. van Riper and Donald Boyer, "The Planning and Reporting of Clinical Trials," *New York State Journal of Medicine* (October 1, 1961), 3337–3342. Corporate support for the new standards nonetheless varied considerably. See Lasagna, "Gripesmanship" (n. 110), 466. For pessimistic accounts of the slow rate of "progress," see Badgley, "An Assessment of Research Methods" (n. 87), 246–250; Schor, "Statistical Evaluation of Medical Journal Manuscripts" (n. 87), 145–150.

120 The opposition of George Burch, a participant in Irving Wright's comprehensive evaluation of anticoagulants, to granting Wright's study the official endorsement of the American Heart Association speaks directly to the continuing limitations of controlled trials in setting authoritative practice standards. See Executive Committee of the Scientific Council, American Heart Association, *Minutes*, March 13, 1954, Howard Sprague papers, Countway Library.

uation were the stock-in-trade of specialists in chronic disease, whose authority rested on their claim to formulate complex, unquantifiable judgments about the myriad factors that determined why one patient responded to treatment and another did not.

Contests among scientific disciplines for social authority and intellectual influence are common enough. Yet the social tensions between clinical researchers and statisticians brought to the fore a critical ambiguity in the standard framework of statistical inference: what was the role of experience in interpreting experimental data? For many statisticians, prior experience had no legitimate place in the formal analysis of experimental data. Few statisticians were naive enough to believe that the interpretation of therapeutic experiments was purely an exercise in mathematics. In practice, an experiment whose results conflicted with experience or biochemical theory might deserve closer scrutiny. But standard statistical theory offered no clues to the clinical researcher interested in incorporating his own beliefs about the pathogenesis of disease or the mechanisms by which a drug acted in interpreting a given experimental result.[121]

Until the 1960s, such questions remained concerns only for the high panjandrums of statistical theory debating the foundations of statistical inference. Even more so than Fisher's ideas about randomization, these debates remained theoretical arcana unknown to most medical audiences in this country.[122] Not until 1965

---

121 John C. Bailar III points out to me that Bayesian methods are intended precisely to accommodate these concerns. However, prior to the 1970s, there were few Bayesians working in clinical research, and even fewer methods available for them to use. For early discussion, see Jerome Cornfield's papers: "A Bayesian Test of Some Classical Hypotheses – With Applications to Sequential Clinical Trials," *Journal of the American Statistical Association* 61 (September, 1966), 577–594; and "The Bayesian Outlook and Its Application," *Biometrics* (September 1969), 617–642. On the limited influence of formal Bayesian methods, see Fred Ederer's remarks on Cornfield's sequential designs for clinical trials in Ederer, "Jerome Cornfield's Contributions" (n. 80), 30.

122 For a useful introduction to the postwar debates, see the paper by Frank Anscombe and the ensuing discussion: F. J. Anscombe, "The Validity of Comparative Experiments," *Journal of the Royal Statistical Society* 111 (1948), 181–200. While American statisticians were aware of (and participated in) these debates, only Lancelot Hogben and Raymond Wrighton in Britain developed their implications for randomized experiments in medicine. See Lancelot Hogben and Raymond Wrighton, "Statistical Theory of Prophylactic and Therapeutic Trials: I," *British Journal of Social Medicine* 6 (1952), 89–117; Raymond Wrighton, "The Theoretical Basis of the Therapeutic Trial," *Acta Genetica et Statistica Medica* 4 (1953), 312–343. I know of only one, brief, American mention of the British work: see Lasagna and Meier, "Clinical Evaluation of Drugs" (n. 110), 349–350. In the 1950s, Irwin Bross and the British statistician Peter Armitage began devising experimental designs for sequential medical trials in another departure from the traditional hypothesis-testing framework. Familiar to industrial statisticians, these innovations were rarely employed by medical researchers prior to the 1980s. See Irwin Bross, "Sequential Medical Plans," *Biometrics* 8 (1952), 188–205; Peter Armitage, *Sequential Medical Trials* (Springfield, IL: Charles C. Thomas, 1960). On the reaction to Armitage's ideas, see F. J. Anscombe, "Sequential Medical Trials," *Journal of the American Statistical Association* 58 (1963), 365–383; John C. Bailar III, "Patient Assignment Algorithims: An Overview," in *Proceedings: 9th International Biometric Conference* (Raleigh, NC: Biometric Society, 1978), vol. 1, pp. 189–206. On the wartime development of sequential methods, see G. A. Barnard and R. L. Blackett, "Statistics in the United Kingdom, 1939–1945," in Anthony C. Atkinson and Stephen E. Fienberg, eds., *A Celebration of Statistics: The ISI Centenary Volume* (New York: Springer-Verlag, 1985), pp. 41–49.

did statisticians begin publicly discussing their conviction that "drawing a scientific inference from a set of data is not the formal exercise one finds taught in statistical classrooms."[123]

The following two chapters take up in greater detail the intellectual and social challenges faced by advocates of clinical trials. The first explores the history of the Diet-Heart study, an experiment that, biomedical researchers ultimately concluded, was too costly and too logistically complex to undertake. The second examines the long and furious debate over a randomized controlled trial of drugs to prevent the complications of diabetes: the University Group Diabetes Program study.

123 Marvin Zelen in S. J. Cutler, S. W. Greenhouse, J. Cornfield, M. A. Schneiderman et al., "The Role of Hypothesis Testing in Clinical Trials," *JCD* 19 (1966), 857–882 (quotation from 873). This conference of NIH and non-NIH statisticians was the first full and public discussion of challenges to the standard account of experimental design and statistical inference offered in the medical literature and classroom. For a similar story in psychology, see Gigerenzer, "Probabilistic Thinking and the Fight against Subjectivity" (n. 89), pp. 11–33.

6

You gotta have heart

Today, over most of the earth, want is the rule and atherosclerosis is being prevented by chill penury. Where a luxus diet prevails, diabetes and atherosclerosis flourish.[1]

"Luxury living," "high standard of living," and "prosperity" are medically meaningless terms. One must find and designate more clearly the responsible factor or factors in these broad terms.[2]

In 1950, heart disease and diseases of the circulatory system accounted for nearly 40 of every 100 deaths recorded by the U.S. vital statistics system.[3] The death rate for cardiovascular disease had been rising since the early 1900s, owing, contemporaries believed, to the combination of an aging population, a decline in infectious disease mortality, improved diagnosis, and vital statistics reporting.[4]

While some observers deemed the increase in cardiovascular mortality evidence of past medical progress in conquering infectious disease, for Louis Dublin, senior statistician at the Metropolitan Life Insurance Company, it pointed to a more ominous change in American habits: "Because of our prosperity and abundance, a large number of our people are literally eating themselves to death."[5] Once an

---

1 William Dock, "The Causes of Arteriosclerosis," *Bull NY Acad Med* 26 (1950), 188.
2 Norman Joliffe, "Fats, Cholesterol and Coronary Heart Disease: A Review of Recent Progress," *Circulation* 20 (July 1959), 112.
3 "Disease of the heart" accounted for 36.9 percent of all deaths; other circulatory disorders (including hypertension and aortic aneurism) for an additional 3 percent of all deaths. National Office of Vital Statistics, *Vital Statistics of the United States. 1950* (Washington, DC: Government Printing Office, 1954), vol. 1, p. 171; vol. 3, pp. 66–67.
4 Theodore D. Woolsey and I. M. Moriyama, "Statistical Studies of Heart Disease: II. Important Factors in Heart Disease Mortality Trends," *Public Health Reports* 63 (1948), 1247–1267; Alfred E. Cohn and Claire Lingg, *The Burden of Diseases in the United States* (New York: Oxford University Press, 1950), pp. 55–58. Incorporated in these changes were a decline in the relative importance of heart disease from infectious causes: Paul D. White, "Changes in Relative Prevalence of Various Types of Heart Disease in New England: Contrast between 1925 and 1950," *JAMA* 152 (May 23, 1953), 303–304.
5 Louis I. Dublin and Mortimer Spiegelman, "Factors in the Higher Mortality of Our Older Age Groups," *AJPH* 42 (April 1952), 428.

active, agricultural people, we were now a nation of sedentary city dwellers who overate. The result, Dublin intimated, was a cardiovascular mortality rate for middle-aged men in excess of that found anywhere else among the "leading nations" of the world.[6] To correct it, Dublin called for a "campaign of education against overeating, which is one of the besetting sins of our country."[7]

Dublin's views on the "epidemic" of heart disease were based on decades of actuarial research, adequate enough to convince insurance executives that overweight, middle-aged men were poor risks.[8] Medical researchers were harder to persuade. A long tradition of dietary fads and fashions, much of it based on conflicting nutritional assumptions, had left many academic physicians skeptical about dietary advice.[9] While few physicians advised their cardiac patients to gain weight, few were willing to state what benefits, if any, lay in dieting. Moreover, if the American diet played a role in heart disease, few researchers in 1950 were certain which dietary constituents were harmful, and even fewer thought that the answers lay in international comparisons of mortality rates.[10] Yet by the end of the decade, federally funded investigators from six prominent medical institutions were planning the pilot study for an ambitious social experiment to lower the rate of cardiac mortality by giving thousands of middle-aged American men specially prepared diets.

The Diet-Heart study was one of the earliest of a series of ambitious clinical trials in the prevention and treatment of heart disease launched by the National Heart and Lung Institute in the 1960s and 1970s. Unlike some of its better known contemporaries – the Coronary Drug Project or the Multiple Risk Intervention Trial – the full Diet-Heart study was never authorized. Nonetheless, the story of the Diet-Heart study provides a useful window on the changing places of laboratory research, epidemiological studies, and clinical trials in the American academic medical world of the 1960s.

---

6 Ibid., 424–428.
7 Louis I. Dublin, "Public Health and the Diseases of Old Age," in James Stevens Simmons, ed., *Public Health in the World Today* (Cambridge: Harvard University Press, 1949), p. 235.
8 On the history of insurance investigations on obesity, see Hillel Schwartz, *Never Satisfied: A Cultural History of Diets, Fantasies and Fat* (New York: Free Press, 1986), pp. 155–159, 216; David P. Barr, "Health and Obesity," *NEJM* 248 (June 4, 1953), 968. On actuarial practices, see Louis I. Dublin, "Relation of Obesity to Longevity," *NEJM* 248 (June 4, 1953), 971.
9 On dietary fads and their regulation, see Schwartz, *Never Satisfied* (n. 8); Roberta Pollack Seid, *Never Too Thin: Why Women Are at War with Their Bodies* (New York: Prentice-Hall, 1989), pp. 81–103; James Harvey Young, *Medical Messiahs: A Social History of Health Quackery in Twentieth-Century America* (Princeton: Princeton University Press, 1967), pp. 333–345, 357.
10 Samuel Proger, "Obesity and Heart Disease," *Medical Clinics of North America* 35 (September 1951), 1351–1359; Sigmund Wilems, "Some Nutritional Factors Concerned in the Development and Regression of Arteriosclerotic Lesions," in National Institute of Health, *Seminar on the Degenerative Lesions of Metabolism. October 5, 1947* (mimeographed transcript), pp. 35b–37; Samuel A. Levine, "Heart Disease: Its Medical Aspects," *Ann Int Med* 39 (September 1950), 573; "Diseases of the Coronary Arteries," in *Proceedings: First National Conference on Cardiovascular Disease* (New York: American Heart Association, 1950), p. 85. For a critique of insurance-based data of diet and cause of death, see Ancel Keys, "Nutrition in Relation to the Etiology and the Course of Degenerative Diseases," *Journal of the American Dietetic Association* 24 (1948), 282.

The following section analyzes the history of ideas about arteriosclerosis and heart disease before World War II. It is followed by a section on the contested role of epidemiological evidence in demonstrating the role of dietary fat in coronary heart disease. The remaining sections analyze the political and intellectual travails of an experiment that never was: the Diet-Heart study.

ARTERIOSCLEROSIS: THE MAKING OF A DISEASE

The consensus of many clinicians is that intimal arteriosclerosis is an inevitable consequence of the aging process and that the study of this condition will not result in significant advances in its prevention or treatment.[11]

It cannot be said, any more, that vascular stenosis is a disease of the decresence of life, an idea which had dominated medical thinking up to a comparatively short time ago.[12]

In 1913, the pathologist Nicolai Anitschkow reported to European audiences on a series of studies in which Russian investigators had fed rabbits a diet rich in eggs. The arterial wall [intima] of the rabbits' aortas had become lined with fatty deposits, which were, Anitschkow contended, identical with cholesterol. This work provided the basis for Anitschkow's lifelong contention that deposits of excess cholesterol in the arterial wall were the main culprit in the development of human atherosclerosis.[13]

While Anitschkow was ultimately acclaimed as a "farsighted" and even a "revolutionary" scientist, for the next thirty years his findings were treated as a laboratory curiosity whose interpretation was disputed and whose clinical significance was doubtful.[14] For informed practitioners, the condition Anitschkow

---

11 Alfred Steiner, "Cholesterol in Arteriosclerosis, with Special Reference to Coronary Arteriosclerosis," *Medical Clinics of North America* 34 (May 1950), 674.

12 Joseph H. Barach, in NIH, *Seminar on the Degenerative Lesions of Metabolism* (n. 10), p. 1.

13 Anitschkow's paper served as a corrective to earlier work by A. I. Ignatowski, who maintained that egg protein was the responsible agent for the pathological changes. Ignatowski is, however, generally credited with developing the (rabbit) animal model for studying atherosclerosis. Anitschkow's 1913 paper was recently reprinted in English: N. Anitschkow and S. Chalatow, "On Experimental Cholesterin Stearosis and Its Significance in the Origin of Some Pathological Processes," *Arteriosclerosis* 3 (March–April 1983), 178–182. On Anitschkow, see T. N. Khavkin, "Nikolai Nikolaevich Anitschkow (in Commemoration of the 90th Anniversary of His Birthday," *Beitrage zur Pathologie* 156 (1975), 301–312. See also N. Anitschkow, "Experimental Arteriosclerosis in Animals," in Edmund V. Cowdry, ed., *Arteriosclerosis: A Survey of the Problem* (New York: Macmillan, 1933), pp. 271–322.

14 For retrospective judgments of Anitschkow's work, see the worshipful assessment of William Dock, who deemed Anitschkow's early work as comparable with that of Harvey and Lavoisier. William Dock, "Research in Arteriosclerosis – The First Fifty Years," *Ann Int Med* 49 (September 1958), 699–705; see also Richard J. Bing, "Atherosclerosis," in Richard J. Bing, ed., *Cardiology: The Evolution of the Science and the Art* (USA: Harwood Academic Publishers, 1992), pp. 130–133.

For contemporary skepticism regarding the role of cholesterol in arteriosclerosis, and Anitschkow's work in particular, see Soma Weiss and George R. Minot, "Nutrition in Relation to Arteriosclerosis," and W. Ophuls, "The Pathogenesis of Arteriosclerosis," both in Cowdry, *Arterio-*

found in his experimental animals remained the "cholesterol disease of rabbits," despite the efforts of American researchers in the 1930s to extend his conclusions to human disease.[15] According to one authority, "The oft-expressed hope of preventing arteriosclerosis is actually a hope of preventing the body from growing old as years pass, and there is as yet little basis for it."[16]

Given prevailing medical concepts of heart disease, most physicians remained indifferent to Anitschkow's contention that arteriosclerosis was a preventable metabolic disorder. In the 1930s and 1940s, textbook authors emphasized the acute management of heart attacks, and the convalescent care of cardiac patients (known as "cardiacs"). While textbooks might briefly review speculations about the factors that predisposed patients to heart disease, the prevention section in such texts was nonexistent.[17] Moreover, textbook writers presented a model of heart attacks that drew minimal attention to the long-term changes in the coronary arteries associated with arteriosclerosis.

Physicians in these decades thought of the heart as a hardworking pump "which empties and fills itself like a bellows – a hollow pump made of muscle."[18] A heart

sclerosis (n. 13), pp. 233–248, esp. 236–7, 242; and pp. 256–257; Eli Moschcowitz, "Arteriosclerosis," in William D. Stroud, ed., *The Diagnosis and Treatment of Cardiovascular Disease* (Philadelphia: F. A. Davis, 1943), vol. II, pp. 1553–1555. See also the lengthy review article by G. Lyman Duff, "Experimental Cholesterol Arteriosclerosis and Its Relationship to Human Arteriosclerosis," *Archives of Pathology* 20 (1935), 81–123, 259–304.

15 Timothy Leary, "Atherosclerosis, the Important Form of Arteriosclerosis, a Metabolic Disease," *JAMA* 105 (August 17, 1935), 476. Leary, a Boston pathologist, was the principal exponent of Anitschkow's cholesterol hypothesis in this country during the 1930s and 1940s. See idem, "Arteriosclerosis with Special Reference to Coronary Sclerosis: Parts I and II," *Modern Concepts of Cardiovascular Disease* 11 (October–November 1942); idem, "Arteriosclerosis: A Metabolic Disease," in *Seminar on the Degenerative Lesions of Metabolism* (n. 10), pp. 27–32. On Leary, see "Timothy Leary (1887–1954)," *NEJM* 251 (December 30, 1954), 1115–1116.

16 H. M. Marvin, "The Prevention and Relief of Heart Disease As a Public Health Problem," in Stroud, *The Diagnosis and Treatment of Cardiovascular Disease* (n. 14), vol. II, pp. 1025–1026. See also John Wyckoff, "The Treatment of Arteriosclerosis," in Cowdry, *Arteriosclerosis* (n. 13), pp. 570–572.

17 Among the factors discussed were heredity (family history of heart disease), overwork and stress, occupation and body type. See Samuel A. Levine, *Clinical Heart Disease* (Philadelphia: W. B. Saunders, 1936), p. 135; Paul Dudley White, *Heart Disease,* 3rd ed. (New York: Macmillan, 1944), pp. 479, 482–483; Howard B. Sprague, "Coronary Artery Disease, Coronary Occlusion and Myocardial Infarction," in Robert L. Levy, ed., *Disorders of the Heart and Circulation* (New York: Thomas Nelson and Sons, 1951), pp. 450–451. See, however, Bishop's view of heart disease as due to an underlying chronic food intoxication and/or sensitivity: Louis Fagueres Bishop, *Arteriosclerosis: A Consideration of the Prolongation of Life and Efficiency after Forty* (London: Oxford University Press, 1914), pp. 119–124; idem, *Heart Troubles: Their Prevention and Relief* (New York: Funk and Wagnalls, 1920), pp. 274–275, 285–296.

18 J. H. Irvine, "Heart Disease and What to Do about It," *Hygeia* 24 (1946), 32. For an extended development of the pump metaphor, see the account of a heart attack victim's son in Eugene F. Snyder, *From a Doctor's Heart* (New York: Philosophical Library, 1951), pp. 50–54. On the development and teaching of the physiological concept of the heart that underwrote the pump metaphor, see Joel Howell, " 'Soldier's Heart': The Redefinition of Heart Disease and Specialty Formation in Early Twentieth Century Britain," in William F. Bynum, Christopher Lawrence and Vivian Nutton, eds., *The Emergence of Modern Cardiology* (London: Wellcome Institute for the History of Medicine, 1985), pp. 34–52; idem, "Cardiac Physiology and Clinical Medicine: Two Case Studies," in Gerald L. Geison, ed., *Physiology in the American Context, 1850–1940* (Bethesda, MD: American Physiological Society, 1987), pp. 279–292.

attack was said to occur when a "thrombus" (clot) blocked the arteries supplying the heart with oxygenated blood. The resulting damage to the heart muscle impaired the pump's ability to perform.[19]

In the acute stages of a heart attack, experts advised, the main problem was to reduce the pump's workload – through sedatives, bed rest, and, if necessary, diuretics to relieve excess fluid.[20] By the late 1940s, some specialists recommended treatment with anticoagulants during the acute phases as well.[21] Recommendations for longer-term management called for a reduction of activity, including a possible change of jobs.[22]

Dietary prescriptions were similarly conceived to reduce the strain on overworked, damaged pumps. Cardiologists recommended low-sodium diets during the acute stages of a heart attack, to reduce blood volume and pressure. Low-protein, low-calorie diets were administered in the hospital with similar physiological objectives in mind.[23] Some physicians advocated a "semi-starvation diet" of

19 Levine, *Clinical Heart Disease* (n. 17), pp. 134–137. Of the early texts, Henry Christian's pays the most attention to the finding of arteriosclerosis in autopsied cases of infarction, and to Anitschkow's work. See Henry A. Christian, *The Diagnosis and Treatment of Diseases of the Heart* (New York: Oxford University Press, 1935), pp. 262–263. By the 1940s, Paul Dudley White's text was also emphasizing Leary's work. Compare Paul Dudley White, *Heart Disease* (New York: Macmillan, 1931), pp. 421–425, and idem, *Heart Disease,* 3rd ed. (n. 17), pp. 479–481. On the development of the notion of coronary thrombosis, see Christopher Lawrence, " 'Definite and Material': Coronary Thrombosis and Cardiologists in the 1920s," in Charles E. Rosenberg and Janet Golden, eds., *Framing Disease: Studies in Cultural History* (New Brunswick, NJ: Rutgers University Press, 1992), pp. 50–82. Compare W. Bruce Fye, "The Delayed Diagnosis of Myocardial Infarction: It Took Half a Century!," *Circulation* 72 (August 1985), 262–271.

20 In addition, morphine was generally advised for pain relief. On acute management of cardiac patients, see Paul D. White, "The Treatment of Heart Disease Other Than by Drugs," *JAMA* 89 (August 6, 1927), 436–437; Levine, *Clinical Heart Disease* (n. 17), pp. 148–149; David Scharf and Linn J. Boyd, *Cardiovascular Diseases: Their Diagnosis and Treatment* (St. Louis: C. V. Mosby, 1939), pp. 216–218; Fred M. Smith, "Coronary Artery Disease," in Stroud, *The Diagnosis and Treatment of Cardiovascular Disease* (n. 14), vol. I, pp. 398, 426; Samuel A. Levine, *Clinical Heart Disease,* 3rd ed. (Philadelphia: W. B. Saunders, 1945), pp. 119–124; A. Carlton Ernstene, *Coronary Heart Disease* (Springfield, IL: Charles C. Thomas, 1948), pp. 50–56; *Proceedings: First National Conference* (n. 10), pp. 84–85. By the late 1940s, specialists began to reduce the extent of bed rest recommended.

21 Compare the recommendations of a national committee of heart specialists to include anticoagulants as "standard treatment" in "Diseases of the Coronary Arteries," *Proceedings: First National Conference* (n. 10), p. 85, with the views in Levine, *Clinical Heart Disease,* 3rd ed. (n. 20), pp. 124–125.

22 On long-term changes in activity, see Louis F. Bishop Jr. and Ruth V. Bennett, "Live with Heart Disease – and *Like* It!," *Hygeia* 15 (1937), 221–222, 352–353, 355; S. Calvin Smith, *Heart Patients: Their Study and Care* (Philadelphia: Lea and Febiger, 1939), pp. 139, 156–157; William J. Leaman Jr., *Management of the Cardiac Patient* (Philadelphia: J. B. Lippincott, 1940), p. 270; Levine, *Clinical Heart Disease* [1936] (n. 17), p. 153.

23 On dietary restrictions, see White, "Treatment of Heart Disease" (n. 20), 438–439; George A. Harrop Jr., *Diet in Disease* (Philadelphia: P. Blakiston Son, 1930), p. 246; C. Sidney Burwell, "The Relation of Diet to Heart Disease," *Southern Medical Journal* 25 (December 1932), 1218; F. A. Willius, "A Talk on the Regulation of Diet in Heart Disease," *Proceedings of the Staff Meetings of the Mayo Clinic* 11 (March 25, 1936), 202–203; Levine, *Clinical Heart Disease* [1936] (n. 17), pp. 152–153; George C. Griffith, "Diet in the Treatment of Heart Disease," *Medical Clinics of North America* 21 (July 1937), pp. 1085–1093; Scharf and Boyd, *Cardiovascular Diseases* [1939] (n. 20), 248–249; Levine, *Clinical Heart Disease,* 3rd ed. (n. 20), p. 123; *Proceedings: First National Conference* (n. 10), p. 85.

under 800 calories to "diminish" the "work of the heart."[24] After an attack, some doctors advised their patients to lose weight, on the commonsensical view that the heart works harder when the body carries ten, twenty, or thirty extra pounds: "The fat contains many blood vessels through which blood must be forced, and the heart work necessary for this must be added to that of carrying the weight."[25] Treatment and aftercare shared a common goal: spare the damaged, hardworking pump.

By the late 1940s, a different paradigm of heart disease was emerging, one in which the acute emergency of a heart attack had an extended biological history. Textbook authors increasingly emphasized the central role of long-term arteriosclerosis in the development of heart disease. According to Paul Dudley White, coronary heart disease was virtually synonymous with the effects of diseased coronary arteries, and "practically the totality of coronary artery disease is atherosclerotic in type."[26] The heart remained a pump, but one that hopefully might be spared through prevention rather than salvaged by treatment: "At the risk of over simplification, it may be stated that the [means for] prophylaxis of coronary occlusion is the postponement of the onset of arteriosclerosis."[27]

The principal hopes for prophylaxis lay in altering the high levels of cholesterol found in the blood of heart attack victims.[28] By 1950, some specialists were

24 See Samuel A. Levine, *Clinical Heart Disease,* 2nd ed. (Philadelphia: W. B. Saunders, 1942), p. 147; Snyder, *From a Doctor's Heart* (n. 18), pp. 89–90. Similar recommendations for weight loss were made in cases of angina: Levine, ibid., p. 118; *Proceedings: First National Conference* (n. 10), p. 84.

25 Harold Pardee, *What You Should Know about Heart Disease,* 2nd ed. (Philadelphia: Lea and Febiger, 1935), p. 82. See also Leaman, *Management of the Cardiac Patient* (n. 22), p. 539; Frederick A. Willius, *Cardiac Clinics: A Mayo Clinic Monograph* (St. Louis: C. V. Mosby, 1941), pp. 205–209; Joseph M. Stein, *Your Heart* (New York: Alliance Book Corporation, 1941), p. 49; Smith, "Coronary Artery Disease" [1943] (n. 20), vol. I, pp. 400–403; Irvine, "Heart Disease and What to Do about It" (n. 18), 70.

26 White, *Heart Disease,* 3rd ed. (n. 17), pp. 474–475 (quotation from p. 474); Sprague, "Coronary Heart Disease, Coronary Occlusion and Myocardial Infarction" (n. 17), p. 437; Ernest P. Boas and Norman F. Boas, *Coronary Artery Disease* (Chicago: Year Book Publishers, 1949), pp. 188–189, 54–61. Note also William Stroud's decision to add a section on "arteriosclerosis" to his annual review for internists of significant research on heart disease – a sign that arteriosclerosis had arrived: William D. Stroud, "Diseases of the Heart and Blood Vessels," in *The 1942 Year Book of General Medicine* (Chicago: Year Book Publishers, 1942), pp. 515–517.

Although texts from the 1930s or early 1940s mention the presence of "atheromas" in the arteries of patients who died of coronary thrombosis, only Henry Christian's text makes the development of arteriosclerosis central to his account of the pathogenesis of coronary heart disease. See Christian, *The Diagnosis and Treatment* (n. 19), pp. 262–263. The Bishops join Christian as among the earlier clinical advocates emphasizing the unity of arteriosclerosis and coronary heart disease. See Louis Fagueres Bishop and Louis Fagueres Bishop Jr., "Coronary Disease and Its Relation to the Increase of Cardiac Morbidity," *New York State Journal of Medicine* 34 (May 1934), 393–399.

27 Charles T. Stone, in "Cardiology: Panel Discussion," *Chicago Medical Society Bulletin* 52 (December 31, 1949), 543.

28 Alfred Steiner, "Cholesterol in Arteriosclerosis, with Special Reference to Coronary Arteriosclerosis," *Medical Clinics of North America* 34 (May 1950), 678–679.

The association between blood cholesterol levels and arteriosclerosis was far from uniform, and contested by some researchers. See Menard M. Gertler, Stanley Marion Garn, and Paul Dudley White, "Diet, Serum Cholesterol and Coronary Artery Diseases," *Circulation* 2 (1950), 703; Mau-

suggesting that the development of arteriosclerosis might be retarded, prevented, or possibly even reversed by adoption of a low-calorie and/or low-fat diet.[29] Yet even those who advocated such diets for patients with high blood cholesterol levels (hypercholesterolemia) confessed that the "relationship of hypercholesterolemia to arteriosclerosis" remained something of a puzzle.[30]

A growing body of experimental research on the mechanisms that generated arteriosclerosis and on the ways in which the body produced, used, and disposed of cholesterol, added to clinicians' perplexities. Experimenters offered not one but several competing mechanisms for the development of arteriosclerosis: high cholesterol was but one of several putative culprits.[31] Even those who accepted that high cholesterol levels produced arteriosclerosis disagreed about the sources of that cholesterol: Was it due to consumption of a diet rich in animal fat, or to some metabolic defect that prevented some individuals from getting rid of the cholesterol their bodies produced? Some researchers reported that high-cholesterol diets had little effect on blood cholesterol levels, whereas others asserted that the cholesterol content of diet had a substantial influence on blood cholesterol.[32]

Animal experiments presented similar ambiguities. The blood cholesterol levels of some animals, like Anitschkow's rabbits, went up when they were fed pure cholesterol diets. Cholesterol levels went down in dogs given a comparable regimen.[33] What kind of animals were humans? No one knew.

By the 1950s, decades of experimental research on animals, along with the study of human arteries by pathologists, had produced a consensus that arteriosclerosis was a disease, not an inevitable concomitant of aging. Biochemical study had

rice Bruger and Elliot Oppenheim, "Experimental and Human Atherosclerosis: Possible Relationships and Present Status," *Bull NY Acad Med* 17 (September 1951), 549; Jeremiah Stamler, "Pathogenesis and Therapy of Atherosclerosis," *Medical Clinics of North America* 36 (January 1952), 179; Thomas M. Durant, "Insurance Hazards of Overweight Dietary Factors in the Development of Atherosclerosis," *Transactions of the Association of Life Insurance Medical Directors of America* 35 (1952), 273. The issue was further confounded by John Gofman's contention that the harmful role was played by so called low-density lipoproteins: John W. Gofman, "Diet and Lipotrophic Agents in Atherosclerosis," *Bull NY Acad Med* 28 (May 1952), 279–293.

29 Tinsley R. Harrison, "Diseases of the Heart and Blood Vessels," in *The 1948 Year Book of General Medicine* (Chicago: Year Book Publishers, 1948), p. 514; Stone, "Cardiology: Panel Discussion" (n. 27), 543–544.

30 Stone, "Cardiology: Panel Discussion" (n. 27), 546.

31 The principal contenders were "physical" models of arteriosclerosis, in which initial damage to the arterial intima, sometimes secondary to hypertension, was the cause of subsequent pathology. For a thorough review of the various theories of pathogenesis, see W. C. Hueper, "Arteriosclerosis," *Archives of Pathology* 38 (1944), 162–181, 245–285, 350–364. See also L. N. Katz and D. V. Dauber, "The Pathogenesis of Arteriosclerosis," *Journal of the Mt. Sinai Hospital* 12 (1945–1946), 382–410. For a briefer, more up-to-date assessment, see William Dock, "Causes of Arteriosclerosis" [1950] (n. 1), 182–188.

32 See Dock, "Causes of Arteriosclerosis" (n. 1), 186–187. Further perplexity was introduced by researchers experimenting with various combinations of high-fat, high-protein, and high-calorie diets, each of which was asserted to have considerable influence on blood cholesterol.

33 An effective dog model for cholesterol feeding experiments was developed in the late 1940s by Alfred Steiner and his associates, who found that when dogs were fed a high-cholesterol diet along with thiouracil, they developed arteriosclerosis comparable with that of humans. See Steiner, "Cholesterol in Arteriosclerosis" (n. 28), 675–677.

begun to sort out the various components of dietary fat and their pathways in the body. Yet the patient's fundamental question – why me? – remained unanswered:

We can produce the lesion, and modify its evolution, experimentally, just as we do with tuberculosis. We know its etiology, but, as in the case of most infections, we have only a vague idea as to pathogenesis. Why one man develops meningitis and a dozen others remain carriers is as mysterious as why one man with hypercholesteremia is dead of a myocardial infarct at twenty, another is hale, but spotted with xanthomata, at sixty.[34]

In the face of uncertainty, therapeutic regimens were hotly contested. For every two experts who advocated turning to a low-fat diet, there was one who insisted on the basis of the latest biochemical research that cholesterol, not fat, was the culprit. The majority sided with the Cornell University's David Barr:

It may be fairly said that the beneficial effect of dietary restriction of cholesterol alone is not as yet established. The role of such restriction when the ingestion of both fat and cholesterol are greatly limited is undetermined. Under these circumstances one must ask whether there is justification for placing patients who are thought to have atherosclerosis on cholesterol free diets which are extremely distasteful and entirely contrary to human habit and appetite.[35]

Neither clinical uncertainty nor scientific disagreement, however, prevented researchers from insisting that more research would resolve clinical dilemmas.[36] In 1948, the U.S. Congress had authorized the creation of the National Heart Institute, intended to channel federal dollars to university researchers eager to further explore the mysteries of heart disease. Congressional appropriations for the Heart Institute (NHI), initially held in check by the demands placed on the federal budget by the war in Korea, climbed to $15 million by 1954, and until 1963 roughly doubled every two to three years.[37] Like much of the effort funded by the National Institutes of Health in these years, the monies went disproportion-

---

34 Dock, "Causes of Arteriosclerosis" (n. 1), 184.
35 David Barr, in "Conference on Therapy: Low Cholesterol Diet in the Treatment of Atherosclerosis," *American Journal of Medicine* 12 (March 1952), 362. The opinions expressed in this symposium provide a fair range of the contemporary difference of opinion on this question. For other expressions of agnosticism, see Jack D. Davidson, "Diet and Lipotropic Agents in Arteriosclerosis," *American Journal of Medicine* 11 (December 1951), 747; Irvine H. Page, "Low Cholesterol–Low Fat Diets in Prevention and Treatment of Atherosclerosis," *Medical Clinics of North America* 36 (January 1952), 199; Stamler, "Pathogenesis and Therapy of Atherosclerosis" (n. 28), 193; Bruger and Oppenheim, "Experimental and Human Atherosclerosis" (n. 28), 552; Aaron Kellner, "Lipid Metabolism and Atherosclerosis," *Bull NY Acad Med* 28 (January 1952), 11–27. For advocacy of a low-fat diet, see Thomas M. Durant, "Nutritional Factors in Cardiac Disease," *Ann Int Med* 35 (August 1951), 404–407; Ancel Keys, "Human Atherosclerosis and the Diet," *Circulation* 5 (1952), 117. For criticisms of Keys that place a greater emphasis on cholesterol, see the remarks of William Dock in "Conference on Therapy: Low Cholesterol Diet," 358.
36 See the emphasis placed on research in the remarks of Paul D. White, T. Duckett Jones, and Louis Katz in *Proceedings: First National Conference* (n. 10), pp. 11–18.
37 *NIH Factbook* (Chicago: Marquis Academic Publishing, 1967), p. 99. On the creation of the NHI, see Stephen P. Strickland, *Politics, Science and Dread Disease: A Short History of United States Medical Research Policy* (Cambridge: Harvard University Press, 1972), pp. 50–53; on the slowdown in financing during the Korean War, and the subsequent expansion, pp. 64, 89–133.

ately to laboratory research, reflecting the prevailing opinion that "laboratory study . . . appears to be the most promising approach" for studying heart disease in general, and arteriosclerosis in particular.[38]

Nonetheless, in the 1950s some laboratory-trained researchers began turning away from experimental work as the key to explaining patterns of heart disease. They turned instead to investigating human heart disease, not just in cardiology clinics, where the progression of arteriosclerosis in the sick could be studied, but in free-living communities of healthy middle-aged men who might someday be expected to develop heart disease.

EPIDEMIOLOGY AND THE EXPERIMENTS OF NATURE

To an experimentalist it is distressing to have to admit that major reliance must be placed on methods which are non-experimental, or at least provide no close experimental control. This is an area which, at present, it is apparently necessary to devote a great deal of attention to the experiments of nature.[39]

Epidemiology is apt not to be a decisive method for resolution of these problems of chronic disease despite the current popularity of this endeavour. At best the method may supply a few clues and enough encouragement to gifted people who, by intuitive knowledge and industry, will find the answer in the laboratory.[40]

As early as the 1920s, investigators had noted with interest that certain populations in Asia and Africa had far lower rates of heart disease than were found in the urban, industrialized nations of western Europe and the United States.[41] By the late 1940s, researchers were calling for investigations into the diets of poor non-Europeans: "If it could be shown that diets such as those described in certain areas of China lead to a diminished amount of arteriosclerosis, we ought to know about it in great detail."[42]

38 See the spirited defense of laboratory studies by George V. Mann, "Experimental Studies of Atherosclerosis," in Ancel Keys and Paul D. White, eds., *Cardiovascular Epidemiology: World Trends in Cardiology I* (New York: Hoeber-Harper, 1954), p. 158. On the postwar emphasis on laboratory studies at NIH and more generally, see Harold F. Dorn, *Social Sciences in the Research Program of the National Institutes of Health,* n.d., Research Planning Council, March–December 1950, Box 37, Accession 90-60A-0560, W-NRC; Alvan R. Feinstein, Neal Koss, and John H. M. Austin, "The Changing Emphasis in Clinical Research: I. Topics under Investigation. An Analysis of the Submitted Abstracts and Selected Programs at the Annual 'Atlantic City Meetings' during 1953 through 1965," *Ann Int Med* 66 (February 1967), 396–419.
39 Keys, "Nutrition in Relation to . . . Degenerative Diseases" [1948] (n. 10), 283.
40 George V. Mann, "The Epidemiology of Coronary Heart Disease," *American Journal of Medicine* 23 (1957), 478.
41 Soma Weiss and George Minot, "Nutrition in Relation to Arteriosclerosis," in Cowdry, *Arteriosclerosis* (n. 13), pp. 239–242; George A. Harrop Jr., *Diet in Disease* (Philadelphia: P. Blakiston Son, 1930), pp. 12–14, 22–23.
42 David Seegal, "Limitations in Our Knowledge Concerning the Diagnosis, Treatment and Prevention of Human Arteriosclerosis," in *Seminar on the Degenerative Lesions of Metabolism* (n. 10), p. 43.

Interest in comparative study was greatest among those who believed that the "luxus diet" prevailing in the United States was a major cause of the nation's high rates of heart disease. Perhaps, critics of the American diet suggested, the high-fat diets that prevailed in the "land of plenty" were themselves pathological.[43] If all Americans overate, then even "the figures that have been so painfully collected to show" "the average weight" of "North American or European population[s]" should be ignored, and Americans at risk of heart disease guided toward a "physiologic diet," which would maintain them at their "ideal weight" of age eighteen.[44]

Skeptics countered that many factors other than diet could account for the lower rates of heart disease observed outside the industrialized West: "heredity, climate, economic conditions and modes of living may be of [greater] importance."[45] Others questioned the reliability of the data about diet and cause of death in places like China.[46] Among the skeptics was the physiologist Ancel Keys: "Arguments about the incidence of atherosclerosis and the customary intake of cholesterol in the Far East are based on no real data on either atherosclerosis incidence or the character of the diet."[47]

Keys, along with most of his generation of physiologists, took the carefully controlled, rigorously quantified, environment of the physiological laboratory as a standard of scientific excellence.[48] Early in his career, however, he began working with physiologists who aimed at reproducing the rigors of the experimental laboratory in settings outside the laboratory. Trained in the 1920s at the University of California, Keys had worked at the Harvard Fatigue Lab where he conducted field studies on high altitude physiology prior to and during World War II. Other wartime studies on the nutritional requirements of soldiers resulted in the development of the "k-ration." In all this work, Keys's characteristic approach was

43 The phrase "luxus diet" and the notion that the American diet was "unphysiologic" come from the internist William Dock: see "The Causes of Arteriosclerosis" (n. 1), 188, and "Prophylaxis and Therapy of Arteriosclerosis," *Transactions of the Association of Life Insurance Medical Directors of America* 34 (1950), 10–15. Thomas Durant refers to the negative effects of living in the "land of plenty" while documenting the increase in fats in the American diet in "Nutritional Factors in Cardiac Disease" (n. 35), 404.
44 Dock, "Prophylaxis and Therapy of Arteriosclerosis" (n. 43), 11.
45 Wilems, "Some Nutritional Factors" (n. 10), p. 37b.
46 Gertler et al. "Diet, Serum Cholesterol and Coronary Artery Disease" (n. 28), 697–698, 702–703.
47 Ancel Keys, "Human Atherosclerosis and the Diet," *Circulation* 5 (1952), 117. See also Keys's reservations about the quality of the dietary and medical data derived from insurance records in Keys's "Nutrition in Relation to Etiology" [1948] (n. 10), 282; Keys had already begun to advocate prospective comparative studies at this point (284).
48 Of all the biomedical disciplines, physiology was the first and more extensively quantified: Halbert L. Dunn, "Application of Statistical Methods in Physiology," *Physiological Reviews* 9 (1929), 275–398; Frederic L. Holmes, "The Intake–Output Method of Quantification in Physiology," *Historical Studies in the Physical and Biological Sciences* 17 (1987), 235–270. On the uses of controlled environments in metabolic studies, see my discussion in Chapter 2. Keys's own interest in the scientific problem of individual variation led him to an unusual and profound understanding of the methodological requirements of studying metabolic variation. See Ancel Keys, "The Physiology of the Individual As an Approach to a More Quantitative Biology of Man," *Federation Proceedings* 8 (1949), 523–529.

to combine field studies with investigations performed under the more controlled conditions of the metabolic laboratory. The laboratory studies enabled Keys to develop precise measurements of physiological mechanisms, while the field research enabled him to see how metabolism behaved in more naturalistic settings. Following the war, Keys applied the same methods in studying the sources of heightened cardiovascular mortality.[49]

Intrigued by the high rate of mortality from heart disease among "prominent" middle-class men, Keys despaired of finding its causes from studies of laboratory rats:

Only in the most limited sense can it be said that x days in the life of the rat can be counted as y years of useful human life. What is the caloric equivalent for a rat of a hard day of human labor? What is the human counterpart of a microgram of ascorbic acid ingested by a rat? These experiments have only remote relevance to the situation in man; they may be suggestive but it is fatuous to proceed to direct quantitative analogies.[50]

The answer to questions about human heart disease, Keys argued, did not lie in animal studies but in making studies of human disease as rigorous as possible: "An obvious approach is to select a considerable number of individuals who can be examined in detail with regard to nutritional status, habits and biological characteristics and to follow them over the years with repeated examinations."[51]

Keys's earliest epidemiological studies were conducted in the United States, following a cohort of Minnesota business and professional men over several decades to see which ones developed heart disease and which did not.[52] In 1952,

---

49 During the war, Keys also directed a landmark study on the effects of dietary deprivation, conducted with conscientious objectors: Ancel Keys et al., *The Biology of Human Starvation*, 2 vols. (Minneapolis: University of Minnesota Press, 1950).

The following biographical accounts of Keys by his students and associates are useful in detailing events and intellectual influences: Henry Blackburn, "Introduction to Ancel Keys Lecture: Ancel Keys, Pioneer," *Circulation* 84 (September 1991), 1402–1404; E. S. Buskirk, "From Harvard to Minnesota: Keys to Our History," *Exercise and Sports Sciences Review* 20 (1992), 1–26. See also Ancel Keys, "Recollections of Pioneers in Nutrition: From Starvation to Cholesterol," *Journal of the American College of Nutrition* 9 (1990), 288–291; Ancel Keys, "From Naples to Seven Countries: A Sentimental Journey," *Progress in Biochemical Pharmacology* 19 (1983), 1–30. The combination of laboratory and field studies was a research tradition at the Harvard Fatigue Laboratory, where Keys trained. See Steven M. Horvath and Elizabeth C. Horvath, *The Harvard Fatigue Laboratory: Its History and Traditions* (Englewood Cliffs, NJ: Prentice-Hall, 1973); Carleton B. Chapman, "The Long Reach of Harvard's Fatigue Laboratory, 1926–1947," *Perspectives in Biology and Medicine* 34 (Autumn 1990), 17–33.

50 Keys, "Nutrition in Relation to Etiology" (n. 10), 282.

51 Ibid. Keys proposed three types of studies: the first was a prospective cohort study of healthy middle-class men; the second was an experimental dietary study of institutionalized populations; the third was comparative studies of diet in areas around the world.

52 The Minnesota study, begun in 1947, antedates and inspired the better-known Framingham study of risk factors for heart disease. See Ancel Keys, "Mode of Life and the Development of Heart Disease: Research for a Preventive Hygiene," *Chicago Heart Association Bulletin* 26 (1948), 3–6; idem, "The Inception and Pilot Surveys," in Daan Kromhout, Alessandro Menotti, and Henry Blackburn, eds., *The Seven Countries Study: A Scientific Adventure in Cardiovascular Epidemiology* (privately printed, 1990), pp. 15–16; idem, "The Diet and the Development of Coronary Heart Disease," *JCD* 4 (1956), 364–380. As was customary with Keys, these field studies were done in

while on a visit to Italy, he observed that "in Naples the only coronary patients were rich men in private hospitals. Their serum cholesterol values were distinctly higher than in the city clerks, policemen and other men whose diets were very low in meats and dairy products."[53] Keys made similar observations in Spain, South Africa, Japan, and Finland over the next four years, all the while publicizing his findings among researchers in the United States. Two consistent patterns emerged: rates of heart disease were lower in countries substantially poorer than the United States, but among middle-class foreigners who consumed an "American-type" diet, rates of heart disease were comparable with domestic patterns.[54]

Keys's earliest comparative studies – employing ad hoc samples, with limited data on dietary intake – fell far short of his own methodological ideals.[55] Nonetheless, the "ethnopathological" approach increasingly provided the strongest case for those who believed that the American diet was inherently pathological. According to Jeremiah Stamler, Americans ate more fat, had higher serum cholesterol levels, and died of heart disease at greater rates than populations anywhere else in the world.[56]

Stamler, recipient of a prestigious American Heart Association career investigator award, had followed Keys's path from the laboratory to epidemiological studies. After a decade's research with cardiologist Louis Katz, developing a chick model for studying atherosclerosis, Stamler began studying Chicago communities, where he found that, "contrary to prevalent notions the professional-executive-managerial group" had the lowest coronary death rates and "unskilled workers" the highest.[57] For Stamler, the apparent anomaly was easily explainable:

parallel with a set of laboratory studies on normal volunteers in which the effects of dietary modification on serum cholesterol were measured. See Ancel Keys, Olaf Mickelsen, E. V. O. Miller, and Carleton B. Chapman, "The Relation in Man between Cholesterol Levels in the Diet and in the Blood," *Science* 112 (July 21, 1950), 79–81. A related set of studies on hospitalized mental patients was also begun in the early 1950s. See Ancel Keys, "Atherosclerosis: A Problem in the Newer Public Health," *Journal of the Mt. Sinai Hospital* 20 (1953), 127–129.

53 Keys, "Recollections of Pioneers" (n. 49), 289; Keys, "Prediction and Possible Prevention of Coronary Disease," *AJPH* 43 (November 1953), 1401–1402.

54 Keys, "Inception and Pilot Surveys" (n. 52), pp. 16–21; Keys, "Sentimental Journey" (n. 49), 3–7; Keys, "Prediction and Possible Prevention" [1953] (n. 53), 1401–1406; Keys, "Atherosclerosis: A Problem in the Newer Public Health" [1953] (n. 52), 119–121, 131–134; Ancel Keys, Francisco Vivanco, J. L. Rodriquez Minon, Margaret Haney Keys, and H. Castro Mendoza, "Studies on the Diet, Body Fatness and Serum Cholesterol in Madrid, Spain," *Metabolism. Clinical and Experimental* 3 (May 1954), 195–212; Keys, "Diet and the Development of Coronary Heart Disease" [1956] (n. 52), 364–380. Much of the early work by Keys and his collaborators is reported in Keys and White, *Cardiovascular Epidemiology* (n. 38). Keys himself thought these early findings had little influence on specialists' beliefs. See Keys, "Recollections of Pioneers" (n. 49), 289.

55 Keys, "Sentimental Journey" (n. 49), 2–3, 7–8.

56 Jeremiah Stamler, "Research Findings on the Etiology of Atherosclerosis," *Nebraska Medical Journal* 41 (March 1958), 75–78; see also L. N. Katz, J. Stamler, and R. Pick, "Nutrition and Atherosclerosis," *Federation Proceedings* 15 (September 1956), esp. 887–889. Stamler used the term "ethnopathological" in an earlier (1952) article on "Pathogenesis and Therapy of Arteriosclerosis" (n. 28), 178. He soon turned to describing these studies as "epidemiological."

57 Stamler, "Research Findings" (n. 56), 77.

there is good reason to believe that millions of Americans, especially poor Americans, consume an unbalanced, obesity-producing diet that is a pernicious combination of over-nutrition and undernutrition. . . .

Hence it is oversimplified, one-sided and inaccurate to characterize the present-day American diet as a "luxus" diet, particularly if one is speaking of the American poor. Theirs is a diet that is "luxus" in certain constituents only, i.e. starches, sugars, fats, oils, calories.[58]

The mounting epidemiological evidence on the hazards of the current American diet drew increasing attention in the medical press.[59] Following President Eisenhower's widely publicized heart attack in 1955, the dangers of high-fat diets were widely discussed (and debated) in the general press as well.[60] With increased recognition came intensified criticism: the mortality statistics produced by foreign doctors could not be trusted; information on diet obtained from questionnaires was scientifically suspect, as was Stamler's historical data on increases in American fat consumption; the arguments from epidemiological data ignored laboratory and clinical studies indicating that dietary fat was just one factor among many leading to arteriosclerosis.[61]

58 Ibid., 78. (I have reversed the order of these two passages in Stamler's text.) For more on Stamler's views of the "luxus" notion, see ibid., 77–79. Both Stamler and Keys took their distance from earlier critical analyses of the American diet, which they were inclined to reject as "unscientific." Stamler's remarks on the "luxus" diet are probably aimed at William Dock, who used the term frequently, while Keys's bête noir was insurance analysts like Louis Dublin who had overemphasized, in his view, the contribution of obesity to heart disease. See Keys, "Sentimental Journey" (n. 49), 17–18; Keys, "Diet and the Development of Coronary Heart Disease" [1956] (n. 52), 368–372.

59 For favorable mentions of the epidemiological work, including European studies of the positive effects of wartime privation on cardiovascular mortality, see G. E. Wakerlin, "Recent Advances in the Pathogenesis and Treatment of Atherosclerosis," *Ann Int Med* 37 (August 1952), 314–315; Forrest E. Kendall in "Current Concepts in the Management of Arteriosclerosis: Transcription of a Panel Meeting on Therapeutics," *Bull NY Acad Med* 31 (March 1955), 199; Louis N. Katz, "The Role of Diet and Hormones in the Prevention of Myocardial Infarction," *Ann Int Med* 43 (1955), 931–933; Paul Dudley White, "The Cardiologist Enlists the Epidemiologist," *AJPH* 47 (April 1957), part 2, 2; idem, "International Cardiovascular Epidemiology," in Keys and White, *Cardiovascular Epidemiology* (n. 38), p. 3.

60 On Eisenhower's heart attack, see "Heart Attack," *Life* (October 10, 1955), 150–159; Ogelsby Paul, *Take Heart: The Life and Prescription for Living of Dr. Paul Dudley White* (Boston: Francis A. Countway Library of Medicine, 1986), pp. 149–183. For the subsequent publicity given dietary factors in heart disease, see "The Specialized Nubbin," *Time* 66 (October 31, 1955), 62–64, 67–69 (which highlights Irvine Page's work); "Fats and Heart Disease," *Time* 68 (November 12, 1956), 59; Francis Drake and Katherine Drake, "New Weapons against Heart Disease," *Reader's Digest* (May 1957), 49–52; Harrison Kinney, "Exclusive! White House Chef Reveals President Eisenhower's Special Diet," *McCall's* (December 1957), 37, 100–101. Keys's work was given exceptional prominence in Steven M. Spencer, "Are You Eating Your Way to a Heart Attack?," *Saturday Evening Post* (December 1, 1956), 24–26, 99–102; and in Blake Clark, "Is This the No. 1 Villain in Heart Disease?," *Reader's Digest* (November 1955), 109–113. His critics were given more attention in Francis Bello, "The Murderous Riddle of Coronary Disease," *Fortune* (September 1958), 142–146, 162, 164, 169–170.

61 Herman Hilleboe, "Some Epidemiological Aspects of Coronary Heart Disease," in New York Heart Association, *Conference on Atherosclerosis and Coronary Heart Disease. January 15, 1957* (New York: New York Heart Association, 1957), pp. 85–89; J. Yerushalmy and Herman E. Hilleboe, "Fat in the Diet and Mortality from Heart Disease: A Methodologic Note," *New York State Journal of Medicine* 57 (1957), 2343–54; Theodore B. van Itallie, "Dietary Constituents and Atherosclerosis,"

In the 1950s, chronic disease epidemiology was a novel and fragile science. Traditional epidemiology studied outbreaks of infectious disease, in search of patterns that would help explain the appearance and disappearance of infections in specific populations. With infectious disease waning as a public health concern, epidemiology's medically qualified practitioners sought to apply the discipline's quantitative methods to the noninfectious diseases now dominant in the industrialized West.[62]

Like their mathematically adept cousins, the biostatisticians, medical epidemiologists interested in noninfectious disease tread gingerly on the prerogatives of more well established laboratory and clinical disciplines. Epidemiology, its spokesmen argued, was an ancillary medical science, a handmaiden of medicine whose task was to offer up hypotheses – suggestions about the world – which would ultimately be proved or disproved in the securer grounds of the laboratory or the clinic. Epidemiological analysis, its practitioners obsessively insisted, can only demonstrate "associations"; it cannot establish causes.[63] Epidemiologists, possibly

Journal of the American Dietetic Association 33 (1957), 355; Paul Densen, Herman Hilleboe, Charles D. Marple, Ogelsby Paul, Jeremiah Stamler, William H. Stewart, and Felix E. Moore, "Etiologic Leads Provided from Population Studies: Suggested Leads for Future Studies. Atherosclerosis," in American Heart Association and National Heart Institute, *Conference on the Epidemiology of Atherosclerosis and Hypertension* (New York: American Heart Association, 1956), pp. 48, 53; Dale Groom, "Population Studies of Atherosclerosis," *Ann Int Med* 55 (July 1961), 51–62. Most of these criticisms were reiterated by an official report of the American Heart Association: Irvine H. Page, Fredrick J. Stare, A. C. Corcoran, Herbert Pollack, and Charles F. Wilkinson, "Atherosclerosis and the Fat Content of the Diet," *Circulation* 16 (August 1957), 163–174. Another implicit criticism was that Keys's studies were conducted on ad hoc samples which provided no valid basis for epidemiological inference. See Mann, "Epidemiology of CHD" (n. 40), 473–474; Thomas Francis Jr., E. Gurney Clark, Stanley Cobb, and Felix Moore, "Potential Contribution of the Epidemiological Approach," in *Conference on the Epidemiology of Atherosclerosis*, pp. 31–32.

62 Elizabeth Fee and Barbara Rosenkrantz, "Professional Education for Public Health in the United States," in Elizabeth Fee and Roy M. Acheson, eds., *A History of Education in Public Health: Health That Mocks the Doctors' Rules* (New York: Oxford University Press, 1991), pp. 244–245; Elizabeth Fee, "Adapting to Specialization: The Founding, Growth and Transformation of the *American Journal of Hygiene,*" *American Journal of Epidemiology* 134 (November 15, 1991), 1036–1037; Mervyn Susser, "Epidemiology in the United States after World War II: The Evolution of Technique," *Epidemiologic Reviews* 7 (1985), 147–177. Professional epidemiologists were relatively late on the scene in expressing their interests in chronic disease – a concept developed by clinicians and actuaries in the 1920s and 1930s. See Daniel M. Fox, "Health Policy and Changing Epidemiology in the United States: Chronic Disease in the Twentieth Century," in Russell C. Maulitz, ed., *Unnatural Causes: The Three Leading Killer Diseases in America* (New Brunswick, NJ: Rutgers University Press, 1989), pp. 11–31.

63 See William G. Cochran, "Methodological Problems in the Study of Human Populations," *Ann NY Acad Sci* 107 (May 22, 1963), 486–487; Harold F. Dorn, "Philosophy of Inferences from Retrospective Studies," *AJPH* 43 (June 1953), 677–683; Philip E. Sartwell, "Some Approaches to the Epidemiologic Study of Chronic Diseases," *AJPH* 45 (May 1955), 613–614; Thomas Francis Jr., "Correlations in Clinical and Epidemiological Investigation," *American Journal of the Medical Sciences* 226 (1953), 380–382; Brian MacMahon, Thomas F. Pugh, and Johannes Ipsen, *Epidemiologic Methods* (Boston: Little Brown, 1960), pp. 11–21. For parallel remarks specifically for cardiovascular disease, see Francis, Clark, Cobb and Moore, "Potential Contribution of the Epidemiological Approach" (n. 61), pp. 29–32; Thomas R. Dawber, William B. Kannell, and Lorna P. Lyell, "An Approach to Longitudinal Studies in a Community: The Framingham Study," *Ann NY Acad Sci* 107 (1963), 540–541. Laboratory workers and traditional clinical investigators, of course, repeatedly articulated the limits of epidemiology in determining causes. See Edward H. Ahrens Jr., "Nutri-

anxious lest too much be claimed for their tender, young science, were among Keys's most prominent critics:

Is the epidemiological evidence substantial enough to convince clinicians and public health workers to change their present attack on coronary artery disease because of recent research findings? Is the medical profession justified in recommending a revolutionary change in our eating habits on the scientific evidence presented? After reviewing the published data, the epidemiologist's answer to both questions is an unequivocal "no."[64]

Keys was a far more thoughtful and careful analyst of epidemiological data than his critics implied. His published replies to criticism indicate that he had a good grasp of the strengths (and weaknesses) of his epidemiological studies. Keys repeatedly argued that any errors in vital statistics would have to be far more massive than his critics imagined to undermine the international comparisons.[65] But more was at stake than the rigor of Keys's methods or the professional standing of epidemiology.

As early as 1952 – well before much of Keys's work was published – cardiologists had begun to debate whether physicians should recommend wholesale changes in the American diet on the basis of existing knowledge about the role of diet in heart disease.[66] By the middle of the decade, debates among the scientific authorities were hot news. Exchanges of opinion took place as often in the pages of *Time* and *Newsweek* as in the abstruse abstracts reported in *Circulation*.[67] In the glare of publicity, critics of the dietary hypothesis cautioned against changing public health policy before all the evidence was in:

tional Factors and Serum Lipid Levels," *American Journal of Medicine* 23 (December 1957), 928; Bernard Lown and Frederick J. Stare, "Editorial: Atherosclerosis, Infarction, and Nutrition," *Circulation* 22 (August 1959), 165. See also Henry Blackburn and Frederick H. Epstein, "History of the Council on Epidemiology and Prevention, American Heart Association. The Pursuit of Epidemiology within the American Heart Association: Prehistory and Early Organization," *Circulation* 91 (February 15, 1995), esp. 1253–1257. The problem of epidemiology's disciplinary identity in this era is a complex one: epidemiologists from the Johns Hopkins School of Hygiene and Public Health were attempting to establish epidemiology's independence from laboratory studies, and define criteria of rigor that do not give the last word to the laboratory.

64 Hilleboe, "Some Epidemiological Aspects of Coronary Heart Disease" (n. 61), 102.

65 Keys, "Prediction and Possible Prevention" [1953] (n. 53), 1403–1405; Keys, "Diet and CHD" [1956] (n. 52), 366–367. As a laboratory trained researcher, Keys in fact agreed that epidemiological evidence could not establish cause-and-effect relations, but thought the argument "trivial." See Ancel Keys, "Diet and Coronary Disease throughout the World," *Cardiologia Practica* 13 (February 1962), 227–228. For additional responses to the critics of epidemiological evidence, see also Jeremiah Stamler, "Diet and Atherosclerotic Disease: IV. Epidemiology of Coronary Heart Disease in the United States," *Journal of the American Dietetic Association* 34 (1958), 1053–1055; Joliffe, "Fats, Cholesterol and Heart Disease" [1959] (n. 2), 114–118, 121.

66 See Wakerlin, "Recent Advances" (n. 59), 321; Irvine H. Page, "Low Cholesterol–Low Fat Diets in Prevention and Treatment of Atherosclerosis," *Medical Clinics of North America* 36 (January 1952), 199.

67 See, in addition to the sources cited in n. 60: Eugene D. Fleming, "Which Diets Are Best for You?," *Cosmopolitan* (February 1957), 58–61; "Eat What You Like But. . . . Exclusive Interview with Dr. Frederick J. Stare, Harvard School of Public Health," *U.S. News and World Report* 42 (March 29, 1957), 48–54; "Dieting and the Heart," *Newsweek* (November 11, 1957), 113.

Scientific knowledge is not complete enough at present to postulate with certainty the evolution of fatty diets to blood lipids to atherosclerosis to coronary artery disease. Until more links are forged and fastened together to complete the chain of cause-and-effect in coronary artery disease, those of us who have the responsibility to apply new knowledge in public health practice must not proceed too far too fast.[68]

Bruised by earlier episodes of conflict with physicians over venereal disease treatment (and national health insurance), by the 1950s public health authorities in the United States had developed a conservative approach to public health policy. Working in close concert with researchers and clinical specialists from academic medicine, the Surgeon General of the United States would defer actions until his academic consultants had reached a substantial consensus.[69] In the case of arteriosclerosis, researchers were divided about the merits and weight of the scientific evidence.

Clinicians were, if anything, even more concerned about the lack of a suitable diet to use in prevention. Existing low-fat diets, used for patients with a family and personal history of heart disease, were unpalatable as well as inconvenient for doctor and patient alike:

Successful clinical use of the low fat diet is one of the most difficult forms of treatment a physician can undertake for his patient. . . . [The patient] must be made to realize that he is not alone in his efforts and that the treatment program offers a series of opportunities to grasp rather than a series of penalties inflicted.

To accomplish this so that the patient is happy in his newly created dietary environment requires careful patient selection initially, intense indoctrination, repeated visits to maintain his enthusiasm, continuous dietary support, opportunity to become acquainted with fellow dieters, and most important of all, a general understanding of the disease process from

68 Hilleboe, "Some Epidemiological Aspects" (n. 61), 102. For other contemporary statements urging caution in the face of scientific uncertainty, see also Lown and Stare, "Editorial: Atherosclerosis, Infarction, and Nutrition" (n. 63), 161–167, esp. 165; Herbert Pollack, "Dietary Fats and Their Relationship to Atherosclerosis," *Circulation* 16 (August 1957), 161–162; Charles D. May, "Fats in the Diet in Relation to Atherosclerosis," *JAMA* 162 (December 15, 1962), 1468–1469; van Itallie, "Dietary Constituents and Atherosclerosis" (n. 61), 354–355.

Keys had begun to publicly advocate low-fat diets several years before Stamler, but he could hardly be called an advocate of official action at this time. See Ancel Keys, "Human Atherosclerosis and the Diet," *Circulation* 5 (1952), 117. Compare Stamler, "Pathogenesis and Therapy of Athero-sclerosis" [1952] (n. 28), 193, with Katz, Stamler and Pick, "Nutrition and Atherosclerosis" (n. 56), 893.

69 Thus, the Surgeon General took a largely hands-off approach to the National Foundation for Infantile Paralysis's 1954 evaluation of the Salk polio vaccine. While insisting on certain safeguards in preparation of the vaccine, officials at NIH's Bureau of Biologics nonetheless treated the vaccine as the NFIP's affair until after safety was demonstrated. See Marcia Lynn Meldrum, *"Departures from the Design": The Randomized Clinical Trial in Historical Context, 1946–1970* (Ph.D. thesis, State University of New York at Stony Brook, 1994), pp. 121–123. Similarly, in issuing the Surgeon General's report on smoking, Public Health Service officials relied heavily on obtaining consensual advice. See A. Lee Fritschler, *Smoking and Politics: Policymaking and the Federal Bureaucracy* (Engle-wood Cliffs, NJ: Prentice-Hall, 1969), pp. 42–49. For a different interpretation, see John C. Burnham, "American Physicians and Tobacco Use: Two Surgeons General, 1929 and 1964," *BHM* 63 (1989), 1–31.

which he suffers and a knowledge of how to live successfully with it. This requires TIME from the physician, dietitian and fellow patients.[70]

Few patients were considered appropriate candidates for dietary management: ample "intelligence and imagination," along with a suitable "home life," were required.[71]

Medical politics and the difficulties of diet aside, any public statement critical of the standard American diet attacked one of the most prominent symbols of postwar American prosperity. As both Stamler and Keys were aware, conclusions drawn from comparative studies showing the unhealthful effects of the "normal" American diet could readily be seen as "un-American," a potent charge in the Cold War era:

It may seem quite strange to many of us that our American diet may not be as "perfect" as we like to think it is. We are rightly proud of our national wealth, our standard of living. But this pride should not be permitted to lull us into a false sense of security. Let us put the basic question to ourselves: Do we know what is an optimal diet for optimal health for an optimal life span? Our answer must be a categorical No.[72]

For Stamler, as for Keys, science would provide an answer to the question of an optimal diet. But what kind of science?

By the late 1950s, the two researchers had established to their own satisfaction that the normal American diet was unhealthy. For Keys and Stamler, if not for all their critics, comparative epidemiology had done its work.[73] Most researchers had long ago turned to conventional clinical investigations on small groups of patients and/or normal volunteers, in order to disentangle which dietary components were the culpable elements. A key issue was whether different kinds of dietary fat (e.g., animal or vegetable) had a distinctive role in altering serum cholesterol levels.[74] Yet neither clinical investigation coupled with biochemical research nor

---

70 A. M. Nelson, "Treatment of Atherosclerosis by Diet," *Northwest Medicine* 55 (August 1956), 874. See also Van Itallie, "Dietary Constituents" (n. 61), 354; Margaret Edwards, Anne E. Caldwell, and Margaret Zealand, "Diet and Atherosclerosis," *Journal of the Medical Society of New Jersey* 56 (June 1959), 300–303. See also Irvine Page's account of his own self-experimentation with a low-fat diet which resulted in weight loss but also "depression and irritability." Irvine H. Page, "Atherosclerosis: An Introduction," *Circulation* 10 (July 1954), 21.

71 Nelson, "Treatment of Atherosclerosis by Diet" (n. 70), 874; Page, "Low Cholesterol–Low Fat Diets" (n. 66), 198.

72 Stamler, "Research Findings" (n. 56), 76. See also Keys, "Diet and CHD" (n. 52), 366.

73 See, for example, Keys's two assessments of the research findings in the early 1960s, which both defend the body of epidemiologic evidence and articulate its limitations for clarifying further questions, either scientific or of public health policy: Ancel Keys, "The Risk of Coronary Disease," *Circulation* 23 (June 1961), 805–812; "Diet and Coronary Disease throughout the World" (n. 65), 225–244.

74 Researchers raising this question tended to be nutritionists and/or clinical investigators who relied heavily on traditional biochemical and metabolic studies of closely observed, numerically small groups, in tandem with animal research. In addition, such researchers were inclined to be cautious about recommendations to alter the diet until more was known about the effects of specific dietary constituents. See Eleanor L. Lawry, George V. Mann, Ann Peterson, Alice P. Wysocki, Rita O'Connell, and Fredrick J. Stare, "Cholesterol and Beta Lipoproteins in the Serums of Americans:

further epidemiological studies would answer the most important question, Would a change in diet lower the rate of heart disease?[75]

By the end of the decade, various investigators around the country, including Keys and Stamler, had begun experimenting on a small scale with dietary change.[76] Given the medical concerns over the difficulties of dietary management, such studies were intended principally to see if it was possible to change the dietary habits of middle-aged men at high risk of developing heart disease, in the hopes of lowering their cholesterol levels. Unlike conventional clinical investigations, these studies aimed at changing the diet, not studying it further. Yet, like more traditional clinical investigations, none of the pilot studies was large enough or long enough to establish whether dietary alterations, if "successful," would thereby reduce the number of deaths from heart disease.[77]

While these pilot studies were just beginning, several groups of investigators began meeting to plan the next stage of research: a large-scale controlled clinical trial of dietary change, to test whether diet was capable of reducing the rates of heart disease.

THE EXPERIMENT THAT NEVER WAS: THE DIET-HEART STUDY

In 1959, several researchers "independently recommended to the National Heart Institute . . . that a national cooperative study" be organized to study the effects "of dietary change on incidence of heart disease."[78] Two of the three – Irvine H. Page and Jeremiah Stamler – were nationally recognized authorities on heart

Well Persons and Those with Coronary Disease," *American Journal of Medicine* 22 (April 1957), 605–623; Grace A. Goldsmith, "Highlights on the Cholesterol-Fats, Diets and Atherosclerosis Problem," *JAMA* 176 (June 3, 1961), 783–790; D. H. Hegsted, Anna Gotsis, Fredrick J. Stare, and Jane Worcester, "Interrelations between the Kind and Amount of Dietary Fat and Dietary Cholesterol in Experimental Cholesterolemia," *American Journal of Clinical Nutrition* 7 (1959), 5–12.

75 Although Keys in collaboration with his wife prepared a cookbook based on the "Mediterranean diet" in 1959, he remained agnostic about the effects of dietary change in reversing arteriosclerosis. Keys's underlying model of the disease presupposed a long-term relation between dietary intake and metabolism, which led him to be skeptical about the potential for reversal based on an intervention in middle age. See Keys, "Diet and Coronary Disease throughout the World" (n. 65), 240–241.

76 Keys had begun experimenting with modified diets on human subjects in a laboratory setting in the early 1950s. See Keys, "Atherosclerosis: A Problem in Newer Public Health" (n. 52), 128–129. By 1959, Stamler and others had begun studies on the effects of dietary alterations in the community setting. See the sources cited in n. 77.

77 Jeremiah Stamler, "Current Status of the Dietary Prevention and Treatment of Atherosclerotic Coronary Heart Disease," *Progress in Cardiovascular Diseases* 3 (July 1960), 62–85; J. Stamler, D. Berkson, Q. D. Young, Y. Hall, and W. Miller, "Approaches to the Primary Prevention of Clinical Coronary Heart Disease in High-Risk, Middle Aged Men," *Ann NY Acad Sci* 97 (August 29, 1963), 932–951; Norman Joliffe, Seymour H. Rinzler, and Morton Archer, "The Anti-Coronary Club; Including a Discussion of the Effects of a Prudent Diet on the Serum Cholesterol Level of Middle-Aged Men," *American Journal of Clinical Nutrition* 7 (July–August 1959), 451–452.

78 Jeremiah Stamler, *History of the National Diet Heart Study and the Deliberations of the Executive Committee on Diet and Heart Disease* [1968], p. 2, Box 127, Irvine Page papers, Cleveland Clinic archives, Cleveland [hereafter Page papers].

disease.[79] As befits national authorities, each had taken different positions on the question of dietary influences on arteriosclerosis.

Page, the senior of the two, began his long research career in the 1930s at the Rockefeller Institute, followed by a productive decade as a researcher for Eli Lilly, where he and his colleagues isolated angiotensin, a substance that regulates blood pressure. A world authority on hypertension, Page also had a long-standing interest in the question of diet and heart disease. Trained in the laboratory tradition of clinical investigation, Page's research interests were in analyzing the chemical and physical mechanisms of arteriosclerosis. As research director at the Cleveland Clinic since 1945, Page had been one of the leading skeptics during the 1950s concerning the role of dietary fat in the development of arteriosclerosis.[80]

In the second half of the decade, Page gave greater credence to evidence on the dietary sources of heart disease. As the chair of successive American Heart Association committees on arteriosclerosis, and as an oft-quoted authority in the general press, Page was especially sensitive to the mounting demand for authoritative advice on diet. Despite his orientation toward studies of physiological mechanisms, by 1959 he was ready to put the dietary theory to the test of a controlled clinical trial.[81] Like Page, Stamler, who had already begun his own pilot study of dietary intervention, felt that only a large, controlled clinical trial could provide the kind of authoritative proof required to change the American diet: "deliberate, planned, controlled intervention and alteration in specific aspects of the mode of life, with evaluation of the resulting effects on occurrence of disease – [have] become the critical tests of the validity of hypotheses and theories."[82]

79 The third researcher, Ivan D. Frantz, a biochemically trained physician/nutritionist at the University of Minnesota, and a sometime collaborator of Ancel Keys, had recently proposed to NHI a study on a closed, prison population, to "test the possibility of altering the development of atherosclerosis by dietary means." Ivan D. Frantz to Dr. J. Franklin Yeager [NHI], December 29, 1959, Folder "Yeager," Box 253, Page papers. For an overview of Frantz's previous work, see Ivan D. Frantz Jr., "Cholesterol Metabolism," *Minnesota Medicine* 38 (November 1955), 779–783.

80 Nancy Hoffman, "Irvine H. Page, MD: Not One Man, but Many," *JAMA* 244 (October 17, 1980), 1765–1772. For a discussion which places Page's work on hypertension in context, see Louis J. Acierno, *The History of Cardiology* (New York: Parthenon Publishing Group, 1994), pp. 324–334. For Page's reservations regarding the epidemiological data, and Jerry Stamler's work in particular, see Irvine H. Page to E. C. Andrus, May 29, 1957, Box 243, Page papers. See also Page, Stare, Corcoran, Pollack, and Wilkinson, "Atherosclerosis and the Fat Content of the Diet" (n. 61). For illustrations of Page's research "style" and emphases in arteriosclerosis, see Page, "Atherosclerosis: An Introduction" (n. 70), 1–27. Page's interest in the topic dates back to the 1930s: Irvine H. Page and William G. Bernhard, "Cholesterol Induced Atherosclerosis: Its Prevention in Rabbits by the Feeding of an Organic Iodine Compound," *Archives of Pathology* 19 (1935), 530–536.

81 Page et al., "Atherosclerosis and the Fat Content of the Diet" [1957] (n. 61), 163–178; "Dietary Fat and Its Relation to Heart Attacks and Strokes: Report by the Central Committee for Medical and Community Programs of the American Heart Association," *JAMA* 175 (1961), 389–391. Terms of the latter statement were being prepared in 1959: see Emmet Bays to Fredrick Stare, February 12, 1959, Box 251, Page papers. After making the cover of *Time* magazine in 1955, the quotable Page was a standard news source. See "The Specialized Nubbin," *Time* 66 (October 31, 1955), 62–64, 67–69, and Irvine H. Page, "How to Avoid Heart Trouble," *U.S. News and World Report* 46 (February 27, 1959), 74.

82 Jeremiah Stamler, "Diet and Atherosclerotic Disease: III. Epidemiologic Findings," *Journal of the American Dietetic Association* 34 (1958), 929.

As early as 1951, researchers had been calling for controlled clinical trials of the dietary theory, reflecting the controlled experiment's postwar role as the "gold standard" of therapeutic research.[83] The increased publicity given to controversies on the causes of arteriosclerosis only heightened researchers' anxieties about raising "false hopes" in patients or "unduly frightening" them.[84] For Stamler and Page, a controlled trial offered a suitably scientific way of resolving the growing public controversy over dietary advice. With the official encouragement of the National Advisory Heart Council (NAHC), of which Page was a former member, Page convened a larger group to begin planning a cooperative study.[85] The NAHC was the appointed advisory group for the National Heart Institute, which funded much of the nation's research into heart disease. Like Page and Stamler, the academic cardiologists on the NAHC may have seen a clinical trial as the most suitable way to resolve the controversy among their peers. Moreover, by the late 1950s, Congress was beginning to ask more pointed questions about why so many Americans kept dying of heart disease, despite the more than $176 million poured into NHI since 1950.[86] If the NIH could not yet produce cures, perhaps it could produce more consistent advice.

The planning group for the Diet-Heart study began meeting in the spring of 1960. In addition to Stamler, Page invited Ancel Keys; Jerome Cornfield, NIH's most eminent biostatistician; Frederick Stare, the prominent Harvard nutritionist who, like Page, had been skeptical of Key's epidemiological work; Ivan D. Frantz, a biochemically trained physician and nutritionist at the University of Minnesota, and author of one of the three original proposals to NIH; Vanderbilt University's George V. Mann, an outspoken advocate of laboratory studies of arteriosclerosis; Felix Moore from the University of Michigan, previously the chief statistician at the National Heart Institute; and Jerome Green, an NIH staff member and cardiological researcher. These additions further widened the range of opinions, backgrounds, and motives, which had to be accommodated if the proposed study was to proceed.

According to the theory of clinical trials, investigators who are undecided about the merits of a proposed treatment come together to give the therapy an objective test. In practice, the ideal of "equipoise" is rarely met. A planning group may include researchers who are more or less persuaded of a therapy's merit, researchers who are in equal measure skeptical, and a handful of the prescribed agnostics who are truly undecided.

In the case of the Diet-Heart study, participants ranged from Ancel Keys, who

83 Durant, "Nutritional Factors" [1951] (n. 35), 405; Wakerlin, "Recent Advances" [1952] (n. 59), 320–321.

84 Emmet Bays to Fredrick Stare, February 12, 1959, Box 251, Page papers. See also E. Silber, R. Pick, and L. N. Katz, "Clinical Management of Atherosclerosis," *Circulation* 16 (June 1960), 1193.

85 See Irvine H. Page to George Mann, June 18 1961, Box 127, Page papers.

86 On congressional concerns, see Strickland; Irvine H. Page to George V. Mann, June 18, 1961, Box 127, Page papers. The figure of $176 million represents the total appropriations for the National Heart Institute, 1950–1959. *NIH Factbook* (n. 37), p. 99.

had been advocating low-fat diets since the mid 1950s, to men like Stare and Page who were among Keys's early critics. The statisticians Moore and Cornfield, uncommitted to any particular theory of heart disease, nonetheless brought their own opinions on research methodology to the table.[87]

The proposed study differed from the majority of studies with which the researchers were familiar. Neither previous public health trials nor clinical trials of drugs provided a model: "It cannot be patterned along the lines of the Salk vaccine, fluoridation, lipoprotein, or estrogen studies, because much more cooperation, especially of a subjective nature, is needed from the participants."[88] Nor could it be modeled on the "small, well-controlled clinical investigation [that] may reveal basic scientific information concerning mechanisms [of arteriosclerosis] but may not confirm or deny the hypothesis that a change in diet will be effective in the general population."[89] Rather, something new was needed, a "large-scale public health field trial" to see whether people's eating habits could be changed, and whether that made a difference in preventing heart disease.

The purposes of conducting such a study seemed clear enough: "Before any firm recommendations can be made for change in the American diet, a large-scale, public health field trial must be done to prove conclusively that such a change will reduce the incidence of heart attacks."[90]

Agreement over the overall goals of a "large-scale clinical trial," however, did not guarantee agreement about the means or methods of such a study. Those, like Ivan Frantz, who were most concerned to analyze the effects of dietary change on serum cholesterol, argued for studying a closed institutional population, where dietary intake could be closely measured and controlled.[91] Others, like the NIH's Jerome Green, insisted that studies of institutional inmates missed the point. If the

---

87 Despite his advocacy of a low-fat diet, Keys regarded it as an open question whether dietary intervention in middle age could *reverse* the effects of a lifetime high-fat diet. See Keys, "Diet and Coronary Heart Disease throughout the World" [1962] (n. 65), 240–241. On Moore's views, see Felix E. Moore, "Committee on Design and Analysis of Studies," *AJPH* 50 (October 1960), part II, 10–19, and George V. Mann to Irvine Page, September 8, 1960, Box 127, Page papers. For Cornfield, see Jerome Cornfield, "Principles of Research," *American Journal of Mental Deficiency* 64 (September 1959), 240–252; Fred Ederer, "Jerome Cornfield's Contributions to the Conduct of Clinical Trials," *Biometrics* 39 (March 1982), Supplement, 25–32. On Stare's views, quite critical of the "dietary hypothesis" in general, and of epidemiological evidence in particular, see Lown and Stare, "Atherosclerosis, Infarction and Nutrition" [1959] (n. 63), 164. On Stare's background, see Fredrick J. Stare, *Harvard's Department of Nutrition, 1942–1986* (Boston: Harvard School of Public Health, 1987), pp. xvii–xxi; idem, "Nutrition Research from Respiration and Vitamins to Cholesterol and Atherosclerosis," *Annual Review of Nutrition* 11 (1991), 1–20.

88 Irvine H. Page, *A Plan for the Study of Diet, Plasma Lipids and Myocardial Infarction: A Report to the National Advisory Heart Council,* Box 127, Page papers. This document is undated but was composed sometime between April 1960, when the investigators met, and June 1960, when the report was presented to the National Advisory Heart Council.

89 Ibid.

90 Ibid.

91 Ivan D. Frantz to Irvine H. Page, March 16, 1960. Frantz nonetheless agreed not to "oppose" a study of a free-living population. See also Page to George V. Mann, June 18, 1961. Both documents Box 127, Page papers. At some point, Frantz switched his proposal for a prison study to one planned in collaboration with Keys, at the state mental hospital in St. Peter, Minnesota: Ivan D.

study were to provide a basis for public health recommendations, Green argued, it should be conducted on a group living under circumstances similar to those of the general population: "Certainly the studies in mental institutions will be much easier to perform but the great public health significance of this type of investigation must ultimately rest with a demonstration of feasibility and efficacy [in] a free living population."[92]

Similar disagreements over aims and means surfaced in a divisive debate over experimental design initiated by the statistician Jerry Cornfield. The Diet-Heart study was one of the first large clinical trials in which the NIH statisticians played a major role. Cornfield, an uncompromising advocate of double-blind trials, insisted on the need to conceal treatment assignment from both patient and treating physician if the study was to meet prevailing scientific standards of evidence. Ancel Keys and others responded that it was difficult enough for treating physicians to motivate patients to diet, without keeping the physician in the dark as to whether his patient was actually getting a modified diet.[93] Only when Cornfield threatened to resign over the issue did the other investigators agree to attempt a double-blind study.[94]

The diet-heart researchers found themselves trying to reconcile in one study the tensions between two intellectual traditions: one, a pragmatic public health tradition aimed, in the final analysis, at changing public policy and social behavior; the other, a research tradition intended to establish a rigorous scientific basis for all therapeutic practices.[95] Anxieties about motivating participants in a double-blind trial underscore the investigators' dilemma: how to satisfy the methodological requirements of a controlled clinical trial while conducting a mass public health trial aimed at changing the behavior of large groups of people?

The Diet-Heart study called for an unusual effort in social engineering, to which researchers brought their own social assumptions about American life. Not only did the study require the cooperation of food companies in the preparation and distribution of specially produced foods, but it called for an unprecedented effort to change the behavior of study participants. Any clinical trial requires the

Frantz, *Protocol for a Pilot Study of the Effect of Diet on the Incidence of Manifestations of Atherosclerosis in a Closed Population,* May 13, 1961, Box 13, Helen Brown papers, Cleveland Clinic Archives.

92 Jerome Green to Jeremiah Stamler, April 10, 1961, Jerome Green papers [hereafter Green papers]. These papers are in the custody of the Division of Research Grants, NIH. I am grateful to Dr. Green for facilitating access.

93 Jerome Cornfield to Irvine H. Page, December 4, 1961; Diet and Heart Disease, *Minutes of the Meeting of the Investigators and Biostatisticians,* December 18, 1961. Concerns about motivating participants also permeate the group's report to the NAHC: *A Plan for the Study of Diet, Plasma Lipids and Myocardial Infarction.* All documents Box 127, Page papers.

94 For Cornfield, the group's lack of commitment to the double-blind principle augured poorly for the scientific standing of the future trial. See Cornfield to Page, December 4, 1961; Jeremiah Stamler, *History of the National Diet-Heart Study and the Deliberations of the Executive Committee on Diet and Disease.* Both documents, Box 127, Page papers.

95 It is of interest that two of the precursors to the Diet-Heart study – Norman Joliffe's New York "Anti-Coronary Club" study and Stamler's Chicago study – were conducted under the auspices of the respective municipal health departments.

cooperation of patients, who must not only enroll in the study but ideally remain in it to the end, all the while sticking to their assigned treatment.[96] Ensuring that patients take their medicine is always a problem, but when the treatment involves changing the eating habits of middle-aged men over the course of several years, the difficulties are compounded a hundredfold. Not only must the men be motivated, but, in an era when preparing the family's food was still regarded as women's work, investigators deemed it essential to enlist their wives as well. Eligibility was confined to married men; the idea that the diets of single men could be effectively managed to provide a test of the theory was apparently never discussed.[97]

Researchers deemed such social engineering necessary if the study was to provide a fair test of the dietary hypothesis. The same criteria applied to the more technical aspects of study design. Dietary advocates like Stamler and Keys feared that a double-blind study might hamper physicians' efforts to motivate their patients. Suppose the study found no differences between experimental and control groups, Stamler asked. Would that prove that dietary change did not prevent heart disease, or would it simply show that these investigators had failed to change the eating habits of their subjects? The compliance issue colored other discussions of the diet experiment: for example, how "severe" should the dietary change be? Too great a departure from the customary American diet would lead to massive noncompliance, whereas too little a change might fail to test the dietary theory.[98]

Other issues of study design, while less controversial, pointed to additional difficulties of the proposed prevention trial. It would be easiest (and cheapest) to show an effect for diet if one enrolled a population at high risk of heart disease. With a high-risk population, one could enroll fewer subjects and still demonstrate

96 Statisticians were just beginning to think through the issue of "compliance" or patient adherence to therapy in clinical trials at this time. The Diet-Heart study was one source for these discussions. See M. Anthony Schork and Richard D. Remington, "The Determination of Sample Size in Treatment–Control Comparisons for Chronic Disease Studies in Which Drop-Out or Non-Adherence Is a Problem," *JCD* 20 (1967), 233–239; Max Halperin, Eugene Rogot, Joan Gurian, and Fred Ederer, "Sample Sizes for Medical Trials with Special Reference to Long-Term Therapy," *JCD* 21 (1968), 13–24. For a pioneering discussion in an actual clinical trial, see the Coronary Drug Research Project Group, "Influence of Adherence to Treatment and Response of Cholesterol on Mortality in the Coronary Drug Project," *NEJM* 303 (October 30, 1980), 1038–1041.

97 Nor was the eligibility of women discussed: prior to the 1980s, the only person to raise the exclusion of women as a key issue in clinical trials of heart disease was the philanthropist and lobbyist Mary Lasker, in connection with the Coronary Drug Project. See her *Memorandum Recommending Atromid Drug Trial,* attachment to Mary Lasker to John W. Gardner [HEW Secretary], July 14, 1967, National Heart Institute, Intramural 6-10, OD, NIH. Another social criterion, that subjects have an acceptable credit rating, was imposed at the request of the commercial food distributors enlisted in the study.

98 *Diet and Heart Disease. Protocol for Pilot Studies in a Free-Living Population,* May 1961, Box 13, Helen Brown papers, Cleveland Clinic Archives; *Minutes of the Diet and Nutrition Committee,* January 17, 1961, Box 127, Page papers.

an advantage for diet (if one existed). On the other hand, choosing a high-risk group meant choosing a population that least resembled the general public.[99]

As the planning group deliberated, their uncertainties grew. Routine issues of study design – How many subjects were needed? – depended on unanswered questions: How many seemingly healthy men would volunteer for a study of dietary change? How would compliance be measured? How much compliance could they expect? How many people would quit the study? What kinds of diets would produce the maximum effect while remaining acceptable to participants? Ultimately, the investigators concluded, the uncertainties were too great. Before attempting a full-scale study, they would initiate a briefer multiclinic feasibility study.[100]

The group's proposals were extensively reviewed by outside researchers and NIH officials between 1961 and 1962. Reviewers raised concerns similar to those discussed by the planning group. In particular, they insisted, the investigators must commit themselves to the double-blind approach "in view of the bias which some of these [researchers] have already demonstrated in favor of the thesis which they are testing."[101] In addition to reviewers' concerns about study methodology, NIH officials had an overriding concern about the scale and cost of a full study once the feasibility studies were done. Overruling objections by subordinates that NIH should not commit itself to the pilot studies "unless and until it can commit itself to the full-scale study in the event feasibility is demonstrated," NIH director James Shannon approved the initial grants without making any promises about the future.[102]

99 *Minutes of the Design Committee*, February 24, 1961; *Minutes of the Diet and Nutrition Committee*, January 17, 1961. Both Box 127, Page papers. In general, the statisticians on the design committee emphasized the costs and logistical difficulties of a larger, lower-risk population, while the cardiologists and nutritionists on the diet committee insisted on the irrelevance of the high-risk population to the basic issue at hand.

100 See *Minutes of the Design Committee Meeting*, February 24, 1961; *Minutes of the Design and Nutrition Committee Meeting*, January 17, 1961. A firm decision to undertake feasibility studies appears to have been taken in a meeting of the Executive Committee on March 21, 1961, although such plans are implicit in earlier discussions. The final decision was a victory for those in the group – such as George Mann and Felix Moore – who deemed any plans for a full study "premature." See *Diet and Heart Disease Study. Chronology of Some Pertinent Events*, February 13, 1962; George V. Mann to Irvine H. Page, September 8, 1960 and June 7, 1961. All documents in Box 127, Page papers.

101 Special Review Committee: Diet and Heart Feasibility Studies, March, 29, 1962, Extramural Research, 6-1: Diet Heart Feasibility Study, OD, NIH. This panel also insisted on a greater degree of uniformity and centralized control for the six pilot study sites. For outside concerns, see *The Design and Conduct of Feasibility Studies: Diet and Heart Disease*, June 12, 1962, Green papers.

102 David E. Price to James Shannon, April 6, 1962, Extramural Research, 6-1: Diet-Heart Feasibility Study, OD, NIH. NIH's administrative handling of the Diet-Heart study was unusual from the start. The initial technical reviews for the NAHC were done by a committee which included Page and some of the other investigators; after approval [review] by the NAHC, NIH director Shannon intervened, and the higher levels of the NIH bureaucracy were involved in the reviews on an unprecedented scale. See, in addition to Price's memo, Jerome J. Green, *Personal Notes Meetings Held at NIH on Thursday, September 14, 1961*, September 17, 1961; Page to J. Franklin

The Diet-Heart Feasibility Study began enrolling patients at five clinical centers in 1963. Patients were assigned to one of four experimental diets or to a control group intended to mimic the "usual American diet." Patients were to purchase their foods from centers supplied with the special study diets.[103] Investigators in the 6,000-plus person, one-year-long pilot study had no hope of reducing the rates of heart attacks in the experimental group. Rather their aim was to see if the food industry could produce palatable low-fat foods, if sufficient subjects could be enrolled in the study, and if they could be persuaded to consume the specially prepared foods.[104] The best the investigators could hope for was to demonstrate that when subjects adhered to the diet, serum cholesterol levels would drop. Positive results would enable researchers to go ahead in planning a full study, which would show, once and for all, whether dietary change could reduce heart disease.

The good news from the feasibility study was that patients on both experimental diets had an 11 percent lowering in serum cholesterol. Not only did the volunteers eat the specially prepared foods, but the diets worked![105] On the other hand, investigators reported, the control group was "more health-conscious" than the "general population," so that the control patients remained relatively healthy despite their elevated cholesterol levels.[106]

The control group's good news was bad news for the medical researchers. The size of any clinical trial depends on the number of "events" (deaths, heart attacks,

Yeager, November 15, 1961, both Green papers; Page to James Shannon, April 28, 1962, Box 251, Page papers; National Advisory Heart Council, *Minutes of Meeting*[s], June 22–24, 1961, November 18–20, 1961, June 21–23, 1962, Records of the National Heart Institute, Bethesda, MD; and Page to Shannon, April 28, 1962; Dr. H. F. Dorn to Ralph E. Knutti, May 21, 1962; Director, NHI [Ralph Knutti] to Surgeon-General, Public Health Service, through Director, NIH, May 25, 1962; Knutti to Luther Terry, James Shannon, David Price, E. C. Andrus, Irvine Page, Jerome Green, July 2, 1962, all Extramural Research, 6-1: Diet-Heart Feasibility Study, OD, NIH.

103 The preceding is a simplification of the actual experimental design. In each of the five cities, patients were assigned to one of two experimental diets, or to a control group. To gather information on additional dietary regimens and administrative procedures, the Minnesota researchers experimented with alternative arrangements. An experimental diet with a much higher ratio of polyunsaturated fats was tested in the state mental hospital site. A fourth experimental diet was tested on an open population group: patients in this study were not blinded to the diet they were receiving. These modifications were presumably a response to concerns raised by the two Minnesota investigators – Ivan Frantz and Ancel Keys – in the planning stages. The feasibility studies were further modified by the decision at some sites to extend the study another six months (the "Extended Study') and to recruit an additional group of subjects (the "Second Study'). These changes were meant to resolve further questions about dietary modifications, recruitment rates, and dropout rates, including, in the Second Study, measuring the effects on participation of "frankly acknowledg[ing]" the use of random assignments. For details of the protocol, see National Diet-Heart Study Research Group, "The National Diet-Heart Study Final Report," *Circulation* 37 (March 1968), Supplement I, I2–I8, I28–I36.

104 Ibid., I1–I2.

105 Ibid., I12–I13.

106 Ibid., I4.

etc.) researchers expect to find. The rarer the event, the larger the study must be. To show a difference between dietary and control groups in a full-scale study, either the researchers would have to enroll much higher risk subjects, or they would need many more subjects than the 100,000 previously estimated.[107] As NIH officials had feared, a full-scale study would either be much more costly than the investigators had imagined, or it was going to tell public health officials far less about avoiding heart disease in "healthy" men.

Nor did the feasibility study resolve differences of opinion in the group regarding the pro's and con's of a double-blind study. The published report came down on the side of Keys and others who had argued against a double-blind design.[108] Yes, the subjects in the feasibility study adhered to their diets, despite being kept in the dark about whether the diets made a difference. The report nonetheless cautioned that the lessons of a one-year study may not apply in a longer test:

It may be difficult if not impossible, to recruit and hold large numbers of men for a five year study on a double-blind basis, in which the men would not be informed of their diet group or serum cholesterol responses for five years. A double-blind design may be a serious handicap in fully motivating and educating participants and their families for the most effective sustained adherence to a dietary program.[109]

Not only did the double-blind design have a "corrosive effect" on the staff morale, the report claimed, but, in order to maintain the double-blind, the control group was given dietary instruction and provided with foods similar to that of the experimental groups. The control diet "of the feasibility study was certainly not a fully satisfactory control diet for a mass field trial."[110]

Disagreements among the diet-heart researchers about the scope and methods of a full-scale study were substantial, so much so that at times it seemed as if the group would issue a report with no recommendations. It took two years of active debate and Irvine Page's heart attack before the group's report was ready.[111] But regardless of internal debates over aspects of experimental design, the diet-heart investigators agreed that a full study was now both necessary and possible. They recommended that NIH begin immediately planning a five-year study, in "20 or more major metropolitan areas," of dietary prevention for heart disease.[112]

107 Ibid., 117–118.
108 For discussions of this issue among the investigators, see Ancel Keys to Irvine H. Page, June 15, 1966; *Draft Minutes of December 6, 1966: Diet-Heart Study Meeting,* January 4, 1967; Fred Ederer to Jeremiah Stamler, February 27, 1967, all Green papers.
109 National Diet-Heart Study Research Group, "Final Report" (n. 103), 117.
110 National Diet-Heart Study Research Group, "Final Report" (n. 103), 1256–1257. See also 1141–1142.
111 On Page's heart attack (and anxieties for the study) see Irvine Page to Tinsley Harrison, July 7, 1967, Box 127, Page papers. See also "The Doctor's Heart Attack," *Time* 90 (November 3, 1967), 52. For further evidence of strong internal dissension, and doubts about whether the group could agree on a written report, see Fred Ederer to Joe Bragdon, April 6, 1966; Irvine Page to Bragdon, April 9, 1966; Ancel Keys to Irvine H. Page, June 15, 1966. All Green papers.
112 National Diet-Heart Study Research Group, "Final Report" (n. 103), 121–126.

NIH officials were more cautious. Following the well-established maxim, "when in doubt, defer and consult," in 1967 NHI Director Donald Fredrickson commissioned the first of two review panels to advise NIH on whether a dietary prevention study was feasible and appropriate. The first panel, chaired by Rockefeller University's Edward Ahrens, recommended against a "primary prevention" trial – a trial of otherwise healthy men – in a free-living population, on the grounds that such a study was more expensive and less likely to succeed in producing a definitive answer. In its place, they proposed a study of secondary prevention – a controlled trial of diet among men who had already experienced a heart attack – along with a smaller study of primary prevention in an institutionalized population.[113] The committee's recommendations were no surprise. Ahrens had made his scientific reputation combining biochemical research with metabolic studies in carefully controlled clinical environments.[114]

Two years later, a second review panel also chaired by Ahrens, recommended against "a single large scale diet-heart trial" "at this time."[115] According to the reviewers,

This conclusion was based on three convictions: that one might well fail to obtain the desired definitive scientific answer from this huge undertaking; that the managerial problems of carrying out a well-controlled study within such a large free living population (estimates ranging from 24,000 to 115,000 individuals) . . . for the lengthy period of time (7–10 years) required . . . would make the study difficult to complete; finally, in view of these uncertainties, the projections of manpower and dollar costs (ranging from $500 million to more than one billion dollars) for such a study are formidable.[116]

In the aftermath of the Task Force on Arteriosclerosis, the "national Diet-Heart Study" was dead. But who or what killed it?

113 U.S. National Heart Institute, Diet-Heart Review Panel, *Mass Field Trials of the Diet-Heart Question* (New York: American Heart Association, 1969), xi. The panel's emphasis on the cost implications of the Diet-Heart study contrasts strongly with NHI director Donald Fredrickson's instructions that the panel focus on the scientific validity of the study while leaving "logistical, ethical and financial" issues aside.

114 For examples of Ahrens's earlier work, see Edward H. Ahrens Jr., David H. Blakenhorn, and Theodore T. Tsaltas, "Effect on Human Serum Lipids of Substituting Plant for Animal Fat," *Proceedings of the Society for Experimental Biology and Medicine* 86 (1954), 872–878; idem, "Nutritional Factors and Serum Lipid Levels," *American Journal of Medicine* 23 (December 1957), 928–952, esp. 935; Edward H. Ahrens Jr., Jules Hirsch, William Insull Jr., and Malcolm Peterson, "Effects of Dietary Fats on Serum Lipid Levels in Man," *Transactions of the Association of American Physicians* 70 (1957), 224–233. For his views on dietary fat restrictions, see Edward H. Ahrens Jr., "Symposium on Significance of Lowered Cholesterol Levels," *JAMA* 170 (August 29, 1959), 2198–2199; idem, "Hardening of the Arteries: Can It Be Prevented by Appropriate Diet?," *Journal of Rehabilitation* 32 (March–April 1966), 93–96. See also idem, "Nutritional Factors and Serum Lipid Levels," 928–952. For an articulate expression of Ahrens's reservations regarding the limited relevance of controlled trials to patient management, see E. H. Ahrens Jr., "The Diet-Heart Question in 1985," *Lancet* i (May 11, 1985), 1085–1987.

115 National Heart and Lung Institute, Task Force on Arteriosclerosis, *Arteriosclerosis* (Washington, DC: National Institutes of Health, 1971), vol. II, p. 65.

116 Ibid.

DEATH OF A STUDY

It is difficult to provide a fully satisfactory account of why the "definitive" Diet-Heart study was never done. Part of the difficulty lies in the nature of the documentary trace – the unpublished correspondence, transcripts, and reports which the historian uses to guide his way through the more public opinions, assertions, and refutations of the historical actors. While the problem of documentation exists for any period of historical study, the documentary trace for events of contemporary history is notoriously uneven. In the case of the Diet-Heart study, so many records are in private hands that one cannot even reliably say which materials have been destroyed. Analyzing the actions, much less the motives, of historical actors under such circumstances is a tricky business at best.

In part, the Diet-Heart study was a victim of changed research politics: more medical researchers seeking a limited, if not a diminished pool of federal dollars. By the late 1960s, both laboratory and investigator-initiated research – the centerpieces of NIH research policy in the postwar era – were under increasing congressional attack. Researcher anxieties were especially heightened by NIH's 1969 threat to cut second-year budgets for continuing grants by as much as 20 percent, the year that the diet-heart investigators issued their call for a full study.[117] While in theory the Diet-Heart study might have benefited from the rising congressional interest in applied research, in practice it got caught in the backlash from researchers who thought that the answers to prevention and treatment would be found within the walls of the laboratory, not in a clinical trial whose possibilities for success seemed at best uncertain. For reviewers wondering where their future support was coming from, the financial implications of the Diet-Heart study for the federal research budget were a major consideration, a concern shared by NIH director James Shannon, and his immediate successor, Robert Q. Marston.[118]

117 The National Heart and Lung Institute budget had actually declined in fiscal years 1964 and 1965; it began to grow again in fiscal year 1966, but was in virtually a steady state in fiscal years 1968 and 1969. *NIH Factbook* (n. 37), p. 99. On the politics of the fiscal year 1970 budget, negotiated in the spring and fall of 1969, see Richard A. Rettig, *Cancer Crusade: The Story of the National Cancer Act of 1971* (Princeton: Princeton University Press, 1977), pp. 29–33. Among the threatened programs was the National Heart and Lung Institute's long-standing epidemiological study in Framingham. See also Robert Q. Marston, "Federal Support of Education and Research: Policy Issues and National Needs," *Yale Journal of Biology and Medicine* 42 (August 1969), 8.

118 The Task Force on Arteriosclerosis, which recommended against a diet-heart study, issued an extended plea for a renewed emphasis on "basic, investigator initiated" research (complete with an historical appendix justifying the fruits of undirected, basic research). See National Heart and Lung Institute, Task Force on Arteriosclerosis, *Arteriosclerosis* (n. 115), pp. 245–248, 356–365. For contemporary concerns of the laboratory-oriented researcher in cardiovascular disease, see the address by Daniel Steinberg, chair of the AHA Council on Arteriosclerosis, "Progress, Prospects and Provender," *Circulation* 41 (April 1970), 723–728. While Steinberg endorsed the idea of a full-scale dietary trial in passing, his address was largely a paean to the resourcefulness and utility of basic research. For the NIH perspective, see Testimony of James A. Shannon, U.S. House of Representatives, Committee on Appropriations, *Hearings . . . Departments of Labor, and Health, Education and Welfare Appropriations for 1969. Part V. National Institutes of Health,* 90th Congress, 2nd

Even for those who deemed clinical trials a necessary evil, there were other, more promising candidates for public investment. In the face of congressional demands to see more practical applications from NIH, agency officials had reluctantly committed the agency to a multiyear, multimillion dollar clinical trial of heart disease prevention: the Coronary Drug Project (CDP). Planning for the CDP had initially faced many of the same questions posed to the Diet-Heart study: Would patients enroll for the duration? How many subjects were needed? How much would it cost? Would the "prosaic and tedious" clinical trial divert researchers and funds from "more imaginative and rewarding efforts"? Opposition of senior NIH officials to the CDP ceased only when Congress awarded $650 million for the study in addition to the regular NHI appropriation.[119] The CDP soon became the showpiece of NIH testimony, trotted out for display whenever members of the appropriations committees asked about practical results from the federal effort in medical research.[120]

Studies of cholesterol-lowering drugs certainly had powerful lay advocates both within and outside of Congress which studies of diet lacked.[121] It could be argued further that support for the CDP, in preference to the Diet-Heart study, represents the medical profession's preference for drugs over diet, and treatment over preven-

Session, 22–24; Testimony of Robert Q. Marston, U.S. House of Representatives, Committee on Appropriations, *Hearings . . . Departments of Labor, and Health, Education and Welfare Appropriations for 1970. Part 4. National Institutes of Health*, pp. 315–316, 91st Congress, 1st Session; Testimony of Robert Q. Marston, U.S. Senate, Committee on Appropriations, *Hearings . . . Departments of Labor, and Health, Education and Welfare Appropriations for 1971*, p. 2852, 91st Congress, 2nd Session. For Shannon's view on basic research, see also Strickland, *Politics, Science and Dread Disease* (n. 37), pp. 188–189, 200–203.

119 On the history of congressional financing for the CDP, see William J. Zukel, "Evolution and Funding of the Coronary Drug Project," *Controlled Clinical Trials* 4 (1983), 281–288, 298–312. Funding for the CDP continued to be a sore spot in the annual budgetary wranglings between NIH, Bureau of the Budget, and Congress. For doubts inside and outside the CDP regarding costs and feasibility, see Summary Sheet, Heart Special Projects, Special Review Committee, December 12, 1963; Ad Hoc Committee on Clinical Trial of AntiAtherosclerotic Drugs, March 24, 1961; Cooperative Study of Drugs and Coronary Heart Disease, 3rd Meeting of Consultant Participants, September 13–14, 1962; Cooperative Study of Drugs and CHD, Policy Board, December 6, 1962. All Extramural Research-6 NHI, OD, NIH. See also Director and Deputy Director, NIH, to Ralph Knutti, Director NHI, November 13, 1963, Intramural Research Drugs (1963), OD, NIH; *Memorandum, Subcommittee on Preliminary Estimates of Costs, Committee on Anti-Atherosclerotic Drugs*, June 9, 1961, Green papers.

120 The increasing attention given the CDP over the diet-heart study by NHLI and NIH officials testifying in Congress is noticeable. See Testimony of Donald Fredrickson, U.S. House of Representatives, Committee on Appropriations, *Hearings . . . Departments of Labor, and Health, Education and Welfare Appropriations for 1968. Part 5. National Institutes of Health*, pp. 306, 320–321, 90th Congress, 1st Session; Testimony of Donald Fredrickson, U.S. House of Representatives, Committee on Appropriations, *Hearings . . . Departments of Labor, and Health, Education and Welfare Appropriations for 1969. Part V. National Institutes of Health*, pp. 480–498, 501–503, 90th Congress, 2nd Session; Testimony of Robert Q. Marston, U.S. House of Representatives, Committee on Appropriations, *Hearings . . . Departments of Labor, and Health, Education and Welfare Appropriations for 1970. Part 4. National Institutes of Health*, pp. 315–316, 91st Congress, 1st Session.

121 Strickland, *Politics, Science and Dread Disease* (n. 37), pp. 215–217; James A. Shannon to Sen. Gaylord Nelson, November 8, 1967, Intramural Research 6-10, Atromid-S, OD, NIH; Mary Lasker to John W. Gardner, July 15, 1967, Intramural Research, 6-10, OD, NIH. These materials

tion (if prophylactic drug prescribing can be called "treatment").[122] If so, it is difficult to explain why the 1971 Task Force on Arteriosclerosis, which adamantly rejected a national study of dietary prevention, recommended a multiple intervention prevention trial of diet, smoking cessation, and exercise. In 1972, Congress funded the Multiple Risk Factor Intervention Trial (MRFIT).[123] Professional support for MRFIT suggests the limits of any explanation for the demise of the Diet-Heart study that is grounded solely in medical politics and scientific ideologies.

In part, the Diet-Heart study was a victim of circumstances and history, including the successes of its principal investigators in touting the message of dietary prevention. Ancel Keys had been preaching the virtues of a low-fat diet to medical audiences since the early 1950s, a message addressed directly to the public after 1959, when the Keys's "Mediterranean diet" cookbook first appeared. By the early 1960s, both Keys and Stamler were arguing that the prudent clinician would begin dietary advice now, before any definitive study was accomplished.[124]

By 1970, Irvine Page had joined Stamler and Keys in calling for a national policy of medical screening with "dietary counseling" for individuals found to be at "high risk" for coronary artery disease. The presidential committee chaired by Keys and Page also recommended that the food industry begin a development program to prepare low-fat foods "suitable for manufacture and distribution to the entire American public" in "expectation that the [Diet-Heart] study will demon-

deal with Lasker's specific proposal to expand beyond the CDP for a trial testing Atromid-S in primary prevention of heart disease. For an earlier Lasker effort to get an NIH commitment to clinical trials of new drugs for heart disease, see Mrs. Albert D. Lasker to Douglas Cater [White House], September 10, 1965, General/Legislation/Health, White House Central Files, Subject Files, Lyndon Baines Johnson Library, Austin, Texas.

122 However, any such argument must account for the skepticism of NHI Director Donald Fredrickson, who doubted whether "any means requiring intake of four capsules per day for life is an ideal mass solution to a disease that usually takes 30 to 50 years to announce its presence." See Director [Fredrickson] NHI to Director [Shannon] NIH, April 26, 1967, OD, NIH. Fredrickson's comment is probably in response to Lasker's efforts to promote a new trial of Atromid-S on top of the CDP. For contemporary opinion – mostly skeptical – on the value of cholesterol lowering drugs, see Bernard Lown, Oscar W. Portman, and Fredrick J. Stare, "Some Comments on the Use of Agents Which Lower Serum Cholesterol," *Clinical Pharmacology and Therapeutics* 3 (July–August 1962), 421–424; Karoly G. Pinter and Theodore B. Van Itallie, "Drugs and Atherosclerosis," *Annual Review of Pharmacology* 6 (1966), 251–266; David Kritchevsky, "The Use of Pharmacologic Agents in Atherosclerosis Therapy," *Ann NY Acad Sci* 149 (November 21, 1968), 1058–1068.

123 NHLI, Task Force on Arteriosclerosis, *Arteriosclerosis* (n. 115), 144–147; William J. Zukel, Oglesby Paul, and Harold W. Schnaper, "The Multiple Risk Factor Intervention Trial (MRFIT): I. Historical Perspectives," *Preventive Medicine* 10 (1981), 387–401. Regrettably, this official account adds nothing to the public record concerning the complex discussions and negotiations that must have taken place among the various parties.

124 For Stamler's views, which emphasized dietary counseling for "high-risk" persons but at times blurred the distinction between "high-risk" individuals and the general population: Jeremiah Stamler, "The Problem of Elevated Blood Cholesterol," *AJPH* 50 (March 1960), part II, 14–19; J. Stamler et al., "Approaches to the Primary Prevention" [1963] (n.77), 948–949. For other proposals to act, rather than wait, see Weldon J. Walker and Jacques L. Sherman Jr., "Dietary Fat and the General Public," *American Heart Journal* 66 (1963), 272–273. See also Ancel Keys and Margaret Keys, *Eat Well and Stay Well* (Garden City, NY: Doubleday, 1959).

strate the dietary treatment to be effective."[125] Although the diet–heart researchers never gave up their appeals for a "definitive" scientific study of dietary intervention, increasingly they took the position that neither physicians, public health officials, or the general public could afford to wait while "hundreds of thousands of deaths occur each year from diseases related to arteriosclerosis."[126] Yet the more Americans began changing their diet, the less likely it was that a true "control" group could be found for a clinical trial of the dietary hypothesis.[127]

Self-inflicted wounds aside, the diet–heart researchers suffered in other respects from the complexities of their task and the timing of their initiative. Successive NHI review panels brought in new groups of researchers to the discussion, each with their own ideas about how best to conduct a controlled trial of dietary interventions. New ideas produced new debates: the Task Force on Arteriosclerosis, for example, spent much of its time debating the pros and cons of using a panel of community physicians to provide a control group that received dietary advice, but no specially prepared foods. While one group of reviewers insisted that community physicians were the ideal group with whom to test dietary advice, others argued that the proposal implicitly assumes that we "expect [the family physician] to do a poor job."[128]

New epidemiological research also produced new ideas about preventing heart disease. While experts continued to debate the strengths of the epidemiological evidence linking heart disease and diet, additional epidemiological studies had

125 Ancel Keys and Irvine H. Page, "Adults in an Affluent Society: The Degenerative Diseases of Middle Age," in *White House Conference on Food, Nutrition and Health: Final Report* (Washington, DC: Government Printing Office, 1970), pp. 52–53. See also a committee headed by Stamler, which took a similar stance in recommending changes in diet and food production while awaiting the results of definitive studies. "Report of Inter-Society Commission for Heart Disease Resources: Primary Prevention of Atherosclerotic Disease," *Circulation* 42 (December, 1970), Supplement, A83–87.

126 Keys and Page, "Adults in an Affluent Society" (n. 125), 53. For a virtually identical argument, see "Report of Inter-Society Commission for Heart Disease Resources" (n. 125), A83. At the same time, both reports still call for a federal commitment to plan and fund a study of dietary prevention. See also Jeremiah Stamler to Irvine H. Page, February 26, 1970, Box 251, Page papers; and, in addition, Ivan Frantz's notion that Americans were "one experiment away" from being able to resolve existing doubts about dietary interventions. Ivan Frantz, *The Present Status of the Diet-Heart Question*, September 10, 1970. Copy in author's possession, courtesy of Dr. Ivan Frantz.

127 Keys had articulated this dilemma in 1962; see "Diet and Coronary Heart Disease throughout the World" (n. 65), 231–232. The issue was hotly debated by the Diet-Heart Review Panel, and remained a concern for the Task Force on Arteriosclerosis. See *Meeting, May 21–22, 1968* [Diet-Heart Review Panel], Green papers; Max Halperin and Jerome Cornfield to William J. Zukel, January 29, 1971, Box 23, Folder 8, Diet-Heart Protocol Planning Committee, Jerome Cornfield papers, Department of Special Collections, Parks Library, Iowa State University, Ames, Iowa [hereafter Cornfield papers].

128 Ivan D. Frantz to William Zukel, February 6, 1971, Box 23, Folder 8, Diet-Heart Protocol Planning Committee, Cornfield papers. According to Frantz, unless one assumed that the community physicians would do a poor job, the outcomes in the proposed control group would not differ from those in the group receiving modified diet. Frantz advocated a randomized experiment in which both groups were managed by the clinical investigators. See also Frederick H. Epstein to William J. Zukel, February 2, 1971, Box 23, Folder 8, Diet-Heart Protocol Planning Committee, Cornfield papers.

built up the case for cigarette smoking and exercise as equally important factors. Preventive medicine researchers – a natural constituency for controlled trials of dietary prevention – were unwilling to put all their eggs in the dietary basket, especially if NIH was going to ration support for clinical trials of heart disease prevention. By the early 1970s, public health researchers – Stamler included – had begun advocating multiple intervention trials.[129] NHI statisticians, another natural constituency, had meanwhile backed the CDP as a model for demonstrating the value of clinical trials in setting health policy.[130]

By 1970, short-term clinical trials were well established as a legal standard of therapeutic efficacy and as a standard of excellence in medical research. Although randomized trials were hardly universal in clinical medicine, they were far more common than they had been two decades earlier.[131] The Diet-Heart study is hardly a typical case. Yet both the aspirations and frustrations of the diet-heart investigators are instructive in understanding the social and intellectual contests of the clinical trial in the third quarter of the twentieth century.

The Diet-Heart study was meant to provide a "scientific" test of "hypotheses" concerning the role of diet in heart disease. But the hypotheses being tested varied widely, depending on the individual who was speaking and the occasion on which he spoke. In designing their trial, the diet-heart investigators attempted to define a narrow, single hypothesis: Would dietary change affect the rate of heart disease in the general (male, middle-aged, married) population? Others implicitly regarded the Diet-Heart study as a test of an etiologic theory – Did the American diet "cause" heart disease? – and, depending on their training and professional

---

129 On multiple risk factors for heart disease, see Fredrick H. Epstein, "The Epidemiology of Coronary Heart Disease: A Review," *JCD* 18 (1965), 748–762; Thomas R. Dawber and H. Emerson Thomas Jr., "Prophylaxis of Coronary Heart Disease, Stroke and Peripheral Atherosclerosis," *Ann NY Acad Sci* 149 (November 21, 1968), 1038–1057; "Report of Inter-Society Commission for Heart Disease Resources" (n. 125), A51–A82. Multiple interventions in prevention were an early interest of Stamler's. See Stamler et al., "Approaches to Primary Prevention" [1963] (n. 77), 932–951; Jeremiah Stamler, David M. Berkson, Monte Levinson, et al., "A Long Term Coronary Prevention Evaluation Program," *Ann NY Acad Sci* 149 (November 21, 1968), 1022–1037. In 1967 he had unsuccessfully tried to convince the diet-heart group to recommend a multiple intervention trial, and in 1969 Stamler (along with Fred Stare) applied to NHI with an unsuccessful proposal for a multiple intervention study. See *Draft Minutes of December 6, 1966 Diet-Heart Study Meeting,* January 4, 1967, Green papers; Zukel et al., "The Multiple Risk Factor Intervention Trial" (n. 119), 391–392.

130 See the remarks of Jeremiah Stamler at Cooperative Coronary Heart Disease Drug Project, *Minutes of the Meeting of the Technical Group,* January 23–24, 1967, Records of the Coronary Drug Project, Maryland Medical Research Institute, Baltimore. I am grateful to Drs. Gennell Knatterud and Paul Canner for making these records available to me. On the importance of the CDP to the NIH statisticians, see Max Halperin, David DeMets, and James H. Ware, "Early Methodological Developments for Clinical Trials at the National Heart, Lung and Blood Institute," *Statistics in Medicine* 9 (1980), 882.

131 Thomas C. Chalmers, "The Clinical Trial," *Milbank Memorial Fund Quarterly/Health and Society* 59 (Summer 1981), 326; Robin Badgley, "An Assessment of Research Methods Reported in 103 Scientific Articles from Two Canadian Medical Journals," *Canadian Medical Association Journal* 103 (July 29, 1961), 246–250; Stanley Schor, "Statistical Evaluation of Medical Journal Manuscripts," *JAMA* 195 (March 28, 1966), 145–150.

orientation, agreed or disagreed with the proposal that a controlled clinical trial of diet in a general population could best test this theory. The diet–heart investigators themselves repeatedly alluded to other questions that the proposed study would resolve: What dietary advice should physicians give their patients? What changes should the food industry make in product mix? What advice should the Surgeon General give the American public to reduce the level of heart disease? Again, depending on which of these questions one hoped to answer, one might hold very different opinions about the merits or demerits of the Diet-Heart study.

Implicitly, the diet–heart researchers regarded a controlled clinical trial as analogous to a scientific experiment. But the proposed Diet-Heart study was very unlike the average scientific experiment. In medicine, at least, scientific experiments are not conducted by scores of people and multiple committees, do not involve tens much less hundreds of thousands of people, and do not generally cost millions or tens of millions of dollars. Any clinical trial involves a complex process of social negotiation over intellectual ends and practical means: Which issues can I reasonably address with these colleagues, these institutions, these patients, and these funding levels? What data and data gathering procedures must I have (to resolve my doubts, satisfy my standards, convince my colleagues, and further my career), and which are dispensable? The diet-heart investigators achieved consensus on some of these issues (the need for a randomized study), split the difference on others (open vs. closed populations, choice of dietary regimens), and left some of their colleagues dissatisfied with other decisions (double-blinding). Producing a social consensus on all these issues among a broader and more diverse research community was too much to ask.

7

Anatomy of a controversy:
The University Group Diabetes Program study

> After all, most of what is learned in life is not learned from properly controlled experimentation. To an official body hoping to obtain from an experiment guidance on policy the distinction between an objective demonstration and a plausible personal opinion should be made unmistakably clear.[1]

On May 21, 1970, some 800,000 diabetics were greeted with the news that tolbutamide (Orinase), a drug widely used in the treatment of milder diabetes, was causing "early death" in a substantial number of individuals. Investigators in the "biggest, most sophisticated and probably the longest study of diabetes ever made" had found that patients taking tolbutamide experienced significantly higher cardiovascular mortality than patients receiving a placebo.[2] On the basis of these findings, the U.S. Food and Drug Administration (FDA) was reviewing indications for the use of tolbutamide.[3] For all but a handful of physicians, the *Washington Post* report provided their first introduction to the University Group Diabetes Program (UGDP) study, whose findings were to be the subject of a decade-long controversy concerning the safety and utility of oral hypoglycemic drugs.

One of the earliest, multicenter, long-term clinical trials funded by the National Institutes of Health (NIH), the UGDP was meant to be a model of clinical investigation.[4] Planned and managed by a team of statisticians and clinicians, the study addressed a series of long-standing controversies over the clinical management of diabetes. Intended to demonstrate how a properly designed, randomized,

---

1 R. A. Fisher in "Discussion," *Journal of the Royal Statistical Society* 111 (1948), 203.
2 Morton Mintz, "Antidiabetes Pill Held Causing Early Death," *Washington Post,* May 21, 1970, 1, 7. An earlier announcement appeared on the Dow Jones ticker tape the day before. Curtis L. Meinert and Susan Tonascia, *Clinical Trials: Design, Conduct and Analysis* (New York: Oxford University Press, 1986), p. 53.
3 Harold M. Schmeck Jr. "Scientists Wary on Diabetes Pill," *New York Times,* May 22, 1970, p. 56.
4 The only comparable study I know of is the international collaborative ten-year study of ACTH and cortisone in rheumatic fever, begun in 1951 and jointly funded by the NIH and MRC. "The Treatment of Acute Rheumatic Fever in Children: A Cooperative Clinical Trial of ACTH, Cortisone and Aspirin," *Circulation* 11 (March 1955), 313–371; "The Evolution of Rheumatic Heart Disease in Children: Five-Year Report of a Cooperative Clinical Trial of ACTH, Cortisone and Aspirin," *Circulation* 22 (October 1960), 503–515. I was unable to find substantial administrative and scientific records of this study in the United States.

controlled trial could resolve differences of clinical opinion, the UGDP instead became a symbol of all that was wrong with the statistical enterprise in medicine.

Few recent controversies in medicine are comparable in length and rancor to that over the UGDP.[5] More extended debates – over the treatment of breast cancer or the safety of oral contraceptives – never focused as much attention, for so long, on a single study. And however much suspicions about the integrity of researchers may have figured in privately held judgments in other disputes, the UGDP is unusual in the degree to which such accusations were publicly traded. As an example of a study that tried – and failed – to resolve a controversy about the merits of medical treatment, the UGDP certainly represents an extreme case. But if the intensity of the debate over the UGDP was atypical, the conceptual issues and political dilemmas raised by the study are not.

Within the world of clinical medicine, the UGDP posed various questions about the respective roles of statistical and medical expertise: Which group should determine the methods of treatment and evaluation measures in clinical research? Who should have the final say in interpreting results from controlled studies? At the level of statistical theory, the UGDP posed analogous questions about the proper relation between statistical inference and scientific decisions: What criteria apply in deciding when a clinical experiment should be stopped? How are unanticipated results from a unique study to be interpreted?[6] At the level of policy, the controversy posed questions about the appropriate relation between scientific claims and regulatory decisions: Which studies count as proper evidence? When competing experts disagree about the merits of a study, how are the disagreements adjudicated? How are the results of clinical trials to be translated to medical practice?[7] None of these questions are unique to the UGDP. The persistence of the debate over the UGDP, however, calls attention to a prior question: How is the controversy to be explained?

5 Among its other distinctions, the UGDP is, to my knowledge, the only RCT to be the subject of a Supreme Court case, regarding the ownership of clinical data produced by government-funded research. See Joel Shelby Cecil and Eugene Griffin, "The Role of Legal Policies in Data Sharing," in Committee on National Statistics, National Research Council, *Sharing Research Data* (Washington, DC: National Academy Press, 1985), pp. 172–175. Earlier versions of the present analysis include: Harry M. Marks, *Tolbutamide – When, Where and Why? A Case Study in Clinical Decision-Making* (Boston: Executive Programs in Health Policy and Management, Harvard School of Public Health, 1978); idem, "Medical Science and Clinical Ambiguity: The Role of Randomized Clinical Trials in Therapeutic Controversies," a paper presented at the 109th Annual Meeting of the American Public Health Association, Los Angeles, November 1981; idem, *Ideas As Reforms: Therapeutic Experiments and Medical Practice, 1900–1980* (Ph.D. thesis, Massachusetts Institute of Technology, 1987), pp. 187–234. For other historical accounts of the UGDP controversy, both of which came to my attention well after the present account was completed, see James Wright Presley, *A History of Diabetes Mellitus in the United States, 1880–1990* (Ph.D. thesis, University of Texas at Austin, 1991), pp. 424–455; Meinert and Tonascia, *Clinical Trials* (n. 2), pp. 52–62.

6 Jerome Cornfield, "Recent Methodological Contributions to Clinical Trials," *American Journal of Epidemiology* 104 (1976), 408–421; Paul Meier, "Statistics and Medical Experimentation," *Biometrics* 31 (June 1975), 511–529.

7 Hubert C. Peltier, "Clinical Trials of Drugs from the Viewpoint of the Pharmaceutical Industry," *Clinical Pharmacology and Therapeutics* 18 (November 1975), part 2, 637–642.

To proponents of the UGDP, the persistence of the controversy requires little explanation. They regard the study as a pioneering effort whose conclusions have been repeatedly affirmed as valid in the face of intensive scrutiny.[8] The critics' failure to accept the study can only be explained as due to nonrational factors: ignorance or cupidity. Not surprisingly, the UGDP's critics regard it as a flawed study from which no conclusions can be drawn, and suggest that support for the UGDP is the result of the clan loyalty of statisticians and their camp followers.[9] In each case, there are purportedly two sides, truth and error; of these, only error calls for a social explanation, truth providing its own justification.

Historians and sociologists of science have found that asymmetric arguments of this sort, "I have reasons but you have prejudices," are not uncommon in scientific debate. Such debates are frequently found to entail disagreements not merely about the interpretation of individual experiments, but about the rules by which different experimental evidence is evaluated and weighed. The analyst's first duty is to examine the way in which both parties to a debate have constructed their arguments, and to identify the underlying issues each party believes to be at stake.[10]

In the case of the UGDP, what began as a debate over the merits of a particular clinical finding broadened into a dispute about the relative merits of statistical and clinical expertise in drawing inferences from the study. This scientific debate was exacerbated by the FDA's decision to draw on the UGDP's report in modifying the package labeling for the oral hypoglycemic drugs. The agency's action led critics of the study to publicly challenge both the validity of the UGDP's conclusions and the basis of the FDA's authority for prescribing the labeling of drugs.

To understand the controversy, it is necessary to understand both the clinical context in which it arose and the political context in which it was addressed. In the following section, I describe the state of knowledge about the management of diabetes in the period just before the design of the UGDP. I next describe the study and the development of the controversy. The remaining sections of the chapter analyze the efforts of the FDA and other groups to adjudicate the dispute.

8 Thaddeus E. Prout, Genell L. Knatterud, and Curtis Meinert, "Diabetes Drugs: Clinical Trial" [Letters], *Science* 204 (April 27, 1979), 362–363; Martin Goldner, ibid., 363–365.
9 Holbrooke S. Seltzer, "Efficacy and Safety of Oral Hypoglycemic Agents," *Annual Review of Medicine* 31 (1980), 261–272; Alvan R. Feinstein, "How Good Is the Statistical Evidence against Oral Hypoglycemic Agents?," *Advances in Internal Medicine* 24 (1979), 73–76.
10 G. Nigel Gilbert and Michael Mulkay, "Warranting Scientific Belief," *Social Studies of Science* 12 (1982), 383–408; G. D. L. Travis, "Replicating Replication? Aspects of the Social Construction of Learning in Planarian Worms," *Social Studies of Science* 11 (1981), 11–32. See also Everett Mendelsohn, "The Political Anatomy of Controversy in the Sciences," in H. Tristam Engelhardt and Arthur L. Caplan, eds., *Scientific Controversies: Case Studies in the Resolution and Closure of Disputes in Science and Technology* (Cambridge: Cambridge University Press, 1987), pp. 93–124. My analysis differs from Mendelsohn's principally in that where Mendelsohn takes "interests" to be historically and logically prior to controversies, I regard the production of interests as part of the process through which controversies are created.

DIABETES: TREATMENT AND DISEASE

"Diabetes" refers to a group of metabolic disorders characterized by a common inability to efficiently process and regulate levels of glucose in the blood. Normally, the body processes glucose with the aid of a hormone, insulin. For a variety of reasons, only partially understood, diabetics either fail to produce sufficient quantities of insulin or, in some instances, are unable to employ their insulin effectively in processing glucose.

Specialists at the time distinguished between two broad classes of diabetes, Type I and Type II, each with its own distinctive etiology, symptoms, and prognosis.[11] Type I, or insulin-dependent diabetes mellitus (IDDM, once termed "juvenile diabetes"), usually appears by age forty and entails a total or near total inability to produce insulin. Prior to the introduction of insulin in 1922, the majority of such patients died within five years of diagnosis.[12] Most diabetics, however, were known as Type II diabetics, formerly termed "adult-onset diabetes."[13] "Non-insulin-dependent diabetes mellitus (NIDDM)," as it is now known, represents a less severe condition, in which the body often retains some capacity to produce insulin, but cannot employ it effectively enough to prevent elevated blood glucose

11 This classification and nomenclature were introduced in 1978 by the National Diabetes Data Group, National Institutes of Health. In addition to distinguishing between Type I and II diabetes, they recognized three additional syndromes: gestational diabetes, or diabetes associated with pregnancy; diabetes secondary to other conditions; and impaired glucose tolerance, formerly termed "chemical" or "subclinical" diabetes. The principal significance of the new terminology was to provide a standardized terminology for clinical and epidemiological research, and to negate the customary association between age of onset and type of diabetes, which was embodied in the traditional nomenclature. See National Diabetes Data Group, "Classification and Diagnosis of Diabetes Mellitus and Other Categories of Glucose Intolerance," *Diabetes* 28 (1979), 1039–1057.

12 For descriptions of the dramatic impact of insulin on the lives of young diabetics, see Michael Bliss, *The Discovery of Insulin* (Chicago: University of Chicago Press, 1984). The extent of insulin's effect on diabetes mortality was and remains a complex subject. Mortality rates from diabetic coma had already improved from 64 to 42 percent with the introduction of Allen's "semistarvation" therapy in 1915. See Mayer B. Davidson, "The Continually Changing 'Natural History' of Diabetes Mellitus," *JCD* 34 (1981), 5, and, for a summary of the historical debate, see Presley, *A History of Diabetes* (n. 5), pp. 248–250, 290–314. Mortality aside, many specialists imposed onerous restrictions on the daily lives of young diabetics. See Chris Feudtner, "The Want of Control: Ideas, Innovations, and Ideals in the Modern Management of Diabetes Mellitus," *BHM* 69 (Spring 1995), 66–90.

13 Precise up-to-date numerical estimates of the two types of diabetes are not available; it is known, however, that 81 percent of existing diabetics are forty-five years or older, and that 74 percent of newly diagnosed diabetics are forty-five years or older. These statistics do not refer, however, to the date at which diabetes first manifested itself. *Report of the National Commission on Diabetes to the Congress of the United States,* vol. 3, part 1, *Scope and Impact of Diabetes* (1) (Washington, DC: Department of Health, Education and Welfare [pub] no. [NIH] 77-1021, 1976), pp. 71, 73. The problem is further exacerbated by the fact that the severity and precise nature and development of the impairment in metabolism are more significant than exact age of onset in categorizing types of diabetes. Moreover, estimates of the incidence of NIDDM, in particular, are particularly sensitive to changes in official diagnostic criteria. See L. Joseph Melton III, Pasquale J. Palumbo, and Chu-Pin Chu, "Incidence of Diabetes Mellitus by Clinical Type," *Diabetes Care* 6 (January–February 1983), 82–85.

levels.[14] Such individuals frequently do use insulin but unlike insulin-dependent diabetics, they do not generally require insulin injections to stay alive.

Despite the discovery of insulin, diabetics of both types have substantially lower life expectancy than the nondiabetic population, and remain at elevated risk for a series of life-threatening and disabling complications. Patients with NIDDM in particular are at substantially higher risk for death from cardiovascular disease and stroke, as well as being subject to diabetes-related blindness, nerve disfunction, gangrene, and kidney failure.[15] While physicians can theoretically distinguish, on the basis of laboratory and clinical findings, between the diagnosis of IDDM and NIDDM, the severity of the disease and its long-run complications vary considerably from individual to individual within each group.[16] These complications represent the major threat to the well-being and future life expectancy of adult diabetics. Whether these complications are preventable has been the subject of a decades-long controversy among specialists.[17]

Effective and appropriate management of diabetes is a complicated and controversial task. What all therapeutic regimens have in common is an attempt to keep the blood glucose levels of the patient somewhere within "normal" range – the means by which this is accomplished and the degree to which blood glucose levels are strictly controlled vary from physician to physician and patient to patient. One school – based at the Joslin Diabetes Clinic – has held that the development of

14 For a recent review on the etiology of NIDDM, see Hannele Yki-Jarvinen, "Pathogenesis of Non-insulin-dependent Diabetes Mellitus," *Lancet* 343 (January 8, 1994), 91–95. For a more complex, less dogmatic, view, see C. Ronald Kahn, "Insulin Action, Diabetogenesis, and the Cause of Type II Diabetes," *Diabetes* 43 (August 1994), 1066–1084. While both articles display a knowledge of molecular mechanisms unavailable, if not unimaginable, to researchers of the UGDP generation, the essential picture of a heterogeneous condition with multiple causes – as yet only partially understood – remains the same.

15 Individuals with NIDDM are not subject to diabetic retinopathy and nephropathy (kidney disease) to the same degree as those with IDDM; they are however, at greater risk than the general population. Davidson, "Changing 'Natural History' " (n. 12), 6–7.

16 Even the group that generated the classification schema acknowledges that discrimination between IDDM and NIDDM may be difficult in certain individuals. National Diabetes Data Group, "Classification and Diagnosis of Diabetes Mellitus" (n. 11), 1044. Of far greater consequence, however, is the heterogeneity of symptoms and prognosis within each class. See Stefan S. Fajans, Michael C. Cloutier, and Robert L. Crowther, "Clinical and Etiological Heterogeneity of Idiopathic Diabetes Mellitus," *Diabetes* 27 (1978), 1112–1125. These underlying differences are compounded by the fact that physicians differ substantially in the proportion of patients they would classify as "diabetic," given a specific laboratory result. See Kelly M. West, "Substantial Differences in the Diagnostic Criteria Used by Diabetes Experts," *Diabetes* 24 (July 1975), 641–644.

17 Since publication of the Diabetes Control and Complications Trial in 1993, in which patients with IDDM showed lower levels of neuropathy and diabetic retinopathy following an "intensive" regimen of glucose control, consensus has shifted to the view that rigorous control does inhibit the development of these two complications. The precise therapeutic implications of this trial for patients with NIDDM, however, are still being debated, however. See The Diabetes Control and Complications Trial Research Group, "The Effect of Intensive Treatment of Diabetes on the Development and Progression of Long-Term Complications in Insulin-Dependent Diabetes Mellitus," *NEJM* 329 (September 30, 1993), 977–986; Roz B. Lasker, "The Diabetes Control and Complications Trial," ibid., 1035–1036; Oscar B. Crofford, "Diabetes Control and Complications," *Annual Review of Medicine* 46 (1995), 267–279.

complications is directly and causally linked to the failure to maintain strict control of blood glucose. Others have maintained that the complications are independent manifestations of the disease process, whose progression is largely unaffected by blood glucose levels.[18]

Efforts to resolve the controversy were hampered by the prevailing traditions in diabetes research. Specialty clinics such as the Joslin, which saw returning patients regularly over the decades, relied on retrospective chart reviews to establish the relation between control and complications. Despite the unusually large case series available to Joslin researchers, their analyses suffered from the problems of all retrospective chart reviews: it was difficult to sort out the confounding effects of duration of disease, severity of disease, and mechanisms of patient selection. The apparent heterogeneity of the underlying disorder aggravated the problem. Some patients develop more complications, and sooner after diagnosis than others. Is the rapid progression of complications in these patients due to uncontrolled glucose levels, or are the complications *and* the difficulties in controlling their blood glucose both evidence that these patients have a more severe form of the disease?[19]

This theoretical dispute has substantial implications for the lives of patients: the more one believes in the long-run medical benefits of control, the more likely one is to advocate aggressive management of diet and life-style and/or the use of insulin, despite its inconveniences and hazards. Patients using insulin must do more than simply inject the drug at regular intervals. Use of insulin, activity, and diet must be kept in an even balance. An error in insulin dosage or a failure to snack between meals can lead to an excess amount of insulin and resulting hypoglycemia.[20]

18 On the Joslin philosophy of control, see Feudtner, "The Want of Control" (n. 12), 66–90. Chicago may have been one medical center where Joslin's ideals of control were disputed: ibid., 79–80. New York was another such site. See Edward Tolstoi, *The Practical Management of Diabetes* (Springfield IL: Charles C. Thomas, 1953). I am grateful to Dr. Jesse Roth for calling Tolstoi's views to my attention.

19 Philip K. Bondy, "Therapeutic Considerations in Diabetes Mellitus," in F. J. Ingelfinger, A. Relman, and M. Finland, eds., *Controversy in Internal Medicine* (Philadelphia: W. B. Saunders Company, 1966), pp. 499–500; Alexander Marble, "Control of Diabetes Lessens or Postpones Vascular Complications," ibid., pp. 493–496. While agreeing on the difficulty of studying the problem, Bondy and Marble take opposing views on the use of "strict" control. For an assessment of the state of knowledge regarding the pathogenesis of vascular complications around the time the UGDP study was designed, see Alexander Marble and George F. Cahill, *The Chemistry and Chemotherapy of Diabetes Mellitus* (Springfield IL: Charles C. Thomas, 1962), pp. 75–76.

20 The rate of errors in insulin dosage or failure to adhere to diet ranges as high as 50 percent in some observational studies. See Julia Watkins, T. Franklin Williams, Don A. Martin, et al., "A Study of Diabetic Patients at Home," *AJPH* 57 (March 1967), 453–455; Kelly M. West, "Diet Therapy of Diabetes: Analysis of a Failure," *Ann Int Med* 79 (1973), 426. The possibility that immunologic responses to insulin bring about further autoimmune damage to the pancreas gave physicians in the 1960s another reason to avoid the use of insulin. George F. Cahill Jr., "Some Thoughts concerning the Treatment of Diabetes Mellitus," in Ingelfinger et al., *Controversy in Internal Medicine* (n. 19), p. 509. For the consequences of strict control in the daily lives of patients, see Feudtner, "The Want of Control" (n. 12), 74–90.

Concerned about these side effects of insulin, physicians welcomed the introduction to the United States in 1956 of tolbutamide, an orally administered drug for diabetics. One of several compounds initially intended as substitutes for insulin in treating juvenile diabetics, tolbutamide was soon found to be of little use in these patients. It was, however, reported effective in a substantial number of patients with adult-onset diabetes, especially in individuals whose diabetes appeared after age forty and those whose daily insulin requirements were under twenty units.[21]

The oral hypoglycemic agents soon became a popular substitute for insulin injections in patients with NIDDM.[22] Their primary advantage was convenience. Not only was the need for injections eliminated, but an end to insulin injections reduced the need for between-meal feedings, formerly necessary to ensure that blood glucose levels did not drop to excessively low levels following the injection.[23] Experts soon recommended tolbutamide as the drug of choice in cases of mild diabetes (i.e., those with no history of ketoacidosis and with insulin use under forty units daily). Tolbutamide's special attractiveness lay in the low rate of toxic reactions and hypoglycemic episodes it provoked.[24] Although both experts and the drug's manufacturer, Upjohn Company, warned that tolbutamide was no substitute for maintaining proper dietary restrictions, its use was associated with a

21 Tolbutamide, which belongs to a class of compounds known as sulfonylureas, was developed in the mid-1950s, after German investigators observed the hypoglycemic effects of chemically related compounds used in the treatment of infections. One of these related compounds, carbutamide, was introduced into use late in 1955 but withdrawn due to toxic side effects by the fall of 1957. See Helmut Mehnert, Rafael Camerini-Davalos, and Alexander Marble, "Results of Long-Term Use of Tolbutamide (Orinase) in Diabetes Mellitus," *JAMA* 167 (June 14, 1958), 818. For a review of the history of research for insulin substitutes, and an overview of the initial American clinical findings, see C. J. O'Donovan, "New Orally Effective Adjuvants in the Management of Diabetes Mellitus," *JCD* 4 (December 1956), 635–643. O'Donovan reports that the German work was preceded by earlier French investigations reporting the hypoglycemic effects of these compounds, but that wartime publication may have inhibited dissemination of the French results.

22 One early study of the use of tolbutamide found that 61.7 percent of over 9,000 patients studied had formerly been managed by a combination of dietary restrictions and insulin. See C. J. O'Donovan, "Analysis of Long Term Experience with Tolbutamide (Orinase) in the Management of Diabetes," *Current Therapeutic Research* 1 (November 1959), 74.

23 Ibid., 85. See also Mehnert et al., "Results of Long-Term Use of Tolbutamide" (n. 21), 826–827. On the preferences of patients for oral drugs over insulin, even against medical advice, see Marble and Cahill, *The Chemistry and Chemotherapy of Diabetes* (n. 19), pp. 141, 158.

24 Craig M. Arnold and Ronald W. Lauener, "Oral Hypoglycemic Drugs," *Canadian Medical Association Journal* 91 (August 22, 1964), 395. Tolbutamide is less likely than other oral hypoglycemic agents to lower blood sugar levels excessively because it has a short "effective span of action." Thus regular doses are less likely to build up to produce hypoglycemia. The low toxicity and rapid excretion were also reported by the American Medical Association's Council on Drugs in its initial assessment of tolbutamide, although it stressed the possibility of acute hypoglycemia when trying to transfer patients from insulin to tolbutamide. See Council on Drugs, "New and Nonofficial Drugs: Tolbutamide," *JAMA* 164 (July 20, 1957), 1333–1335. Researchers from the Joslin Clinic, which had helped to introduce the drug in the United States, did not feel that such acute hypoglycemia was a significant problem. See Mehnert et al., "Results of Long-Term Use of Tolbutamide" (n. 21), 826–827.

further deemphasis on dietary control, in which tolbutamide and other oral hypoglycemic agents "became readily used as substitutes for dietary restrictions."[25]

The increasing use of tolbutamide during the late 1950s generated widespread interest among physicians specializing in diabetes. Particularly intriguing to researchers and clinicians was the suggestion that patients using tolbutamide might develop fewer cardiovascular complications, or develop them later than patients on other treatments.[26] Early in 1959, "members of a study section at the National Institutes of Arthritis and Metabolic Diseases (NIAMD)" began discussing whether a "clinical trial" might resolve the long-standing controversy over the effects of "diabetic control on the course of vascular disease." Shortly thereafter, a group of diabetes specialists, including Max Miller and Harvey Knowles, began formulating plans for a controlled clinical trial of diabetes treatments, tolbutamide included.[27]

The UGDP's proposed multiclinic study represented a new departure in diabetes research, which was strongly influenced by the metabolic tradition of clinical investigation, combining laboratory studies with closely observed clinical cases, and by a reliance on retrospective chart reviews. To help them in negotiating the terra incognita of clinical trials, the investigators recruited Christian Klimt, a young epidemiologist who had previously worked on clinical trials of gamma globulin. At Klimt's suggestion, they decided on a randomized, placebo-controlled design to evaluate the standard treatments then used in treating NIDDM: insulin, tolbutamide, and diet.[28] NIAMD reviewers, welcoming the opportunity to sup-

---

25 R. Camerini-Davalos, O. Lozanzo-Casteneda, and A. Marble, "Five Years' Experience with Tolbutamide," *Diabetes* 11 (1962), Supplement 1, 78; Council on Drugs, "Tolbutamide" (n. 24), 1333–1335; "Orinase [Upjohn Company Flyer]," in W. J. H Butterfield and W. Van Westering, eds., *Tolbutamide . . . After Ten Years* (New York: Excerpta Medica Foundation, 1967), p. 326.

26 Rafael A. Camerini-Davalos and Harold S. Cole, eds., *Early Diabetes: 1st International Symposium on Early Diabetes, 1968* (New York: Academic Press, 1970), pp. 443–470; Rafael A. Camerini-Davalos, "Treatment of Chemical Diabetes," and Robert Felman and Dwight Fitterer, "The Prophylactic Use of Oral Hypoglycemic Drugs in Asymptomatic Diabetes," both in Butterfield, *Tolbutamide . . . After Ten Years* (n. 25), pp. 231–232 and 243–254; Martin Goldner, Genell L. Knatterud, and Thaddeus E. Prout, "Effects of Hypoglycemic Agents on Vascular Complications in Patients with Adult Onset Diabetes," *JAMA* 218 (November 29, 1971), 1400.

27 Harvey C. Knowles Jr., "An Historical View of the Medical-Social Aspects of the UGDP," *Transactions of the American Clinical and Climatological Association* 88 (1976), 150. I owe my awareness of this article to James Wright Presley, *A History of Diabetes* (n. 5).

28 Testimony of Floyd Daft [Director, NIAMD] in U.S. Congress, House of Representatives, Committee on Appropriations, *Hearings. Departments of Labor, and Health, Education and Welfare Appropriation for FY 1960*, p. 751, 86th Congress, 1st Session; Harry M. Marks, Interview with Christian R. Klimt, May 16, 1984. On Klimt's background, see Christian R. Klimt, "Varied Acceptance of Clinical Trial Results," *Controlled Clinical Trials* 10 (1989), Supplement 2, 135S–136S; Genell S. Knatterud and Curtis Meinert, "A Tribute to Christian Robert Klimt (1918–1994)," *Controlled Clinical Trials* 16 (June 1995), 139–142.

port an "almost unique example of a prospective study," endorsed the UGDP plans.[29]

The UGDP was organized as a multicenter trial with three aims:

1. To evaluate the effects of controlling blood glucose levels on the development of vascular (and other) complications;
2. To study the natural history of these complications; and
3. To improve methods in clinical trials.[30]

The study's primary purpose was to resolve the long-standing controversy among physicians as to whether strict and effective control of blood glucose levels would delay or prevent the onset of vascular complications. Much of the evidence in support of this claim was based on the accumulated clinical experiences of individual practitioners, or on retrospective analyses of patients' records from diabetes clinics. Knowles, long a critic of strict diabetic control, argued that a prospective, randomized, and double-blind study could avoid the problems of selection bias and partisan assessment, which had heretofore plagued historically controlled studies.[31]

Equally important to NIAMD reviewers was the study's potential contribution to "the methodology of clinical trials."[32] The UGDP was intended as a model of clinical investigation. Newly diagnosed diabetics from twelve university clinics were randomly assigned to one of four treatment groups: a group receiving insulin at dosages that were adjusted at regular intervals to keep blood glucose levels at targeted levels (IVAR); a group receiving a fixed insulin dosage (ISTD); a group receiving the oral hypoglycemic agent, tolbutamide (TOLB); and a group receiving a placebo. While it was impossible to conceal the use of insulin, where possible the study was "double-blinded" so that neither patients nor treating physicians knew who was receiving tolbutamide and who placebo. At the onset of the study,

29 Special Review Committee, General Comments on Application 06876-01, May 15, 1960, on file at Division of Research Grants, National Institute of Arthritis, Diabetes, and Digestive and Kidney Diseases [hereafter cited as DRG, NIADDKD].
30 University Group Diabetes Program, "Study of the Effects of Hypoglycemic Agents on Vascular Complications in Patients with Adult-Onset Diabetes. I. Design, Methods and Baseline Results," *Diabetes* 19 (1970) Supplement 2, 747.
31 Harvey C. Knowles, "The Problem of the Relation of the Control of Diabetes to the Development of Vascular Disease," *Transactions of the American Clinical and Climatological Association* 76 (1964), 142–147. On Knowles's background and views, see Reginald C. Tsang, "Dr. Harvey Knowles's Contributions to the Field of Diabetes and Pregnancy," *American Journal of Perinatology* 5 (October 1988), 309–311. Not all specialists agreed that a prospective trial, however desirable, was feasible. The Joslin Clinic's Alexander Marble raised questions about the feasibility of such a trial for individuals with NIDDM, in whom the effects of treatment on the appearance of vascular complications were potentially confounded by the duration of undiagnosed disease, and by the prevalence of vascular disease unrelated to diabetes in such a middle-aged population. See Marble, "Control of Diabetes" (n. 19), p. 495.
32 The UGDP's role as an "almost unique example of a prospective study" and the "promise of secondary gains in the methodology of clinical trials" were strongly emphasized by the committee that considered their initial application. Special Review Committee, General Comments on Application 06876-01, May 15, 1960, on file at DRG, NIADDKD.

all 1,027 patients received instruction in the use of a standard diet for diabetics, regardless of which treatment group they belonged to.[33] The program of data collection was to be both comprehensive and exemplary: examinations were scheduled upon admission to the trial and at yearly intervals thereafter. The researchers introduced new objective measures of complications such as neuropathy and diabetic retinopathy, in preference to conventional "subjective" clinical assessments.[34]

The investigators' focus was on the incidence of complications, and they had not expected to find substantial differences in mortality among the treatment groups.[35] As the study progressed, however, routine monitoring of mortality began to indicate an unfavorable trend for patients on tolbutamide, particularly for those dying of cardiovascular causes. The statistical director, Christian Klimt, first called the attention of this trend to the other investigators in 1967, and began to search for baseline differences which might explain results, which, if anything, were the opposite of what might have been expected when the trial was conceived.[36] As the higher mortality continued in the group's weekly monitoring of the data, Klimt became increasingly concerned. At the onset, few of the clinicians agreed: "They couldn't conceive, nobody could conceive, a drug which had been by that time, I don't know, eighteen years on the U.S. market . . . could potentially do harm of such a serious nature that you would get a difference in total death. And by derivation, you know, a much greater difference in cardiovascular mortality."[37]

---

33 Insulin dosages were calculated by a formula relating insulin to body surface: in the IVAR group, dosages would be adjusted at intervals according to how well controlled the patient was; in the ISTD group, initial dosages tailored to individuals were selected in the same way, but unless the patient's health was threatened, the dosages were not to be adjusted. Naturally, it was impossible to blind clinicians or patients to the fact that they were injecting insulin; all evaluations, however, were done by laboratories blind to the patient's treatment status. A fifth treatment group, receiving phenformin, another oral hypoglycemic agent, was added in the second year of the study in six of the UGDP's twelve participating clinics. In order to obtain sufficient numbers of patients in the phenformin group, six patients of every fourteen were allocated to phenformin in these clinics, and two each were assigned to IVAR, ISTD, placebo, or tolbutamide. See UGDP, "I. Design, Method and Baseline Results" (n. 30), 748–750. The effect of this procedure was to drastically reduce the number of patients on tolbutamide and placebo in half the UGDP clinics, a decision that subsequently became the source of some controversy in interpreting the results; the number of tolbutamide and placebo patients in the study overall remained equal, however.

34 Ibid., 751–757, 774–776.

35 The study was initially funded for only five years and one criteria of eligibility was that patients enrolled in the study be expected to live at least that long. The investigators did not, therefore, expect to have a sufficient number of deaths to evaluate the effects of treatment on mortality. The primary outcomes were the neurological, retinal, kidney, and vascular complications characteristic of diabetes. Substantial mortality differences began to appear only after the initial grant was renewed and the life of the study extended. Marks, Interview with Klimt, May 16, 1984. See also the renewal application [06876-06] from the UGDP investigators, on file at DRG, NIADDKD.

36 Marks, Interview with Klimt, May 16, 1984. See also Camerini-Davalos and Cole, *Early Diabetes* (n. 26), pp. 443–470; Camerini-Davalos, "Treatment of Chemical Diabetes" (n. 26), pp. 231–232; Felman and Fitterer, "The Prophylactic Use of Oral Hypoglycemic Drugs" (n. 26), pp. 243–254.

37 Marks, Interview with Klimt, May 16, 1984.

The UGDP investigators faced an unprecedented dilemma: How much evidence is needed that a treatment is harming patients before researchers end that treatment? Although the ethics of starting clinical trials had been extensively discussed, the ethics of stopping them had not. Moreover, statisticians had not given much thought to analyzing data from trials that were prematurely ended. Although numerous indications cast suspicion on tolbutamide, traditional statistical procedures provided limited guidance for interpreting such interim results.[38]

Finding themselves in uncharted territory, the UGDP investigators requested that two outside statisticians – NIH's Jerome Cornfield and Stanford University's Byron Brown – review Klimt's findings.[39] Meanwhile, the mortality differences between patients on tolbutamide and placebo continued to mount. By early 1969, Klimt was among those investigators who saw little point in continuing: even if the effect of tolbutamide was not as strong as the data suggested, it was no longer possible to demonstrate a benefit for the drug. Continued use of tolbutamide by the UGDP, in his view, was therefore unethical. Others in the group, less sure of the findings, felt that the study should continue with the treatment, if for no other reason than to demonstrate convincingly tolbutamide's harmful effects to others.[40]

These differences of opinion erupted at a meeting of the UGDP's principal investigators called in June 1969, to discuss the executive committee's recommendation that treatment with tolbutamide be discontinued. After two days of discussion, the majority voted 21–5 to stop using the drug. The FDA and the three

38 Although stopping procedures and protocols for analyzing experimental data from such studies were relatively well developed for industrial research, little use was made of them in medicine prior to the UGDP, which pioneered in the application of procedures for monitoring and analyzing interim data. See UGDP, "Study of the Effects of Hypoglycemic Agents on Vascular Complications in Patients with Adult-Onset Diabetes: II. Mortality Results," *Diabetes* 19 (1970) Supplement 2, 792–796, 819–822. See also Jerome Cornfield and Samuel W. Greenhouse, "On Certain Aspects of Sequential Clinical Trials," in Jerzy Neyman and Lucien M. Le Cam, eds., *Fifth Berkeley Symposium on Mathematical Statistics and Probability* (Berkeley: University of California Press, 1967), vol. 4, pp. 813–829.

39 Baseline differences in cardiovascular disease did not seem to account for the findings: mortality differences between tolbutamide and placebo patients appeared more pronounced for patients who entered the study without signs of cardiovascular disease than for those with prior cardiac problems. Analysis of the data as of September 1968 found that mortality differences were greatest for patients who had been in the study longest and held up best for patients with good adherence to treatment. Nonetheless, the statistical procedures for analyzing such interim mortality results were hardly conclusive: alternative approaches applied to this data gave different indications. Klimt selected Jerome Cornfield and Byron Brown Jr. as outside reviewers; Cornfield was currently doing work on the theory of interim analysis in conjunction with the Coronary Drug Project, on which he and Klimt were working. See *Summary of the September 1968 UGDP Progress Report and the Resolutions Adopted at UGDP Investigators Meeting of October 4, 1968* and Jerome Cornfield to Max Miller, June 12, 1969, Jerome Cornfield papers, Department of Special Collections, Park Library, Iowa State University, Ames, Iowa [hereafter cited as Cornfield papers]. NIH officials approved Klimt's request for outside consultants on November 20, 1968. LeMar Remmert to Christian Klimt, November 20, 1968, DRG, NIADDK.

40 Marks, Interview with Klimt, May 16, 1984. On the ethical dilemma faced by investigators, see also Theodore B. Schwartz, "The Tolbutamide Controversy: A Personal Perspective," *Ann Int Med* 75 (1971), 305–306.

firms contributing drugs to the study were to be notified immediately of the decision.[41]

The UGDP's decision to terminate the use of tolbutamide before completion of the study was a reasonable one, based on the premise that no matter how long the study continued, it was unlikely, although not impossible, that it would demonstrate a net benefit for the drug. Given this assessment, a majority of the investigators agreed that it was unethical to expose patients any longer to the possible risks associated with the drug. Their subsequent presentation to the scientific community succinctly conveyed this rationale:

The findings of this study indicate that the combination of diet and tolbutamide therapy is no more effective than diet alone in prolonging life. Moreover, the findings suggest that tolbutamide and diet may be less effective than diet alone or than diet and insulin at least insofar as cardiovascular mortality is concerned. For this reason, use of tolbutamide has been discontinued in the UGDP.[42]

It is difficult to imagine a more cautiously worded or carefully reasoned conclusion. Even so, agreement entailed several collateral beliefs, which proved not to be universally shared:

1. That the conclusion regarding the potential risks of using tolbutamide was, on balance, likely to be correct;
2. Correspondingly, that alternative explanations of the heightened cardiovascular mortality in the tolbutamide group were implausible;
3. That the study had adequately demonstrated the lack of efficacy, as well as the potential hazards, of tolbutamide;
4. That the study had appropriately measured the potential benefits of using the drug.

In the majority's opinion, the rigorous experimental design of the UGDP contributed greatly to their belief in these premises and their confidence in the decision.

41 See *Minutes,* Executive Committee, UGDP, May 28, 1969; *Minutes,* Principal Investigators Meeting, UGDP, June 5-6, 1969. At the time I consulted them, these materials were in the possession of the late Thomas C. Chalmers. I am greatly indebted to Dr. Chalmers for making them available to me [hereafter cited as Chalmers papers]. According to Angela Bowen, one of the dissident members of the group, the initial votes were more even, and it took extensive lobbying to bring the vote to the 21-5 result (Interview with Bowen, November 10, 1981). The minutes do not contain counts of any previous votes, though they document extensive discussion among participants. The possibility that tolbutamide was *not* toxic remained a real one for some participants. Jerome Cornfield, one of two outside statistical consultants, was reluctant to "unequivocally" conclude that the drug was toxic, although Cornfield made it clear that he personally would refuse the drug. He nonetheless recommended that treatment with tolbutamide be discontinued; see Cornfield to Max Miller, June 12, 1969, Cornfield papers. After the FDA expressed doubts about the strength of the finding, Max Miller, the UGDP's chairman, again raised the possibility of continuing the tolbutamide component of the study to establish a more definitive finding. Miller appears, however, largely to have been looking for NIAMD to take an official stance on the decision. *Minutes, FDA-UGDP Meeting,* June 16, 1969; Dr. Remmert [Diabetes Program Director, NIAMD] to Donald Whedon [Director NIAMD] June 16, 1969. Both in Chalmers papers.
42 UGDP, "II. Mortality Results" (n. 38), 814.

A minority of the UGDP investigators, however, strongly questioned the strength of the evidence presented, on the basis of doubts about these underlying premises.

In particular, investigators whose own experience with the drug had been favorable thought that differences in medical management among the participating clinics might just as well explain the level of mortality in the tolbutamide group. The tolbutamide mortality was heavily concentrated in four of the clinics, leading to the supposition that differences in medical care or patient risk factors, not differences in the drug, accounted for the finding.[43] The possibility that alternative explanations existed for the excess cardiovascular mortality, coupled with an underlying belief in the benefits offered by the drugs, led these participants to quarrel with the decision. Yet had it not been for the events that accompanied the announcement of the UGDP decision the following spring, these differences of opinion might never have led to such a vociferous controversy.

TOLBUTAMIDE: BIRTH OF A CONTROVERSY

Between June 1969 and May 1970, the UGDP investigators were preparing their data for presentation at the American Diabetes Association's (ADA) annual meeting. Meanwhile, only a small group of specialists in diabetes, drug evaluation, and clinical research knew of their suspicions regarding tolbutamide.[44] Several weeks before the UGDP presented its results at the June 1970 meeting, the *Washington Post* and the *New York Times* publicly announced the study's findings.[45] The FDA quickly issued a summary statement, announcing its intention to revise the labeling for tolbutamide and other sulfonylurea drugs.[46]

43 Not all the doubts initially expressed came from those who dissented from the ultimate decision. One investigator requested a reanalysis of the autopsy data, to see if the differences in cardiovascular deaths would be sustained on closer examination. See *Minutes,* Principal Investigators Meeting, UGDP, June 5–6, 1969, Chalmers papers, and Harry M. Marks, Interviews with Robert Reeves and Angela Bowen, November 10, 1981.

44 Apart from the UGDP investigators and their consultants, individuals aware of the findings included Alvan Feinstein, recruited as a consultant for Upjohn Pharmaceutical Company to review the findings early in 1969; representatives of Upjohn; members of the FDA's Medical Advisory Board, who heard a presentation on the UGDP's findings from the FDA's Charles Anello and Edwin Ortiz in June 1969; Donald Whedon, director of NIAMD, and other NIAMD officials; and various specialists in the treatment of diabetes, including Robert Bradley, subsequently chair of the Committee for the Care of the Diabetic, which was highly critical of the UGDP study.

45 Morton Mintz, "Antidiabetes Pill Held Causing Early Death," *Washington Post,* May 21, 1970, pp. 1, 7. The *Post* article was followed by one in the *New York Times,* the following day: Harold M. Schmeck Jr., "Scientists Wary on Diabetes Pill," *New York Times,* May 22, 1970, p. 56. Of the two, the initial *Post* article was the more alarmist. Given the number of individuals with some knowledge of the study at this point, it is not surprising that the individual responsible for the leak has never been identified. Harvey Knowles has speculated that the leak must be due to one of the circulating copies of the ADA program, released in mid-May. See Knowles, "An Historical View" (n. 27), 156. The supplement of *Diabetes* containing the program abstract arrived at the Francis Countway Library of Medicine of Harvard University on May 26, 1970, five days after the national publicity broke.

46 "FDA Statement. Friday, May 22, 1970," *Diabetes* 19 (1970), Supplement 1, 467. For more on the circumstances surrounding the FDA announcement, see subsequent discussion.

For the twenty-six UGDP investigators, the decision to terminate tolbutamide had been difficult. Yet the difficulty they faced paled in comparison with the next step: reassessing tolbutamide for the 800,000 patients estimated to be using the drug.[47] The premature announcement of the UGDP findings left physicians around the country with few answers for diabetics calling to ask about the safety of their current medication.[48] Abstracts of the study published in *Diabetes* at the end of May added only a few paragraphs of information concerning its design and startling conclusion. Max Miller, chairman of the UGDP group, while deploring the premature notice of the findings, felt it "inappropriate" to comment further before the study received peer review.[49] Like their patients, most physicians remained reliant on the various press reports that appeared over the summer of 1970.[50] Criticisms of the study in the medical press were equally fragmentary and even less informative.[51]

Evaluation of a complex study like the UGDP customarily progresses at what seems like a glacial pace, in the relative obscurity of specialist communities. The experts can consider themselves fortunate if anyone pays immediate attention to what they eventually decide. In the UGDP's case, however, attitudes and opinions were formed in the glare of publicity, and exchanged in the popular media alongside discussion in more sheltered forums. More than one disputant discovered an unexplored gift for polemic along the way. The early notoriety given the UGDP did much to upstage and short-circuit the customary processes of peer review. The widespread publicity announcing the study imparted urgency to each deliberation: prompt action was called for to resolve the uncertainties of patients and physicians alike.

In the ensuing debate, much of the subtlety of the UGDP's reasoning concerning the use of tolbutamide was lost. The group's initial decision had been premised on a complex calculus of risk and benefit, issuing in the judgment that, in the absence of benefit, any evidence of risk needed to be heavily weighted. By and large, beliefs about the possible benefits of tolbutamide remained in the background of subsequent discussions, despite the repeated efforts of UGDP supporters to center the debate on this issue. The spotlight focused instead on the critics'

47 Mintz, "Antidiabetes Pill Held Causing Early Death" (n. 45).
48 "The Tolbutamide Debate," *Medical World News* 12 (January 8, 1971), 39.
49 Thaddeus E. Prout and Martin G. Goldner, "The University Group Diabetes Program: The Effects of Hypoglycemic Agents on Vascular Complications in Patients with Adult Onset Diabetes. 2. Findings at Baseline. 3. Course and Mortality," *Diabetes* 19 (1970), Supplement 1, 374–375. For Miller's remark, see "Statement of Chairman of UGDP [May 21, 1970]," *Diabetes* 19 (June 1970), 467–468.
50 Harold M. Schmeck Jr. "Diabetes Drug Use Backed by Council," *New York Times,* June 15, 1970, p. 42; Harold M. Schmeck Jr., "Pills for the Diabetic: Dilemma for Doctors," *New York Times,* June 22, 1970, pp. 1, 25.
51 Robert L. Reeves, "Erroneous Interpretation of Data," *Northwest Medicine* 69 (July 1970), 870; "The Tolbutamide Controversy," *JAMA* 213 (August 3, 1970), 861.

claims that the UGDP's conclusion about excess mortality associated with tolbuta-mide was invalid, bringing issues about experimental design and inference to the fore.[52]

By December 1970, when the UGDP published extensive details of the study's design and findings, its opponents' basic arguments were already well staked out. Echoing concerns of the UGDP's internal dissenters, critics raised questions about the analysis and distribution of cardiovascular disease among patients in the study. Despite the randomization procedure, the tolbutamide group appeared to be sicker, particularly with regard to cardiovascular risk factors. While none of these baseline differences appeared to be statistically significant, questions remained as to their cumulative effect. Critics were particularly concerned about omitted risk factors such as smoking, not taken into account when the study was designed.[53] The second basic challenge to the tolbutamide finding concerned the distribution of deaths within the study. Deaths appeared to be concentrated in a minority of clinics, raising questions about the selection or management of patients in these cities.[54]

Proponents of the UGDP took remarks about baseline inequalities within the study populations as fundamental criticisms, challenges to what is sometimes termed the "internal validity" of a study. Evidence of such inequalities, even in a subset of the clinics, might be taken as grounds for believing that the randomiza-tion procedure had "broken down," allowing physician bias in patient assignment to enter. In their initial report, the UGDP researchers examined this issue at length. Of ten cardiovascular risk factors, there was a statistically significant difference between the tolbutamide and placebo groups for only one – serum cholesterol. Given the number of factors recorded, chance alone might well be responsible for that difference.[55] As for variations in mortality by clinic, the UGDP team had looked extensively for differences in population characteristics or cardiovascular risk factors that could explain these: among the factors they

---

52 The focus on tolbutamide mortality and on the UGDP's lack of validity is emphasized in *Statement on the Treatment of Diabetes,* telegraph to the Commissioner of Food and Drugs, December 1, 1970, from assembled critics of the UGDP, FDA Docket 75N-0062, vol. 2, on file with Office of the Hearing Clerk, Food and Drug Administration, Rockville, MD, hereafter FDA Docket 75N-0062.

53 On the distribution of cardiovascular risk factors, see [Alvan Feinstein], *An Analytic Critique of the UGDP Protocols* [June 1969], pp. 19–20; idem, *A Supplemental Critique of Recent UGDP Reports* [August 1969], pp. 4–6; and E. Keith Borden [Upjohn Company], *Preliminary Evaluation of the UGDP Report of May 9, 1969* [June 1969], pp. 2, 7–9. On the question of omitted risk factors, see Feinstein, *Supplemental Critique,* p. 4. All documents cited are in Cornfield papers. These criticisms were echoed and elaborated in Feinstein's published article: "Clinical Biostatistics VIII. An Analytic Appraisal of the University Group Diabetes Program (UGDP) Study," *Clinical Pharmacology and Therapeutics* 12 (1971), 172–173, 177–178, 185–189. See also Stanley Schor, "The University Group Diabetes Program: A Statistician Looks at the Mortality Results," *JAMA* 217 (September 20, 1971), 1671–1673.

54 Borden, *Preliminary Evaluation of the UGDP* (n. 53), pp. 2–6; Feinstein, "An Analytic Appraisal" (n. 53), 177–178; Schor, "A Statistician Looks" (n. 53), 1673–1674.

55 UGDP, "II. Mortality Results" (n. 38), 799–803.

examined, they found none of statistical significance.[56] Subsequent reviews came to similar conclusions: the variations in mortality among the clinics were no more than might be expected by chance, and the known differences in risk factors could not explain the increased mortality in these clinics.[57]

For statisticians who viewed the UGDP favorably, demonstrating the integrity of the randomization provided equal reassurance about the role of risk factors like smoking, on which the investigators did not collect data. For the study's proponents, critics' arguments about omitted risk factors showed a misunderstanding of the ability of randomization "to achieve approximate comparability with respect to all variables, whether known or not." In their defense of the UGDP, statisticians emphasized the power of randomized experiments to overcome shortcomings in medical knowledge. The basic rationale for introducing randomized allocation in medicine, NIH's Jerome Cornfield reminded critics, was that so many of the factors that might influence outcome are unknown. Since there was no evidence that the randomization procedure had failed, critics' concerns about the distribution of unreported risks in the study were unfounded, according to Cornfield.[58]

The statistician Paul Meier has observed that much of the argument over the UGDP concerns a fundamental difference over the purposes of randomization: some holding with Bradford Hill that the aim is to make the groups "as nearly equal as possible" whereas others, following R. A. Fisher, rely on randomization to "provide a firm basis" for the use of the statistical tests customarily applied. Adherence to the former view, Meier suggested, set the UGDP critics on the prowl for factors that might be unevenly distributed in the two groups, neglecting the contention that such baseline variations rarely alter the robustness of the analysis. What Meier neglected to mention, however, was how much statisticians contributed to the confusion about randomization. In the UGDP debate, his colleague Cornfield's account of randomization sounds as much or more like Hill's than Fisher's.[59]

Critics of the UGDP attached equal or greater importance, however, to a set of clinical issues that were more difficult to articulate and examine within the language and framework of statistical inference. First, they argued that the fixed dosage of tolbutamide used in the study may have been inappropriately high. Their argument was a physiological one, based on experimental and clinical experience with the drug. High initial dosages might lead to a large rate of secondary failures, patients whose blood glucose was excessive after several years of treatment because they no longer responded to the drug. If so, the cardiovascu-

---

56 Ibid., 807–809, 823–826.
57 Jerome Cornfield, "The University Group Diabetes Program: A Further Statistical Analysis of the Mortality Findings," *JAMA* 217 (September 20, 1971), 1676–1687.
58 Ibid., 1676.
59 See Meier, "Statistics and Medical Experimentation" (n. 6), 519.

lar mortality seen might be the result of using tolbutamide inappropriately, rather than an inherent property of the drug itself.[60]

Similarly, critics maintained that the high rate of vascular complications in the study suggested that many of the patients were sicker at the onset than the UGDP investigators assumed. "All they are really saying is that high-risk patients die sooner than low-risk patients." Critics were arguing that many of these patients ought not to have been on oral hypoglycemics in the first place, and that, consequently, the findings were no test of the drug's safety.[61]

UGDP spokesmen responded that the fixed dosages and diagnostic criteria employed approximated those used in the majority of clinical practices in the country; by implication, the findings could reasonably be extrapolated to these patients.[62] In short, they read both criticisms as challenges to the study's external validity. What the critics were implying, however, was not that the UGDP had drawn the wrong conclusion but that it had conducted the wrong study.

METHODENSTREIT

The issue is whether or not medicine is to become a science or is to remain an art.[63]

The issue is not between medicine as a science and medicine as an art, but whether or not we are to accept at face value questionable conclusions from inadequate data.[64]

For most onlookers, the UGDP controversy was concerned with the appropriate treatment of diabetes. To a small handful of participants, the debate raised questions concerning the appropriate role of statistical methods in clinical investigation. Few of the diabetologists with reservations about the UGDP's findings were equipped to challenge the study's distinguished consultants on points of experimental procedure and analysis. But for Yale University's Alvan Feinstein, the UGDP offered an unusual opportunity to voice his reservations about the growing influence of statisticians in epidemiological research.

An advocate of the importance of clinical expertise in medical research, Feinstein attributed the UGDP's difficulties to an overconfidence in statistical procedures and a neglect of "biologic logic" and "clinical judgment" in designing

---

60 Minutes, Ad Hoc Committee Meeting on UGDP, May 21, 1970, FDA Docket 75N-0062, vol. 7.
61 Robert Bradley, quoted in "The Tolbutamide Debate," *Medical World News* 12 (January 8, 1971), 38.
62 Thaddeus Prout, Genell L. Knatterud, Curtis L. Meinert, and Christian Klimt, "The UGDP Controversy: Clinical Trials versus Clinical Impressions," *Diabetes* 21 (October 1972), 1037–1038.
63 Max Miller in "The Tolbutamide Debate," *Medical World News* 12 (January 8, 1971), 37.
64 Robert Bradley in ibid.

and interpreting the study. Initially invited to review the UGDP by the manufacturer of tolbutamide, Feinstein apparently found the study an irresistible example of all that was going awry in clinical investigation.[65] The UGDP, he argued, was not so much clinically invalid as clinically irrelevant.

To be clinically relevant, according to Feinstein, an experiment had to answer two kinds of questions: How are the patients in the study like my patients? How are they different? How are patients' lives affected by the choice of treatment "a" over treatment "b "? To be clinically meaningful, the answers to these questions had to be provided in terms the physician could recognize and readily interpret. The UGDP, in Feinstein's assessment, had failed to record interpretable information about three crucial parameters of diabetes treatment: the initial severity of the disease (including measures of comorbidity); the rates of nonfatal complications associated with each treatment; and the iatrogenic impact of insulin treatment on a patient's comfort and well-being. In the absence of such information, the UGDP was of limited use to clinicians seeking to reassess their current practice, or apply the UGDP findings to their patients.[66]

The UGDP, Feinstein maintained, was a product of its times. Working in the late 1950s, the principal investigators, in an effort to avoid the flaws in experimental design that had compromised earlier controlled studies, had gone overboard. In a misguided quest for objectivity, they had overlooked the very data needed to interpret their findings.[67] For example, the UGDP had taken great care to define the laboratory data by which eligibility for the study was determined but failed to provide any information about those rejected from the study. How were clinicians able to decide whether their own patients resembled the wheat or the chaff?[68] More important, the characterization of those who were accepted was inadequate and incomplete. The UGDP reported in detail on the rates of angina pectoris – an indication of heart disease – but what exactly did the investigators mean by angina, and did the operational definition differ from clinic to clinic?[69]

The UGDP's aspirations to methodological rigor were, Feinstein alleged, a tragic flaw. The investigators had decided that, whenever possible, evidence of complications, was to consist of *objective* measures of pathology and/or functional impairment – physical evidence that could be interpreted by individuals blind to

65 See "An Analytic Appraisal" (n. 53), 167–191; "The Persistent Clinical Failures and Fallacies of the UGDP Study," *Clinical Pharmacology and Therapeutics* 19 (1976), 78–93; "How Good Is the Statistical Evidence against Oral Hypoglycemic Agents," *Advances in Internal Medicine* 23 (1979), 71–95. For his earlier work on the methodology of clinical research, see Alvan R. Feinstein, *Clinical Judgment* (Baltimore: Williams and Wilkins, 1967).

66 Feinstein, "An Analytic Appraisal" (n. 53), 169–175.

67 Ibid., 175–176, 187–189.

68 See [Feinstein], *An Analytical Critique of the UGDP Protocols* (n. 53), pp. 2–4; idem, "An Analytic Appraisal" (n. 53), 171. One of the exclusion criteria was "inability" to follow the protocol, but "inability" was not further defined. In a chronic disease like diabetes, where patients must permanently adopt some form of treatment, this information is potentially quite valuable to the clinician trying to extrapolate research studies to his own patients.

69 Feinstein, "An Analytic Appraisal" (n. 53), 175.

the status of patients, interpretations that could, in turn, be checked by others, to control for the effects of interobserver variation. Many of these measures were introduced on a wide scale for the first time in this study. For example, to assess nerve conduction, the investigators relied on a biothesiometer, an instrument to measure nerve impulse conduction, rather than on the traditional multidimensional clinical assessment of touch, sensitivity to pain, and vibration with which most clinicians were familiar.[70] Several of these innovative measures proved difficult to interpret.[71] Perhaps most important, the UGDP did not systematically collect data on "softer" patient-reported complications, which matter a great deal in the choice of management strategies for the diabetic patient: episodes of "hypoglycemic" shock, infection rates, episodes of weakness, fatigue, headaches.[72] In summary, the UGDP was not able to provide satisfactory data on many of the intermediate (nonfatal) outcomes of diabetes, which are a consideration in choosing therapy.

Ironically, Feinstein shared with the UGDP investigators the belief that the central issue in the debate was the purported benefits of tolbutamide. Where they differed was on the question of how well the UGDP had measured those benefits. In forming judgments about the risks of using tolbutamide, Feinstein argued, physicians must consider the potential benefits it offers in comparison to insulin, with its hazards and inconveniences. As a result of efforts to accommodate the methodologists' notions of science, the clinicians in the UGDP had failed to provide the kind of information physicians needed to make therapeutic decisions. For Feinstein, the UGDP was an object lesson in the dangers of sacrificing "clinical wisdom and scientific judgment" to "rigid doctrines of statistical design" or the "conveniences" offered by computerized data processing.[73]

In the heat of the immediate debate over the mortality associated with tolbutamide, Feinstein's more fundamental criticisms of the UGDP's approach to clinical investigation went unnoticed.[74] For other critics of the study, the issue became not so much "What does the UGDP suggest I ought to do with my patients?" but "Should the FDA make suggestions about what I should do with my patients on the basis of the UGDP?" Following the FDA's decision, in the fall of 1970, to alter the package labeling that accompanied tolbutamide, critics of the study precipitated a fifteen-year-long legal and political campaign to reduce the agency's confidence in the UGDP. Arguments about the scientific merit of the study

70 For a description of the UGDP's measures, see UGDP, "I. Design, Methods and Baseline Results" (n. 30), 755–757.
71 UGDP reported difficulties in distinguishing "true" abnormalities from artifacts in their photographic records of eye examinations; the rates of abnormalities reported were unusually high. Ibid., 766–767. Apart from one preliminary report, the biothesiometer data were never reported.
72 Feinstein, "An Analytic Appraisal" (n. 53), 173–174.
73 [Feinstein], *An Analytic Critique* (n. 53), p. 25.
74 In his 1971 defense of the UGDP, Jerome Cornfield elected to reply only to criticisms that challenged the internal validity of the UGDP. Feinstein's remarks about unknown baseline inequalities were regarded as gnostic utterances which were unintelligible within the framework of statistical inference. See Cornfield "A Further Statistical Analysis" (n. 57), 1676, 1682.

were consequently conducted against the background of an impending regulatory action.

SCIENCE AND REGULATION

In June 1969, the UGDP investigators had notified the FDA of their decision to discontinue use of tolbutamide in the study.[75] So far as the regulatory agency was concerned, the UGDP's reasoning about the drug's lack of benefit was irrelevant. To justify the oral hypoglycemics' claims to efficacy, advocates need not demonstrate that the drugs reduced cardiovascular complications, but merely that they lowered blood glucose. No one was disputing that claim. The regulatory issue was the mortality finding, and the FDA's initial response was reserved. In the opinion of FDA reviewers, the number of tolbutamide deaths was small, and of borderline statistical significance. Additional numbers would make a more persuasive case.[76] The UGDP investigators stood firm in their initial decision to withdraw the drug.

While the UGDP investigators worked on their report, news of their decision reached physicians at the Joslin Clinic, which had pioneered in the use of the oral hypoglycemics. The Joslin researchers were skeptical of the reputed findings. On May 21, 1970, Henry Simmons, newly appointed head of the FDA's Bureau of Drugs, convened a meeting of the UGDP investigators with their critics.[77] On arriving at the FDA, the visiting diabetologists were greeted by an announcement of the UGDP's findings on the front page of the *Washington Post*. While their meeting proceeded as scheduled, the FDA's deliberations were cut short by the unexpected publicity.[78] The following day, the agency announced its intention to revise the labeling for the oral hypoglycemic drugs, meanwhile cautioning physicians that the drugs should only be "used only in patients with symptomatic adult

75 The UGDP investigators *may* have notified the FDA as early as November 1968 of impending problems with the drug. Summary of the September 1968 UGDP Progress Report and the Resolutions Adopted at UGDP Investigators Meeting of October 4, 1968, Cornfield papers. By June 1969, discussions with the FDA about the decision to stop tolbutamide were under way. See n. 76. The FDA, however, is unable to locate any documents concerning the UGDP prior to May 1970, and appears to date its awareness of the UGDP from March 1970. See *Federal Register* 40 (July 7, 1975), 28587.

76 *Minutes. FDA-UGDP Meeting,* June 16, 1969; Diabetes Program Director, Extramural Programs, NIAMD [LeMar F. Remmert] to Director, NIAMD [Donald Whedon], June 18, 1969, Chalmers papers. The FDA's Medical Advisory Board was equally tentative about the UGDP's provisional findings and advised that the FDA await publication of the study results before acting. FDA, Bureau of Medicine, Medical Advisory Board, *Minutes. June 26–27, 1969,* pp. 6–7, Box 6, Harry Dowling papers, MS C 372, NLM.

77 Present at the meeting were Christian Klimt and Jerome Cornfield, statistical experts from the UGDP; Stanley Schor, a statistician critical of the findings; Robert Bradley and George Cahill, from the Joslin Clinic; a group of other prominent diabetologists (T. S. Danowski, Fred Kruger, Albert Winegrad); and Drs. Finkel, Simmons, Ortiz, and Anello from the FDA. *Minutes, Ad Hoc Committee Meeting on UGDP,* May 21, 1970, FDA Docket 75N-0062, vol. 7.

78 Harry M. Marks, Interview with Robert Bradley, May 20, 1985. The FDA notes of the meeting suggest a "consensus favoring support of conclusions of the UGDP." *Minutes, Ad Hoc Committee Meeting on UGDP,* May 21, 1970, FDA Docket 75N-0062, vol. 7.

onset diabetes mellitus who cannot be adequately controlled by diet alone and who are not insulin dependent (i.e. do not require insulin)."[79]

Closely following the "uniquely pernicious" "gun-jumping public release of the UGDP findings," the FDA's sudden action surprised and alarmed the UGDP's critics. Nonetheless, it was hardly irrevocable. Through the summer of 1970, the agency continued to negotiate with interested parties the precise wording of the revised package labeling for the suspect drugs.[80] On October 22, 1970, FDA officials announced their plan to caution doctors against using oral hypoglycemics for mild diabetics, except in cases where insulin is unacceptable and diet does not work. However moderate these guidelines, they did not satisfy the UGDP's critics. Followed by similar recommendations from the AMA and ADA, the FDA's new pronouncement precipitated a crisis for proponents of the oral hypoglycemics.[81] The drugs' advocates charged that the agency's ruling raised the prospect of malpractice suits for physicians who continued to use the drugs routinely.[82] They responded by holding a national press conference, announcing the formation of a Committee on the Care of the Diabetic (CCD) to persuade the FDA to revise its warning notice.[83]

Over the next twenty months (December 1970–July 1972), the CCD and the FDA conducted an intricate war of words over the precise nature of the labeling changes indicated by the UGDP. The FDA proceeded to its time-honored task of guiding therapeutic practice by managing the language accompanying drug products. To FDA officials, the proposed changes in labeling for the oral hypoglycemics were relatively minor and backed by the weight of scientific and medical authority.[84] Although the CCD's grievances were numerous and varied, its primary concern was that the FDA not unduly "expose" the practicing physician to "medicolegal redress."[85] Adequate protection, in its view, required the FDA to

79 "FDA Statement, May 22, 1970," *Diabetes* 19 (June 1970), 467.

80 *Memorandum of Conference,* July 1, 1970, Records of the Food and Drug Administration. On the importance of premature publicity to the UGDP's critics, see Holbrooke Seltzer to Thomas C. Chalmers, May 20, 1971, Chalmers papers.

81 Harold M. Schmeck Jr., "FDA Cites Doubt on Diabetes Pill," *New York Times,* October 22, 1970, pp. 1, 54; "Doctors Cautioned by AMA Council about Diabetes Pill," *New York Times,* October 23, 1970, p. 17; "New Caution Issued on Drug in Diabetes," *New York Times,* October 28, 1970, p. 30.

82 Robert F. Bradley to Henry Simmons, February 26, 1971, FDA Docket 75N-0062, vol. 2.

83 "Forty Diabetes Experts Deplore Warning on Drug by F.D.A.," *New York Times,* December 2, 1970, p. 19; "In Boston: A Diabetes Tea Party Hits FDA," *Medical World News* (December 18, 1970), pp. 13–14.

84 "2 FDA Officials Defend Position As a Consensus," *Medical Tribune* (November 23, 1970), pp. 1, 20. On the background to the FDA's labeling policies, see Chapter 3, and Harry M. Marks, "Revisiting 'The Origins of Compulsory Drug Prescriptions,' " *AJPH* 85 (January 1995), 109–115.

85 Robert F. Bradley to Henry Simmons, February 26, 1971, vol. 2; *Minutes of Meeting on Labeling of Oral Hypoglycemic Agents,* April 5, 1974, vol. 7; *Memorandum of Meeting Held Wednesday, June 11, 1975,* vol. 7. Since the FDA was still drafting the wording of the labeling to be published in the *Federal Register,* its approach was also in flux, with new initiatives prompting new commentary from the CCD and other onlookers. John Jennings to Charles C. Edwards, March 22, 1971, vol. 2. All documents in FDA Docket 75N-0062.

acknowledge officially the differences of opinion in the medical community concerning the strength of the UGDP study. What may have seemed to CCD representatives a matter of minor consequence posed major difficulties for the regulators.

Shortly before learning of the UGDP case, the FDA had completed a major revision of their policies regarding the scientific evidence acceptable in agency procedures. Eight years after the passage of the 1962 Drug Amendments, the FDA had finally issued regulations describing its requirements for the "well-controlled clinical investigations," which by law were to be the basis of new drug approvals.[86] The new standards had been the subject of a protracted legal struggle regarding the FDA's authority to apply them to drugs, like tolbutamide, which had been approved prior to the 1962 amendments.[87] The criticisms being offered of the UGDP, however reasonable to some diabetologists, did not meet the criteria of "substantial evidence" as defined by the regulations; in the FDA's judgment, "an undiluted and unencumbered warning" was "fully warranted by the available evidence."[88] Translated into practical terms, this meant that differences of opinion over the UGDP would not be mentioned in the new labeling.

The FDA's decision to proceed with new labeling for tolbutamide was based less on a detailed consideration of the legal situation, however, than on a belief that the weight of scientific and medical authority endorsed the UGDP. While negotiating with the UGDP's critics over the wording of the proposed warning, FDA officials were also seeking to assure themselves that the UGDP's supporters would "not pull the rug out from them regarding the package insert."[89] Among the scientific authorities they consulted were officials at the NIH.

NIH officials had more than a passing interest in the developing controversy over the UGDP. Donald Whedon, director of NIAMD, which had funded the study, had participated in the UGDP's deliberations to discontinue the drug.[90]

86 *Federal Register* 35 (May 8, 1970), 7250–7053.
87 The cases, which involved the FDA's right to remove approval from pre-1962 drugs without a hearing unless the manufacturer could produce two studies that met the agency's standards of "substantial evidence," are reviewed in Richard A. Merrill and Peter Barton Hutt, *Food and Drug Law: Cases and Materials* (Mineola, NY: Foundation Press, 1980), pp. 374–375. See also "Drug Efficacy and the 1962 Drug Amendments," *Georgetown Law Journal* 60 (1971), 185–224. Earlier efforts to review the status of pre-1962 drugs under the new law had encountered substantial political and legal difficulties, including a protracted lawsuit by Upjohn Company, tolbutamide's manufacturer, against the FDA's proposed policies for pre-1962 drugs. See "Drug Efficacy," 214–221.
88 This is the FDA's paraphrase of a letter from FDA Commissioner Charles Edwards to Neil L. Chayet [Counsel for the CCD], June 5, 1972, as cited in the *Federal Register* 40 (July 7, 1975), 28588. The full letter appears in U.S. Senate, Select Committee on Small Business, Subcommittee on Monopoly, *Hearings on Competitive Problems in the Drug Industry. May 9–10, June 21, and July 1979*, part 22, pp. 8796–8800, 92nd Congress, 2nd Session.
89 Thomas C. Chalmers [NIH] to Deputy Director for Science, NIH, and Associate Director for Program Planning and Evaluation, NIH, March 23, 1971, Chalmers papers.
90 *Minutes*, Principal Investigators Meeting, June 5–6, 1969, Chalmers papers. In response to questioning at this meeting, Whedon had indicated that he thought the decision to discontinue

With an active program of support for clinical trials, senior NIH officials were concerned about the profession's response to the UGDP. When the initial controversy failed to subside, NIH's director, Robert Marston, asked Thomas Chalmers, director of the NIH's Clinical Center, to review the debate.[91]

A physician passionately committed to controlled trials, Chalmers nonetheless produced a balanced assessment of the controversy. In particular, he attempted to distinguish between the investigators' decision to discontinue tolbutamide in the study and the claim "that tolbutamide actually causes an increased death rate." The former was based on the belief that "this study could not possibly have missed a favorable effect" of the oral hypoglycemic drugs. A simple calculation of sample size, Chalmers observed, would demonstrate the reasonableness of this decision. Evaluating the latter claim would require an extensive analysis of the UGDP's procedures and an examination of other studies.[92] Chalmers's carefully drawn distinction was wasted on NIH Director Marston, who reported to the FDA "that the conclusions of the study are valid" and that "the technical objections have been satisfactorily rebutted," both by the UGDP's coordinating center and its "consulting biostatisticians." The FDA's "proposed package insert on tolbutamide," Marston reassured Commissioner Edwards, "seems to us to be a fair representation of the state of our knowledge."[93]

Armed with a favorable report from NIH and the other authorities they consulted, FDA officials proceeded to formulate their warning statement on oral hypoglycemics, while the CCD proceeded to the courts. In July 1973, the CCD obtained the first of a series of restraining orders preventing the FDA from issuing new labeling on tolbutamide. For the rest of the decade, the CCD's lawyers occupied the courts with aspects of the UGDP case. The legal issues in these suits were complex and like the terms of the controversy itself, shifted as old ground was lost or new targets of opportunity arose. Nonetheless, the CCD's lawyers effectively prevented the FDA from taking final action on the drug until 1984.[94]

Meanwhile, diabetes specialists debated the merits of the UGDP's study. To the beleaguered UGDP investigators, it was not the continuation of the debate but its

---

tolbutamide was warranted, and that the investigators could even recommend having the drug taken off the market.

91 Max Miller to Jerome Cornfield, March 5, 1971, Chalmers papers.

92 Thomas C. Chalmers, *The Controversy over Oral Anti-Diabetic Agents* [Memorandum for Robert Q. Marston], March 11, 1971, Chalmers papers. Chalmers was an early convert to the gospel of controlled trials. See H. Popper, "American Gastroenterological Association: Award of Friedenwald Medal to Thomas Clark Chalmers," *Gastroenterology* 83 (October, 1982), 736–737; Edwin D. Kilbourne, "Presentation of the Academy Medal to Thomas C. Chalmers, M.D.," *Bull NY Acad Med* 63 (December 1987), 912–915.

93 Robert Q. Marston to Charles C. Edwards, April 5, 1971, Chalmers papers.

94 *Federal Register* 40 (July 7, 1975), 28589. The issues raised ranged from questions of administrative procedure and due process to more basic challenges concerning the scope of the FDA's authority and the evidentiary standards required of it. Although litigation effectively prevented the FDA from taking any final action, it did not prevent the agency from entering into new rounds of hearings and negotiations in the interstices between the resolution of one suit and the filing of another.

tone that was disturbing. To Jerome Cornfield, critics seemed "more interested in making debater's points than in constructive suggestions for further analysis."[95] In the spring of 1971, NIH officials began looking for an "august" and impartial body to review the UGDP controversy. After exploring several options, they invited the Biometric Society to form a committee to assess "the validity and the conclusions of the UGDP."[96]

An international organization of statisticians specializing in medical research, the Biometric Society seemed to NIH's Chalmers the most appropriate body to review the controversy:

> We believe that the basis for any dispute about the conclusions should lie in the consider-ation of the technical details of design, execution, and statistical analyses of the [UGDP and contrasting] studies. This critique should be carried out by biostatisticians who are experi-enced in the field of clinical trials.[97]

The UGDP controversy broke out in an era when NIH's commitment to clinical trials was hotly contested, within the research community, by Congress, and within NIH itself.[98] As NIH officials reminded the statisticians, the contro-versy had implications "much broader than the clinical problem of long-term therapy in diabetes"; it could have a "distinct effect" on the NIH's approach to the planning and funding of comparable studies.[99] After assuring themselves that they would have complete access to data from the UGDP and a free hand in formulating their report, statisticians from the Biometric Society agreed to review the controversy.[100]

The Biometric Society panel included a mix of senior and junior statisticians with experience in statistical theory, research methodology, and clinical trials practice.[101] NIH's formal charge to the reviewing committee was limited: to

95 Jerome Cornfield to Max Miller, January 11, 1971, Cornfield papers.
96 Before deciding on the Biometric Society, NIH officials considered the Institute of Medicine, the National Research Council, and the American Statistical Association as possible forums for reviewing the UGDP. Thomas Chalmers, draft letter [not mailed] to Dr. [Robert] Glaser, Institute of Medicine from [Robert Marston], Director NIH, March 23, 1971; *Minutes,* July 21, 1971 [Thomas Chalmers, Peter Armitage, Byron Brown, Peter Bennett, Max Miller]; Thomas Chal-mers, "Proposal for Review of UGDP," August 6, 1971; *Minutes,* August 17, 1971 [Thomas Chalmers, Donald Whedon, Peter Armitage, Max Miller]. All Chalmers papers. On the use of advisory committees more generally, see Sheila Jasanoff, *The Fifth Branch: Science Advisers As Policymakers* (Cambridge: Harvard University Press, 1990).
97 Thomas Chalmers to Bertold Schneider [President, Biometric Society], September 14, 1971. Materials relating to the organization and activities of the Biometric Society committee were provided through the courtesy of Professor Marvin Zelen, Harvard School of Public Health, a member of the reviewing panel [hereafter cited as Zelen papers].
98 See the previous chapter on the Diet–Heart study.
99 Thomas Chalmers to Bertold Schneider, September 14, 1971; *Minutes,* Committee for Assessment of Biometric Aspects of Controlled Trials of Hypoglycemic Agents, May 18, 1972, Zelen papers.
100 See Marvin Zelen to Berthold Schneider, November 16, 1971; Thomas Chalmers to Peter Armitage, Rodolfo Saracci, Berthold Schneider, Colin White, and Marvin Zelen, February 8, 1972, Zelen papers.
101 The members included Peter Armitage, Bertold Schneider, Paul Meier, and Marvin Zelen; the committee was chaired by Yale University's Colin White.

evaluate the "scientific quality" and "in particular . . . the biometrical aspects" of the UGDP and "other controlled trials of oral hypoglycemic drugs."[102] Within the limits of this mandate, the committee's effort was extraordinary: it scrutinized in detail the UGDP operating procedures, extensively reanalyzed the data, and undertook to review not only the published critiques of the study but to interview each of the UGDP's principal critics.[103] But in preparing its report, the review committee operated under constraints of time, money, and, most especially, professional competence.

The panel divided objections to the UGDP into two broad categories: those which might affect physicians' willingness to generalize the UGDP's overall results to their own patients and those which might affect the validity of the UGDP's specific conclusions regarding the possible toxicity of tolbutamide. The former, they decided, were more a matter of medical than statistical expertise, and therefore beyond their competence to judge. The committee's statisticians would confine themselves to issue of experimental design, statistical analysis, and the "policeman's task": investigating claims that the investigators had somehow failed to follow the procedures described in their protocols.[104]

In assessing the UGDP's conclusions regarding tolbutamide, members of the committee concentrated on two areas: they carefully examined the UGDP's operating procedures, to assure themselves that the randomization had not broken down; and they reanalyzed the UGDP data to determine whether specific factors mentioned by the critics might singly or by interaction account for the findings. As befitted a blue ribbon panel of experienced statisticians, both efforts were diligent and ingenious, the committee's analyses improving in several respects on the UGDP's original handling of the data.[105] But in translating the critics' objections into the categories of statistical inference – external and internal validity – and into the mathematical procedures necessary to measure the possibility of interaction effects, the committee lost any opportunity to resolve the controversy.[106]

102 Robert Q. Marston to Colin White, June 9, 1972, cited in "Report of the Committee for the Assessment of Biometric Aspects of Controlled Trials of Hypoglycemic Agents," *JAMA* 231 (February 10, 1975), 585.

103 For a report of the committee's activities, see ibid.

104 See, for example, the committee's remarks on the appropriateness of the UGDP's selection criteria for patients in the trial: "Report of the Committee for the Assessment of Biometric Aspects of Controlled Trials of Hypoglycemic Agents" (n. 102), 591–592, 599.

105 Among the problems handled adroitly by the committee were the role of (1) clinic effects, (2) of baseline cardiovascular risk, and the effects of (3) duration of and (4) adherence to treatment on cardiovascular mortality. The committee's analysis of the first two factors was more thorough and more robust than the UGDP's initial tests, whereas the latter two issues had not been addressed directly in the UGDP's original analysis.

106 The committee was abetted in this by the near-inarticulateness of the UGDP's critics when discussing their objections to the study, which focused predominantly on charges that the UGDP had altered its measures of cardiovascular risk midway through the study. One has the impression in reading the critics' subsequent remarks on the Biometric Society's report that they literally did not comprehend how the analyses developed by the committee worked, and to what a considerable degree they addressed the majority of published criticisms of the UGDP.

The committee's conclusions were, like the UGDP's original report, circum-spect: "On the question of cardiovascular mortality due to tolbutamide . . . we consider that the UGDP trial has raised suspicions that cannot be dismissed on the basis of other evidence presently available."[107] The thoroughness of the commit-tee's review reinforced this judgment: "We find most of the criticisms leveled against the UGDP findings on this point unpersuasive. [While] . . . some reserva-tions about the conclusion that the oral hypoglycemics are toxic must remain . . . we consider the evidence of harmfulness moderately strong."[108]

To the UGDP's medical critics, who already deemed statisticians the most dispensable member in any clinical investigation, the Biometric Society's review was largely irrelevant.[109] In their view, the blue-ribbon panel had failed to address a fundamental issue: Had the UGDP in the first instance collected the appropriate data to evaluate the risk of cardiovascular disease in patients receiving tolbuta-mide?[110] The result was an impasse. To critics, the Biometric Society's report was "predictable" but unconvincing; to proponents, the critics' persistence placed them beyond the pale, among those "more interested in making debater's points than in constructive suggestions" for new analyses and research.[111]

KNOWLEDGE AND INTERESTS *REDUX*

The release of the Biometric Society's report marks the point of diminishing returns in the scientific debate over the UGDP.[112] Arguments about the truth of the UGDP's findings gave way to arguments about the motives of those who doubted, or supported, the study. To those familiar with the history of therapeutic reform, these arguments have a familiar ring. To UGDP proponents, physicians'

107 "Report of the Committee for the Assessment of Biometric Aspects of Controlled Trials of Hypoglycemic Agents" (n. 102), 599.

108 Ibid.

109 See the remarks of Holbrooke Seltzer, "Avoiding the Pitfalls of Long-Term Therapeutic Trials: Lessons Learned from the UGDP Study," *Journal of Clinical Pharmacology and New Drugs* 12 (October 1972), 398. It did not help that the Biometric Society report was released prematurely to the press, furthering critics' contention that the UGDP was circumventing peer review in the scientific community. See James M. Moss, "The UGDP Scandal and Cover-up," *JAMA* 232 (May 26, 1975), 806; Presley, *A History of Diabetes* (n. 5), 438–439.

110 Robert F. Bradley, Henry Dolger, Peter H. Forsham, and Holbrooke Seltzer, "Settling the UGDP Controversy?," *JAMA* 232 (May 26, 1975), 813–815; Moss, "The UGDP Scandal and Cover-up" (n. 109), 806–808; Feinstein, "The Persistent Clinical Failures and Fallacies of the UGDP Study" (n. 65), 89–90.

111 Jerome Cornfield to Max Miller, January 11, 1971, Cornfield papers.

112 Neither the study's critics nor the UGDP's supporters seemed willing to sponsor a new trial, although the NIH had considered this in the early stages of the debate. While the study's critics attached considerable importance to the publication of an analysis by Charles Kilo and Joseph Williamson, the article only followed through on an earlier observation that the placebo group in the UGDP seemed unusually healthy, and that the differences in mortality between placebo and tolbutamide patients were due to the unusual healthiness of the former, rather than the iatrogenic disease of the later. See "The Achilles Heel of the University Group Diabetes Program," *JAMA* 243 (February 1, 1980), 450–457.

continued use of the oral hypoglycemics was explicable only in psychological or economic terms, by

the strong desire of both physicians and patients for a way to treat diabetes that does not involve injections, and . . . a natural reluctance to accept any possibility that the drugs might be harmful. This [attitude] has been fostered by one-sided presentations of the controversy by one or more of the so-called throwaway medical journals so widely read by physicians.[113]

Given the frequency with which diabetics, regardless of what treatment they receive, die of cardiovascular disease, physicians in private practice could not be expected to notice the marginally increased risk associated with the use of tolbutamide.[114] But if the average physician's inability to accept the grim conclusions regarding tolbutamide was due to a failure of imagination, the CCD's reluctance to accept the one study large enough to detect such a risk – the UGDP – could not be benignly explained. In the view of the UGDP supporters, its critics' persistence was due to the corrupting influences of the marketplace on the evaluation process: "one of the things that this 'controversy' has brought out in the last 5 years, I guess – it seems longer – is the incredible way in which a group of physicians teamed up with industry to attack the only scientific evidence there is on the use of these agents, at a time when we sorely need it."[115]

  After five years of controversy, the UGDP investigators had hardened their position. Christian Klimt, who directed the UGDP's data analysis, was quite convinced the oral hypoglycemics were "toxic."[116] To his clinical colleagues, the issue at stake was whether " 'clinical impression,' anecdotal stories and wishful opinions" or "substantial evidence from adequate, well-controlled investigations" were to be the basis of therapeutic practice.[117] The reluctance of the UGDP's critics, after five years of inconclusive debate over the failings of the UGDP, to produce evidence of comparable rigor seemed to the study's advocates silent but

113 Thomas Chalmers, "Settling the UGDP Controversy," *JAMA* 231 (February 10, 1975), 624. See also the remarks of John K. Davidson, "The FDA and Hypoglycemic Drugs," *JAMA* 232 (May 26, 1975), 853, and the testimony offered by Chalmers and Max Miller, the UGDP's study chairman, in U.S. Senate, Select Committee on Small Business, Subcommittee on Monopoly, *Hearings . . . on Competitive Problems in the Drug Industry,* part 25, pp. 10798–10780, 10801, 93rd Congress, 2nd Session.

114 See the testimony of Marvin Zelen in U.S. Senate, Select Committee on Small Business, Subcommittee on Monopoly, *Hearings . . . on Competitive Problems in the Drug Industry,* part 28, p. 13271, 94th Congress, 1st Session; and Jerome Cornfield, *Transcript. FDA Hearings on Oral Hypoglycemic Drugs. August 20, 1975,* 176, FDA Docket 75N-0062.

115 Thaddeus Prout, *Transcript. FDA Hearings on Oral Hypoglycemic Drugs. August 20, 1975,* 84, FDA Docket 75N-0062. See also Knowles, "Medical-Social Aspects of UGDP" (n. 27), 153–155; Chalmers, "Settling the UGDP Controversy" (n. 13,) 625–626; Thomas C. Chalmers, "The Control of Bias in Clinical Trials," in Stanley H. Shapiro and Thomas C. Louis, eds., *Clinical Trials: Issues and Approaches* (New York: Marcel Dekker, 1983), pp. 116–117.

116 Testimony of Christian Klimt, U.S. Senate, Select Committee on Small Business, Subcommittee on Monopoly, *Hearings . . . on Competitive Problems in the Drug Industry,* part 25, p. 10767, 93rd Congress, 2nd Session.

117 Max Miller to Hearing Clerk, FDA, August 21, 1975, FDA Docket 75N-0062.

eloquent testimony of bad faith. Meanwhile, the UGDP remained, according to its defenders, "the only scientific evidence" on the use of the oral hypoglycemic drugs.[118]

This formulation of the problem recalls that of the early twentieth-century therapeutic reformers: there are the ignorant and the greedy, and then there are the rational men of science, among whom the UGDP's partisans naturally classed themselves. To Alvan Feinstein, such claims to a monopoly on scientific rationality represented an extreme form of hubris:

Supporting the UGDP contentions are those who believe that a statistical approach to clinical trials, and particularly the assignment of treatment by randomization, is the single most important desideratum in evaluating therapy. On the other side are those who regard randomization as merely a useful component of the evaluation process and who believe that the clinical validity of a clinical trial has primary scientific importance.[119]

But to the UGDP's other critics, the issue of the best approach to scientific inference from clinical trials was secondary. To the CCD, in particular, the paramount issue was whether "the FDA, the National Institutes of Health, or any other administrative group" had a right to dictate medical practice on the basis of a single, controversial study. Such decisions were best left, in their view, to the profession at large.[120]

The CCD's position recalls that of therapeutic reformers in the late 1930s, eager to raise the standards of professional therapeutic practice, yet reluctant to allow the FDA a commanding role in doing so. Despite their animus against medicine "by administrative fiat," the attitude of CCD members toward the practicing physician was ambivalent. Most physicians, they acknowledged, used the oral hypoglycemic drugs poorly and were in need of better advice to use them more appropriately. Such guidance, however, should come from the profession's self-constituted authorities, the specialists in diabetes, and in the form of education, not commands.

In ruling that the issue was not "who decides," but the nature of the evidence on which decisions are made, the FDA sided with the UGDP. Yet the agency's decision was far less radical than its critics implied. The FDA's actions, confined to modifications of the labeling for tolbutamide, were also true to historical form. For the physician who continued to use the drugs inappropriately, the FDA had no sanctions in mind.[121]

If the CCD's opinion of the practicing physician was ambivalent, UGDP proponents were similarly ambivalent about the FDA. Initially, the UGDP investigators stood aloof from the FDA proceedings, distinguishing their limited conclu-

---

118 Thaddeus Prout, *Transcript. FDA Hearings on Oral Hypoglycemic Drugs. August 20, 1975,* 84, FDA Docket 75N-0062.
119 Feinstein, "How Good Is the Statistical Evidence?" (n. 65), 74.
120 Bradley et al., "Settling the UGDP Controversy?" (n. 110), 813–815.
121 See the testimony of Alexander Schmidt, FDA Commissioner, in U.S. Senate, Select Committee on Small Business, Subcommittee on Monopoly, *Hearings . . . on Competitive Problems in the Drug Industry,* part 28, p. 13307, 94th Congress, 1st Session.

sions about tolbutamide from the FDA's more general indictment of the remaining hypoglycemic drugs. As controversy over the UGDP developed, however, they came to see the FDA ruling as vindicating their study, and any hesitations on the FDA's part as a sign that the agency was confusing "evidence with influence."[122] The FDA's ruling had become a measure of the scientific community's judgment. Either the agency issued a warning to physicians, or it did not. The idea that the FDA might have issued a warning *and* acknowledged uncertainty about the study met with studied incomprehension.

A measure of the situation may be taken from the colloquies between Paul Meier, a statistician member of the Biometric Society review panel and Senator Gaylord Nelson. Meier's insistence that the UGDP was well conceived and executed *and* that its conclusions were uncertain was regarded by Nelson either as unintelligible or as typical of scientific agnosticism, the view that no study is good enough for making policy. Although Meier explicitly repudiated any such attitudes, the idea that someone could affirm the UGDP's scientific quality and explicitly acknowledge the uncertainty of its conclusions was literally incomprehensible.[123]

SOCIAL DECISIONS AND PRIVATE JUDGMENTS

Any conclusions to be drawn from the UGDP experience are potentially as controversial as the study itself. To the UGDP's advocates, the controversy demonstrated the ability of a vocal minority to undermine confidence in the conclusions of a responsibly conducted study, and to frustrate the FDA's efforts to protect the health of diabetic patients. To the study's critics, the controversy represented the usurpation of clinical expertise and physician autonomy in favor of statisticians and bureaucratic dictates. Certainly, the disputants' political and intellectual commitments made it difficult for either party to concede, or at times even to comprehend, the arguments of the other. This inability to reach agreement only reinforced each party's convictions that issues greater than the management of diabetes were at stake: the intellectual integrity of the evaluation process for the UGDP's advocates, the clinical autonomy of the physician for the study's critics. Yet merely to observe that ideological commitments played a role is not sufficient. The question remains: How did they gain the upper hand?

Intellectual or political contests conducted in private proceed by different means than the same contests conducted in more public forums.[124] Once news of the UGDP findings was made public, the customary process of seeking consensus through peer review would not work. The advisory process depends on the ability

122 Thaddeus Prout to Julian Santangelo [FDA], undated, Chalmers papers.
123 See U.S. Senate, Select Committee on Small Business, Subcommittee on Monopoly, *Hearings . . . on Competitive Problems in the Drug Industry,* part 28, pp. 13261–13263, 13267–13271, 94th Congress, 1st Session.
124 Marks, "Revisiting 'The Origins of Compulsory Drug Prescriptions' " (n. 84), 109–115.

to negotiate compromises in private. Concessions are easier to make when they are not publicly acknowledged as such. But the CCD began the regulatory debate by insisting on public redress for damages, which, in their view, had already been done. The UGDP representatives came, over time, to much the same position. Only a public act of vindication by the FDA would begin to repair the harm done by the lengthy delays in the relabeling of the drugs. To give up the effort to relabel the drugs would be to leave the matter to the judgments of individual physicians who, as even the CCD acknowledged, showed few signs of using the drugs responsibly.

The UGDP's proponents began with the presumption that both the study's results and its implications for practice would be deliberated among individuals who shared a common understanding of the issues, but who might nonetheless reach different conclusions. As the controversy progressed, they discovered that the UGDP's critics disagreed not only with the study's specific conclusions but with the intellectual framework in which these issues were being discussed. In accepting representatives of the Biometric Society as the most authoritative body to adjudicate the dispute, the UGDP's advocates only confirmed the critics' view of the decision-making process as partial and coercive, a judgment that has nothing to do with the reasonableness of that body's inferences per se.

This statement of the problem suggests that the choice of forum for interpreting the UGDP's conclusions was as much at issue as the validity of the conclusions themselves. But to address this complaint fully would have required both parties to examine the merits of various institutional arrangements for translating the results of experimental findings into clinical practice. Such an examination, calling for statisticians and clinicians alike to move away from the comfortable grounds provided by their scientific expertise toward the uncharted territories of politics, might well have proved difficult. The UGDP's critics would have had to defend their unexamined partiality for the intellectual autonomy of physicians, in the face of their own admission that many physicians manage diabetes poorly. For the UGDP's defenders, it would have meant exploring the ambivalence toward such autonomy within the tradition of therapeutic reform.

Statistical concepts were introduced into medicine with the expectation that they would not only improve the quality of therapeutic experimentation, but would also contribute to improving therapeutic practice. Yet formal accounts of the properties of different experimental designs and statistical tests do not, and cannot, articulate the means by which the results of well-conducted studies should reform therapeutics. Associated with the identical conceptual apparatus are two widely divergent visions of the social means for bringing rational order to contemporary therapeutic practice.

On one account, members of the medical community, accepting the intellectual discipline of statistics as two generations before they had assimilated that of chemistry, adopt a more rigorous approach to evaluating evidence. Formal aspects of experimental design – randomization, power, alpha and beta levels – become incorporated into medicine along with other criteria. Medical practice improves, on this view, through improvements in methodology which elevate the standards by which evidence is judged. Once physicians learn to reason statistically, procedures that are found wanting by these more rigorous standards of evidence would no longer be accepted by the medical community. An alternative view, equally intent on elevating the standards of therapeutic evaluation, proposes to bypass the step of reforming the judges by putting RCTs in place as the gateway through which all practices must pass before being admitted to clinical practice. The problem is thereby reduced to a simple decision: Which therapies do or do not pass the test? Individuals who do not keep pace with the scientific standards being promulgated must nevertheless fall in step.

Each model represents virtues lacking in the other. The first is tolerant, respective of differences in values and in judgments, but it offers no mechanisms for recognizing intellectual deviance and accepts a slow and uneven rate of change. The second paradigm has the potential to bring about quicker and more uniform changes in practices, but may find it more difficult to distinguish deviance from honest dissent. The choice between them is fundamentally an extrascientific problem. The task of the next chapter is to examine what a political account of the problem can contribute that the sciences of statistics and medicine alone cannot.

CODA: 1995

The University Group Diabetes Program should not be willed into oblivion by ignoring it.[125]

In 1984, the FDA issued labeling "guidelines," advising manufacturers to warn physicians that "the administration of oral hypoglycemic agents has been reported to be associated with increased cardiovascular mortality." The guidelines went on to describe the UGDP findings, and indicated that "Despite controversy regarding the interpretation of these results, the findings of the UGDP study provide an adequate basis for the warning."[126] The FDA's twenty-eight page accompanying justification in the *Federal Register* went virtually unnoticed in the medical press, a

---

125 Thomas C. Chalmers, "Type II Diabetes Insulin versus Oral Agents," *NEJM* 315 (November 6, 1986), 1233.

126 Department of Health and Human Services, Food and Drug Administration, *Guideline Labeling for Oral Hypoglycemic Drugs of the Sulfonylurea Class*, March 16, 1984, Docket 83D-0304. The *Federal Register* notice that followed this announcement ranged from the sublime to the ridiculous – the latter including discussions of the distinction between a regulation and a guideline, and justifying the FDA's decision not to require manufacturers to place a "box" around the warning, the former including discussions of statistical analysis that could well have provided the material for one or more papers in a peer-review journal. See *Federal Register* 49 (April 11, 1984), 14303–14331.

remarkable anticlimax after fifteen years of venomous dispute and hostile litigation.[127] Yet professional inattention was not so surprising, if one realizes that use of tolbutamide had been declining since the early 1980s in favor of newer oral agents.[128] Though all these agents were required by law to demonstrate their value (and safety) in controlled clinical trials, no trial on the scale of the UGDP had ever been conducted. As for medical policy toward controlling blood glucose, it is largely based on analogies from an RCT of insulin-dependent diabetes, much as policies for using tolbutamide had been prior to the UGDP.[129]

127 Based on a search of MEDLINE, and visual inspection of the March–May 1984 issues of *Medical World News, Diabetes* and *Diabetes Care*. In 1979, the American Diabetes Association reversed its earlier position in support of a warning, in a statement that strongly sided with the UGDP's critics. Scientific Advisory Panel of the Executive Committee [Fred W. Whitehouse, Ronald A. Arky, Donald Bell, Patricia A. Lawrence, Norbert Freinkel], "Policy Statement: The UGDP Controversy," *Diabetes Care* 2 (January–February 1979), 1–3.

128 The initial decline in the use of tolbutamide began shortly before the publication of the Biometric Society review. See Stan N. Finkelstein, Stephen B. Schechtman, Edward J. Sondik, and Dana Gilbert, "Clinical Trials and Established Medical Practice: Two Examples," in Edward B. Roberts, Robert I. Levy, Stan N. Finkelstein, Jay Moskowitz, and Edward J. Sondik, eds., *Biomedical Innovation* (Cambridge: MIT Press, 1981), pp. 200–215.

129 See Lasker, "The Diabetes Control and Complications Trial" (n. 17), 1035–1036; Crofford, "Diabetes Control and Complications" (n. 17), 267–279; Maureen I. Harris, Richard C. Eastman, and Carolyn Siebert, "The DCCT and Medical Care for Diabetes in the U.S.," *Diabetes Care* 17 (July 1994), 761–764.

8

The dreams of reason:
Retrospect and prospect

When there is a controversy in an account, the parties must by their own accord, set up, for right reason, the reason of some arbitrator, or judge, to whose sentence they will both stand or their controversy must either come to blows or be undecided.... And when men that think themselves wiser than all others, clamour and demand right reason for judge, yet seek no more, but that things should be determined, by no other men's reason but their own, it is as intolerable in the society of men, as it is in play after trump is turned, to use for trump on every occasion, that suite whereof they have most in their hand.[1]

Politics as reason giving is political argument, not geometry. Politics educates judgment.[2]

Historians customarily end their books by reviewing the story's high points for their general readers, while drawing their colleagues' attention to the broader scholarly implications of their work. The more venturesome among us may comment on ways in which the past lives on in the present. The present, of course, never quite resembles the past to those of us who are living in it. There are always new ideas, new programs, and new forces, which give the lie to the historian's morose judgments about the dead hand of history. Debates over therapeutic reform did not stop in 1975, when the UGDP controversy was on its last legs, or in 1987, when I last summarized discussions among health policy analysts concerning therapeutic reform.[3]

Historians like myself, interested in medicine's present body politic, as well as its past, operate with a kind of double vision. Seeing with double vision is tricky business at best. There is always the danger, in getting the present situation more

---

1 Thomas Hobbes, *Leviathan, or the Matter, Forme and Power of A Commonwealth Ecclesiasticall and Civil,* ed. Michael Oakeshott (New York: Collier Books, 1962), p. 42.
2 Stephen L. Elkin, *City and Regime in the American Republic* (Chicago: University of Chicago Press, 1987), p. 150.
3 Harry M. Marks, *Ideas As Reforms: Therapeutic Experiments and Medical Practice, 1900–1980* (Ph.D. thesis, Massachusetts Institute of Technology, 1987).

clearly into focus, of distorting the past.[4] What follows is an "experimental" conclusion: my attempt to interrogate the history of therapeutic reform, in order to persuade those engaged in such reform to think about their task(s) in a different way.

Throughout the twentieth century, therapeutic reformers have worked toward a common end: ensuring that physicians' therapeutic practices are governed by science and not by the "idols of the marketplace" or the vagaries of clinical opinion. In the first half of the century, reformers emphasized institutional means for giving voice to science, creating the Council on Pharmacy and Chemistry to judge the claims researchers and drug companies made about individual products. Since 1950, reformers have emphasized methodological standards rather than institutional means for achieving a rational therapeutics. Reformers have advised physicians to shun all practices that have not been validated by well-designed, randomized controlled trials. In both eras, federal regulators have emulated the approaches advocated by academic reformers. In the 1930s and 1940s, the U.S. Food and Drug Administration (FDA) relied on the advice and clinical judgment of experienced researchers in assessing "wholly new products." Since the early 1970s, the FDA required that all new claims for drugs be supported by "adequate and well-controlled clinical investigations."[5]

Despite differences in their circumstances and philosophies, therapeutic reformers in both eras have shared certain assumptions about the world of medicine. The most enduring of these is the reformers' conviction that medicine is a republic of science: a self-governing community of equals in which science provides the key to responsible citizenship. My aim in the first half of this concluding chapter is to explore the implications of this crucial concept – the republic of science – for contemporary debates over therapeutic reform.[6] In the second half of the chapter,

---

4 Medical history seems to attract an unusually high proportion of scholars with concerns for the present as well as the past. But as readers of Peter Novick's magisterial account of the American historical profession will recognize, the issue endures and chronically recurs for all historians. See Owsei Temkin, "The Double Face of Janus," in *The Double Face of Janus and Other Essays in the History of Medicine* (Baltimore: Johns Hopkins University Press, 1977), pp. 3–37; Elizabeth Fee and Daniel M. Fox, "The Contemporary Historiography of AIDS," *Journal of Social History* 23 (Winter 1989), 303–314; Barbara Gutmann Rosenkrantz, "Case Histories: An Introduction," *Social Research* 55 (Autumn 1988), 397–399; Peter Novick, *That Noble Dream: The "Objectivity Question" and the American Historical Profession* (Cambridge: Cambridge University Press, 1988).

5 Walton Van Winkle Jr. to Paul Dunbar and Robert Herrick, January 30, 1946, Acc. 88-59A-2736, Box 220, 505.1064–509, W-NRC; *Federal Register* 35 (May 8, 1970), 7251. For further discussion of FDA policy, see Chapter 3 and Harry M. Marks, *Historical Perspectives on Clinical Trials,* Working Paper Prepared for the National Research Council, Committee on AIDS Research and the Behavioral, Social and Statistical Sciences, August 1990.

6 See John Zinman, *Public Knowledge: The Social Dimension of Science* (Cambridge: Cambridge University Press, 1968). The specific language of a "republic of science" belongs, as American historians will recognize, to an earlier era, and in its historical form has somewhat different connotations than the ones discussed here. Nonetheless, I believe that the conceit of a republic of science captures the essential characteristics and embodies the crucial dilemmas of the culture of rational therapeutics in twentieth-century medicine.

I will consider the relation between the republic of science and the rest of us – patients, activists, and citizens.

THE REPUBLIC OF SCIENCE

In the opening chapter I introduced the first dilemma of the republic of science: all members are equal but some are more equal than others. Experts with specialized knowledge of specific diseases, the actions of therapeutic compounds, or research methods claim an authority that other physicians lack. All republics face this dilemma, but a republic of science encounters it in a particularly acute form: what makes the republic's ordinary citizen – the practicing physician – a member of the republic of science?

Therapeutic reformers have offered two distinct answers to this question. At times, reformers in both eras spoke as if there was a general, universally comprehensible, scientific method that required no esoteric skills or knowledge. Statistical analysis via the randomized controlled trial represents the contemporary version of this Baconian organon, but reformers earlier in the century spoke of "scientific method" and "experiment" in much the same way. According to this vision, an understanding and use of the principles of "scientific method" or "statistical reasoning" would level the differences among physicians in specialized knowledge and expertise, allowing for a republic of equals. So long as one's therapeutic practice was based on acceptable evidence, and evidence was interpreted and judged according to commonly understood standards, any practitioner was functioning as a full citizen in the republic.

A second kind of answer acknowledged the vast inequalities among physicians in knowledge, experience, and training. Here, membership in the republic of science was offered to those who would acknowledge the constituted authorities within medicine by allowing their deliberations and reflections to serve as a surrogate for the judgments of the individual physician.

Both visions of scientific citizenship share a common, essential virtue: they are noncoercive. Physicians are presumed to accept voluntarily either the rational dictates of scientific method or the judgments of constituted authorities. The dilemmas arise here in defining, interpreting, and managing the limits of acceptable citizenly conduct.

For reformers who believe in a fully democratic republic of science, the first difficulty arises in defining what counts as "unreasonable" behavior. When physicians disagree about the weight of the evidence, the procedures and criteria for interpreting evidence, or the kinds of allowable evidence on which to base clinical practice, at what point do their disagreements become unreasonable? Were the critics of the University Diabetes Group Program acting unreasonably or were they applying different criteria of evidence than their opponents? If they were acting reasonably in 1970, when information about the UGDP was scarce, were they still acting reasonably in 1975, when the Biometric Society endorsed the study? Perhaps some of the critics' actions and beliefs were reasonable and some were not, but by what standards?

Since the UGDP study, the difficulty of defining unreasonable behavior has only grown more acute. Physicians now commonly discuss issues of experimental design and statistical inference which formerly concerned only a few statistical theorists and philosophers. Among the issues now debated are the following: When are nonrandomized studies legitimate to use, and how do they compare with randomized studies? Should all trials be large, simple trials with mortality as the principal end point? When should a clinical trial be stopped? What role, if any, does evidence from outside a study play in arriving at a scientific conclusion? Which of the various means for calculating probability judgments (e.g., p-values, confidence intervals, likelihood ratio) are appropriate in presenting the results of clinical trials? Should formal statistical methods for combining conflicting results from multiple trials be used? Do competing philosophies of statistical inference have a place in routine clinical experimentation? How may the results of clinical trials be generalized to populations more and less similar to those studied?[7]

Specific studies provide an especially charged locus for debating these issues. Were investigators justified in launching a clinical trial of oxygen supplementation

---

7 Each of these issues has generated a large, varied, and complex literature of its own. The following discussions are cited for illustrative purposes only. On issues of experimental design, including discussions of randomized and nonrandomized studies, see Peter Armitage, "The Role of Randomization in Clinical Trials," *Statistics in Medicine* 1 (1982), 345–352; Salim Yusuf, Rory Collins, and Richard Peto, "Why Do We Need Some Large, Simple Randomized Trials?," *Statistics in Medicine* 3 (1984), 409–420; David L. Sackett and Deborah J. Cook, "Can We Learn Anything from Small Trials?," *Ann NY Acad Sci* 703 (December 31, 1993), 25–32; Michael S. Kramer and Stanley H. Shapiro, "Scientific Challenges in the Application of Randomized Trials," *JAMA* 252 (November 16, 1984), 2739–2745; Edmund A. Gehan, "The Evaluation of Therapies: Historical Control Studies," *Statistics in Medicine* 3 (1984), 315–324; Alvan R. Feinstein, "Experimental Requirements and Scientific Principles in Case-Control Studies," *JCD* 38 (1985), 127–133; Sylvan B. Green and David P. Byar, "Using Observational Data from Registries to Compare Treatments: The Fallacy of Omnimetrics," *Statistics in Medicine* 3 (1984), 361–370; Kenneth J. Rothman and Karin B. Michels, "The Continuing Unethical Use of Placebo Controls," *NEJM* 331 (August 11, 1994), 394–398. On the issues involved in early stopping, see Richard Simon, "Some Practical Aspects of the Interim Monitoring of Clinical Trials," *Statistics in Medicine* 13 (1994), 1401–1409; Stuart J. Pocock, "When to Stop a Clinical Trial," *British Medical Journal* 305 (July 25, 1992), 235–240. On the difficulties of generalizing results from clinical trials, see Salim Yusuf, Janet Wittes, Jeffrey Probstfield, and Herman A. Tyroler, "Analysis and Interpretation of Treatment Effects in Subgroups of Patients in Randomized Clinical Trials," *JAMA* 266 (July 3, 1991), 93–98. On combining evidence, see Andrew D. Oxman and Gordon H. Guyatt, "The Science of Reviewing Research," *Ann NY Acad Sci* 703 (December 31, 1993), 125–133; Kristan A. L'Abbé, Allan S. Detsky, and Keith O'Rourke, "Meta-analysis in Clinical Research," *Ann Int Med* 107 (1987), 224–233; John C. Bailar III, "When Research Results Are in Conflict," *NEJM* 313 (October 24, 1985), 1080–1081. On questions of statistical inference and methodology, see Steven N. Goodman and Richard Royall, "Evidence and Scientific Research," *AJPH* 78 (December 1988), 1568–1574; Robert F. Woolson and Joel C. Kleinman, "Perspectives on Statistical Significance Testing," *Annual Review of Public Health* 10 (1989), 423–440; George A. Diamond and James S. Forrester, "Clinical Trials and Statistical Verdicts: Probable Grounds for Appeal," *Ann Int Med* 98 (1983), 385–394; P. Armitage, "The Search for Optimality in Clinical Trials," *International Statistical Review* 53 (1985), 15–24.

for premature newborns largely to convince others that the technology prevented respiratory failure? Should researchers have relied on a review of poorly controlled studies in high-risk pregnancies to play down their own finding that prenatal ultrasound screening was associated with an excess of perinatal deaths in routine pregnancies? What should physicians tell their patients about lowering their cholesterol when both clinical trials and metaanalyses of clinical trials give conflicting results?[8] While some of these discussions may seem amateurish or trivial to professional statisticians, the majority are serious and informed.[9] Collectively, they pose a perennial dilemma of rationalist science: When reasonable people disagree, where do the boundaries of unreasonable behavior begin?

Historically, therapeutic reformers have assumed that they can recognize unreasonable behavior even if they cannot define it. Reformers have presumed that when physicians prescribe drugs without regard to validated therapeutic indications, they are being swayed by irrational forces: advertising, cupidity, or ignorance. Yet reformers know very little in such cases about why physicians prescribe as they do.[10] Is it because they are ignorant, because they are corrupt, or because they are applying a different standard of evidence?

In interpreting dissident or nonconforming behavior as "irrational," reformers had recourse to a venerable habit in European and American culture. Since the sixteenth century (if not earlier), scientists and philosophers have regularly attempted to draw the boundary between the scientific and other forms of inquiry. Anthropologists and sociologists of science have observed that such boundary drawing is arbitrary, itself a product of historically conditioned norms and beliefs.[11] Within the medical culture I have described in this book, those who operate in

---

8 Valerie Miké, Alfred N. Krauss, and Gail S. Ross, "Neonatal Extracorporeal Membrane Oxygenation (ECMO): Clinical Trials and the Ethics of Evidence," *Journal of Medical Ethics* 19 (1993), 212–218; Richard M. Royall, "Ethics and Statistics in Randomized Clinical Trials," *Statistical Science* 6 (February 1991), 52–62; Jean Robinson, "A Lay Person's Perspective on Starting and Stopping Clinical Trials," *Statistics in Medicine* 13 (1994), 1474; S. G. Thompson, "Why Sources of Heterogeneity in Meta-Analysis Should Be Investigated," *British Medical Journal* 309 (November 19, 1995), 1351–1355.

9 For problems with incorporating heterodox or novel statistical methodologies, see David Machin, "Discussion of 'The What, Why and How of Bayesian Clinical Trials Monitoring,' " *Statistics in Medicine* 13 (1994), 1385–1389; Douglas G. Altman, "Statistics in Medical Journals: Developments in the 1980s," *Statistics in Medicine* 10 (1991), 1900–1901, 1908.

10 Most of the studies surveyed by the Institute of Medicine's Committee for Evaluating Medical Technologies rely on time trends to study the effects of clinical trials on subsequent practice. See Harvey V. Fineberg, "Effects of Clinical Evaluation on the Diffusion of Medical Technology," in Institute of Medicine, Committee for Evaluating Medical Technologies in Clinical Use, *Assessing Medical Technologies* (Washington, DC: National Academy Press, 1985), pp. 187–194. Clearly, however, knowledge of or even belief in clinical trial results provides only a partial explanation of prescribing behavior. The research strategy followed by Arabella Melville and Roy Mapes on physicians' awareness of, and responses to, warnings regarding practolol suggests one line of attack on this problem. See their "Anatomy of a Disaster: The Case of Practolol," in Roy Mapes, ed., *Prescribing Practice and Drug Usage* (London: Croom Helm, 1980), pp. 121–144.

11 The now canonical example is Steven Shapin and Simon Schaffer, *Leviathan and the Air-Pump: Hobbes, Boyle and the Experimental Life* (Princeton: Princeton University Press, 1985).

profit-making institutions have been regarded as operating on the edges of, if not outside, the boundary of science:

In their entrance through scientific channels exaggerated therapeutic claims are made at times, as the result of a lack of critical judgment and adequate controls. But in their introduction through commercial channels, financial consideration and lack of true appreciation of the fundamental problems preclude unbiased observations.[12]

Physicians who do not prescribe according to indications set by validated standards of proof are similarly suspect of "interested" behavior: behavior or beliefs distorted by factors other than the evidence.[13]

The difficulty here is that *all* our behaviors – as physicians, as researchers, as parents, as stockholders – are interested behaviors. Statisticians and therapeutic reformers who are concerned about the financial as well as the intellectual health of controlled clinical trials are "interested." Imputing interests to someone or some group tells us nothing about whether what they propose to do, or are doing, is "scientific" or "rational."[14]

Even within the magic penumbra of "science," science does not speak with a single voice. Reformers have presumed that all sciences lead to the same conclusion or, if they do not, that some sciences are superior to others in judging therapeutic value. Reformers in the era of randomized controlled trials insist that laboratory knowledge of physiological or molecular mechanisms is inferior to experimental demonstrations of therapeutic value in the clinic. Laboratory researchers, on the other hand, are skeptical about our ability to judge the effects of interventions when we do not understand the phenomena that produce those effects. Even in the restricted realm of clinical investigation, there are multiple competitors for authority. Randomized clinical trials represent one among several established strategies for clinical research. Researchers from other intellectual traditions have argued for more conventional forms of clinical investigation, which emphasize integrating clinical research with laboratory studies of biological mechanisms, or for a "clinical science" based on the classification of disease through the systematic analysis of signs, symptoms, and the clinical staging of disease.[15]

12 L. G. Rowntree, "The Role and Development of Drug Therapy," *JAMA* 77 (October 1, 1921), 1064.

13 Here, too, contemporary reformers single out commercial advertising as one of the major influences distorting clinical practice. See J. Avorn, M. Chen, and R. Hartley, "Scientific versus Commercial Sources of Influence on the Prescribing Behavior of Physicians," *American Journal of Medicine* 73 (1982), 4–8; Peter Sleight, "The Influence of Mortality Trials on the Evolution of Clinical Practice," *Cardiology* 84 (1994), 413–419.

14 The point applies equally to the new sociology of science, whose practitioners have generally made the large conceptual leap from noting that even "science" is "interested" to presuming that this tells us something about the validity or invalidity of particular scientific procedures or claims.

15 See Edward H. Ahrens Jr., "Institutional Obstacles to Clinical Research," *Perspectives in Biology and Medicine* 36 (Winter 1993), 194–209; idem, *The Crisis in Clinical Research: Overcoming Institutional Obstacles* (New York: Oxford University Press, 1992); Alvan R. Feinstein, "An Additional Basic Science for Clinical Medicine: Parts I–IV," *Ann Int Med* 99 (1983), 393–397, 554–550, 705–712, 843–848; idem, *Clinimetrics* (New Haven: Yale University Press, 1987).

Disagreements about how best to measure therapeutic value are nothing new. As long ago as the 1760s, the mathematicians Daniel Bernouilli and Jean D'Alembert were arguing about the appropriate way to measure the value of smallpox inoculation.[16] Contests over the proper roles of clinical and laboratory investigation have nearly as long a history.[17] A characteristic solution to such contests over intellectual authority is to create a body capable of weighing and reconciling the various kinds of evidence available.

In the early decades of the century, reformers created the Council on Pharmacy and Chemistry to judge the merits of therapeutic products offered for sale. The council did not eliminate disciplinary or personal differences of opinion regarding the value of specific products. The pharmacologists and clinicians on the council often disagreed about the relative weight to give laboratory and clinical evidence in evaluating new drugs. Moreover, as with any political institution, in arriving at their decisions council members occasionally gave equal or greater priority to preserving the institution's integrity and reputation.[18] Nonetheless, the council's deliberations enabled it to issue collective pronouncements about the merits of therapeutic products.

The council's authority rested on its members' claims to expertise and integrity. The FDA similarly assumed that the opinions of some researchers are more valuable than those of others. As the century progressed, reformers found it progressively more difficult to put their faith in the character and skills of any group of individuals.[19] Under exceptional circumstances, such as war or temporary scarcity, medicine's elite was willing to put drug evaluations in the hands of a select committee or even a single trusted individual, such as "penicillin czar" Chester Keefer, who rationed supplies of "experimental" drugs to researchers willing to abide by a standardized research protocol. Such arrangements proved by

16 Lorraine J. Daston, *Classical Probability in the Enlightenment* (Princeton: Princeton University Press, 1988), 82–91; Harry M. Marks, *Measuring Outcomes: The 18th Century Inoculation Debates,* a paper presented to Seminar on Clinical Trials, Johns Hopkins University, March 8, 1995.

17 William Coleman, "Experimental Physiology and Statistical Inference: The Therapeutic Trial in Nineteenth-Century Germany," in Lorenz Krüger, Gerd Gigerenzer, and Mary S. Morgan, eds., *The Probabilistic Revolution* (Cambridge: MIT Press, 1987), vol. 2, pp. 201–228; John E. Lesch, *Science and Medicine in France: The Emergence of Experimental Physiology, 1790–1855* (Cambridge: Harvard University Press, 1984), pp. 99–165; John Harley Warner, "Ideals of Science and Their Discontents in Late Nineteenth-Century American Medicine," *Isis* 82 (September 1991), 454–478.

18 See the many discussions of consistency in council policy.

19 On the continued importance of local reputation and authority in the practice setting, see John Betz Brown, Diana Shye, and Bentson McFarland, "The Paradox of Guideline Implementation: How AHCPR's Depression Guideline Was Adapted at Kaiser Permanente Northwest Region," *Journal of Quality Improvement* 21 (January 1995), 5–21. Peter Caws argues that such "fiduciary knowledge," as he terms it, grounded in detailed knowledge and experience of scientific authorities, offers a reasonable basis for relying on such authorities. See Peter Caws, "Committees and Consensus: How Many Heads Are Better Than One?," *Journal of Medicine and Philosophy* 16 (August 1991), 375–391. For a discussion concerned with the political efficacy of such advisory committees, see Sheila Jasanoff, *The Fifth Branch: Advisers as Policymakers* (Cambridge: Harvard University Press, 1990).

their nature difficult to sustain. As the cases of streptomycin, cortisone, and even penicillin show, centralized control over drug evaluation was undermined by researchers, drug companies, and practicing physicians who believed that they had equally legitimate claims on the use of experimental drugs.[20]

Following the Second World War, therapeutic reformers increasingly put their faith in methods, not men, engendering all the dilemmas of a rationalist polity discussed here. Since the early 1980s, the difficulties of determining when disagreement becomes irrational deviance or self-interested promotion have been compounded as the financial stakes of defining acceptable clinical practice have risen. As hospitals, insurers, and government agencies have sought a defensible basis for rationing care, groups inside and outside the profession have attempted to set the standards for clinical practice in the name of medical science.[21] This proliferation of standard-setting authorities has done little to reinforce professional confidence in a rational therapeutics. Individual guidelines have been challenged as "imprudent," as "a giant step backwards," as cause for "concern," and as offering "cookbook recipes."[22]

The move in recent decades toward larger, more Taylorized health care organizations, or "managed care," has strengthened the hand of social scientists – statisticians and economists – in current disputes about the roles of evidence and clinical judgment in arriving at a rational therapeutics.[23] The outlines of social

20 On streptomycin rationing, see Chapter 4. On cortisone, see Harry M. Marks, "Cortisone, 1949: A Year in the Political Life of a Drug," *BHM* 66 (Fall 1992), 419–439. For penicilin, see David P. Adams, *"The Greatest Good to the Greatest Number": Penicillin Rationing on the American Home Front, 1940–1945* (New York: Peter Lang, 1991); Gladys L. Hobby, *Penicillin: Meeting the Challenge* (New Haven: Yale University Press, 1985), pp. 165–169. For successful examples of prewar rationing, see Jonathan Liebenau, "The MRC and the Pharmaceutical Industry: The Model of Insulin," in Joan Austoker and Linda Bryder, eds., *Historical Perspectives on the Role of the MRC* (New York: Oxford University Press, 1989), pp. 163–180; John P. Swann, *Academic Scientists and the Pharmaceutical Industry: Cooperative Research in Twentieth-Century America* (Baltimore: Johns Hopkins University Press, 1988), pp. 125–148.

21 On the clinical guidelines movement, see David M. Eddy, "Clinical Decision-Making: From Theory to Practice," *JAMA* 263 (January 12, 1990), 287–290; John D. Ayres, "The Use and Abuse of Medical Practice Guidelines," *Journal of Legal Medicine* 15 (1994), 421–433. By one count, groups have issued over 1,200 practice guidelines in North America. See Jonathan Lomas, "Making Clinical Policy Explicit: Legislative Policy Making and Lessons for Developing Practice Guidelines," *International Journal of Health Technology Assessment* 9 (1993), 11.

22 Jack Froom and Paul Froom, " 'Prudence' in Disease Prevention," *Journal of Clinical Epidemiology* 44 (1991), 1127–1130; Jeffrey J. Rabinovitz and Earl R. Washburn, "Bilirubin Guidelines Are a Setback!," *Pediatrics* 95 (April 1995), 616; Ellen R. Wald and Barry Dashefsky, "Ribavirin: Red Book Committee Recommendations Questioned," *Pediatrics* 93 (April 1994), 672–673; William W. Parmley, "Clinical Practice Guidelines: Does the Cookbook Have Enough Recipes?," *JAMA* 272 (November 2, 1994), 1374–1375. See also Sean R. Tunis, Robert S. A. Hayward, Mark C. Wilson, Haya R. Rubin, Eric B. Bass, Mary Johnston, and Earl P. Steinberg, "Internists' Attitudes about Clinical Practice Guidelines," *Ann Int Med* 120 (June 1, 1994), 956–963; Sandra J. Tanenbaum, "Knowing and Acting in Medical Practice: The Epistemological Politics of Outcomes Research," *Journal of Health Politics, Policy and Law* 19 (Spring 1994), 27–44.

23 For two, very different, views of the evolution of managerial technologies for governing clinical practice, see Daniel M. Fox, "Health Policy and the Politics of Research in the United States," *Journal of Health Politics, Policy and Law* 15 (Fall 1990), 481–499; Marc Berg, "Turning a Practice

and intellectual conflict over rational therapeutics nonetheless retain a familiar shape: town versus gown (practitioner versus academic medical cultures), competing disciplinary traditions within academic medicine, interspecialty conflicts, clinical autonomy and judgment versus managerial approaches to therapeutic practice.[24]

Not surprisingly, contemporary therapeutic reformers reinvent institutions like the Council on Pharmacy and Chemistry at regular intervals.[25] However, their concern with methodological progress has left contemporary therapeutic reformers particularly ill-equipped to adjudicate the claims of competing institutions or social groups for therapeutic authority. While the pluralism of contests for authority comes as no surprise to contemporary social scientists, they too operate with an impoverished vocabulary when it comes to adjudicating the qualities of competing medical institutions: markets, disciplines, and professions.[26]

In contrast to social scientists, social activists have had a more dramatic and original impact on the relatively insular professional world of clinical research. AIDS activists have won a place at the table where clinical trials are planned and organized by clinical researchers and statisticians, while the U.S. Congress has mandated that researchers include women and minorities in NIH-sponsored clinical trials.[27] AIDS activists have persuaded the FDA to modify its procedures and standards for judging the clinical efficacy of new drugs through innovations such as "fast-tracking" and "parallel track," intended to increase access to experimental drugs. They have urged further modifications of customary clinical trial procedure in advocating the abandonment of placebo-controlled trials, the use of

into a Science: Reconceptualizing Postwar Medical Practice," *Social Studies of Science* 25 (August 1995), 437–476.

24 Although the particular institutional and social choices are deeply embedded in the culture of late twentieth-century medicine, the struggle for the autonomy of clinical judgment has a long history. See Judy Sadler, "Ideologies of 'Art' and 'Science' in Medicine: The Transition from Medical Care to the Application of Technology," in Wolfgang Krohn, Edwin Layton Jr., and Peter Weingart, eds., *The Dynamics of Science and Technology: Social Values, Technical Norms and Scientific Criteria in the Development of Knowledge* (Dordrecht: Reidel, 1978), pp. 177–215; Christopher Lawrence, "Incommunicable Knowledge: Science, Technology and the Clinical Art in Britain, 1850–1914," *Journal of Contemporary History* 20 (1985), 503–520.

25 For two proposals in recent decades, see John P. Bunker, Jinnet Fowles, and Ralph Schaffarzick, "Evaluation of Medical Technology Strategies: Proposal for an Institute for Health-Care Evaluation," *NEJM* 306 (March 18, 1982), 687–692; Wayne A. Ray, Marie R. Griffin, and Jerry Avorn, "Evaluating Drugs after Their Approval for Clinical Use," *NEJM* 329 (December 30, 1993), 2029–2032. See also Seymour Perry, "The Brief Life of the National Center for Health Care Technology," *NEJM* 307 (October 21, 1982), 1095–1100.

26 For a general discussion, see Elkin, *City and Regime* (n. 2), pp. 1–17.

27 On new policies for the inclusion of women and minorities in clinical trials, see "Inclusion of Women in Clinical Trials – Policies for Population Subgroups," and Ruth B. Merkatz, Robert Temple, Solomon Sobel, Karyn Feiden, David A. Kessler, and the Working Group on Women in Clinical Trials, "Women in Clinical Trials of New Drugs: A Change in Food and Drug Administration Policy," both in *NEJM* 329 (July 22, 1993), 288–292 and 292–296; Public Law 103-43, June 10, 1993; *Federal Register* 59 (March 28, 1994), 14508–14513; Linda Ann Sherman, Robert Temple, and Ruth B. Merkatz, "Women in Clinical Trials: An FDA Perspective," *Science* 269 (August 11, 1995), 793–795.

surrogate end points to measure treatment effects, and the development of newer, more flexible experimental designs.[28]

Career clinical investigators have charged that these changes represent the triumph of politics over science. In the following section I examine this charge. What does it mean and what does it matter?

SCIENCE AND POLITICS

> To look upon politics from the perspective of truth means to take one's stand outside the political realm. This standpoint is the standpoint of the truthteller, who forfeits his position – and with it, the validity of what he has to say – if he tries to interfere directly in human affairs and to speak the language of persuasion and violence.[29]

> Though the knowledge science has to offer is always more than technical knowledge, what it has to offer to politics is never more than a technique.[30]

The contention that science and politics represent two distinct realms, one concerned with truth and the other with power, has deep roots in Western culture. There is a long (if hardly unbroken) tradition of philosophers since Plato who have argued that the two are and *must be* kept distinct, lest one contaminate the other. Politics, Hannah Arendt argues in the essay just cited, relies on persuasion and, inevitably, coercion to achieve its ends. The enterprise of politics is therefore distinct from, and inimical to, the enterprise of seeking knowledge, or truth.[31] In the traditional canon, philosophy was truth's guardian. Presently, science has taken that role, despite the long-standing philosophical contention that the knowledge

28 While none of these innovations is unique to AIDS trials, they have been given considerably more attention in this disease than in most others. For an overview, see Susan S. Ellenberg, Dianne M. Finkelstein, and David A. Schoenfeld, "Statistical Issues Arising in AIDS Clinical Trials," *Journal of the American Statistical Association* 87 (June 1992), 562–569, and the ensuing discussion in "Comment," 569–583. On AIDS activists and clinical trials, see Steven Gary Epstein, *Impure Science: AIDS, Activism and the Politics of Knowledge* (Ph.D. thesis, University of California at Berkeley, 1993), pp. 360–511; [Deborah Cotton and Allan M. Brandt], "Clinical Research and Drug Regulation," in Committee on AIDS Research and the Behavioral, Social and Statistical Sciences, National Research Council, *The Social Impact of AIDS in the United States* (Washington, DC: National Academy Press, 1993), pp. 90–116; Jeffrey Levi, "Unproven AIDS Therapies: The Food and Drug Administration and ddI," Committee to Study Biomedical Decision Making, Institute of Medicine, *Biomedical Politics* (Washington, DC: National Academy Press, 1991), pp. 9–37; Harold Edgar and David J. Rothman, "New Rules for New Drugs: The Challenge of AIDS to the Regulatory Process," *Milbank Quarterly* 68 (1990), Supplement 1, 111–142.

29 Hannah Arendt, "Truth and Politics," in *Between Past and Future: Eight Exercises in Political Thought* (New York: Penguin Books, 1977), p. 259.

30 Michael Oakeshott, "Rationalism in Politics," in his *Rationalism in Politics and Other Essays* (New York: Methuen, 1981), p. 22.

31 Arendt, "Truth and Politics" (n. 29), pp. 227–264. Arendt's argument, which reflects in part reactions to the reception of her *Eichmann in Jerusalem,* makes additional distinctions between philosophical and factual truths, which need not concern us here.

produced by the empirical sciences is less certain and secure than the truths produced by philosophical inquiry.[32]

Few clinical researchers would take as ascetic and absolutist a line as Arendt's in policing the boundaries between knowledge and politics. Medicine's practical aims and humane concerns – the relief of suffering as well as the cure of disease – make such abstraction difficult for any physician to sustain, even in the name of science. Medicine or even medical science must accommodate values and morality in a way that "pure" science (or even purer philosophy), in their concerns for the truth, need not.[33]

Since the late 1960s, physicians – especially within academic medicine – have increasingly acknowledged the limitations of either medical science or clinical judgment in making decisions about their patients' lives (and deaths). In response to political criticism from feminist organizations, patients' rights activists, and lawyers, physicians have created a series of institutions to oversee the ethical conduct of both routine clinical decisions and medical research. Yet, as Renée Fox argues, the institutions of "bioethics" have served largely to insulate medicine from politics.[34]

In the domain of medical research, institutions receiving federal research support must have an institutional review board (IRB) to scrutinize all research proposals involving human subjects. IRBs have generally emphasized the relatively narrow questions of patients' rights and informed consent. Does the research pose unnecessary risks to patients, and are patients properly made aware of those risks? By and large, they have left evidentiary questions – Is this research worth doing and is the planned research design capable of answering the questions? – to others. Moreover, by creating a special set of standards for research, ethicists have reinforced the notion that research is an exceptional domain from the rest of clinical medicine, requiring special rules and procedures.[35] It has always been a puzzle to me why the customary recourse to unwanted injury – "sue the bastards" – was not deemed sufficient protection. It is equally puzzling why the rules

32 See Don K. Price, *America's Unwritten Constitution: Science, Religion and Social Responsibility* (Baton Rouge: Louisiana State University Press, 1983). For a discussion of statistical inference that makes a strong case along these lines for distinguishing between decisions and inference, see Isaac Levi, "Must the Scientist Make Value Judgments," *Journal of Philosophy* 57 (1960), 345–357; idem, "Consensus As Shared Agreement and Outcome of Inquiry," *Synthese* 62 (1985), 3–11.

33 Eric J. Cassell, *The Nature of Suffering and the Goals of Medicine* (New York: Oxford University Press, 1991).

34 Renée C. Fox, "The Evolution of American Bioethics: A Sociological Perspective," in George Weisz, ed., *Social Science Perspectives on Medical Ethics* (Philadelphia: University of Pennsylvania Press, 1991), pp. 201–220. See also David J. Rothman, *Strangers at the Bedside: A History of How Law and Bioethics Transformed Medical Decision Making* (New York: Basic Books, 1991).

35 Harry M. Marks, *Ethics and Epistemology: A Durkheimian Perspective on Human Experimentation,* a paper presented to the conference on Regulating Human Experimentation in the United States: The Lessons of History, February 23 and 24, 1995, Columbia University, New York. On the workings of IRBs, see Bernard Barber, *Informed Consent in Medical Therapy and Research* (New Brunswick, NJ: Rutgers University Press, 1980); Robert J. Levine, *Ethics and Regulation of Clinical Research,* 2nd ed. (New Haven: Yale University Press, 1988), pp. 321–363.

of informed consent should not apply in everyday medical encounters even more than in the research setting.[36]

In contrast to bioethicists, activist groups have sought a voice in how science is conducted and applied in clinical practice. Activists have shaped the plans of researchers regarding drugs to be tested, populations to be studied, the study protocols and experimental design employed, and the standards by which trial results affect clinical practice. Their efforts have involved politics – the exercise of power and persuasion – as much as science. While some researchers have welcomed the addition of new participants in research planning, others have opposed the new developments as signs of undue (and unwanted) political influence on science.

Clinical researchers' complaints about politics incorporate three distinguishable elements. The first element is territorial: the investigators' terrain has been invaded by new immigrants who do not behave according to local custom and procedure. AIDS activists have staged demonstrations and relied on guerrilla theater to influence researchers, while feminist groups have bypassed researcher-controlled institutions, going directly to Congress to achieve their goals.[37] Even worse, from the researchers' perspective, the new inhabitants seem somehow to have gained the upper hand and are transforming local custom beyond recognition. Moreover, researchers contend that science – in this case, the science of therapeutic evaluation – is a special and distinctive activity, which operates differently from other activities such as politics, from which it must be insulated and protected. Let us examine this view more closely.

For much of this book, I have been arguing that clinical research is intrinsically a social process. The most routine of clinical investigations involves seemingly endless negotiations: negotiations to persuade participating researchers to abide by a uniform protocol even when there are more "interesting" questions to pursue; negotiations with referring clinicians to send patients to the study; efforts to persuade patients to join such studies; negotiations with editors and coauthors about where to publish, how many tables to publish, and how many authors to credit. In all these activities, researchers have to persuade others – scientists, physicians, and patients – that their questions are worth asking; that their research plans (study design, treatment protocol, outcome measures) and their resources (clinical population, clinical staff, ancillary support) are adequate for the job; that their analyses are sound; and that what they have found should alter or affirm existing practice. All of these efforts entail the use of persuasion and power. Is

---

36 For an intriguing if naive argument for reducing the divide between clinical research and routine chronic care, see Andrew Feenberg, "On Being a Human Subject: Interest and Obligation in the Experimental Treatment of Human Disease," *Philosophical Forum* 23 (Spring 1992), 213–230.

37 See Paula A. Treichler, "How to Have Theory in an Epidemic: The Evolution of AIDS Treatment Activism," in Constance Penley and Andrew Ross, eds., *Technoculture* (Minneapolis: University of Minnesota Press, 1991), pp. 57–106.

then all science another form of politics, in the sense argued by many historians and sociologists of science – an exercise of persuasion and power akin to other such exercises?

Before addressing this question, I would like to consider an additional element in professional charges against the politicization of clinical research: that activists' proposals are unreasonable and ill-informed. According to this argument, uninformed scientific policies are arbitrary exercises of political will, which have no place in scientific discussions. Thus, clinical researchers object to recent congressional policies mandating the inclusion of women and minority populations in clinical trials because, they argue, such policies are based on the mistaken premise that there are powerful biological differences between the effects of therapy on men and women or among racial groups [sic], which cannot be detected in studies on a predominantly male population of European ancestry. Researchers invoke their extensive experience in analyzing clinical trial results, indicating that such subgroup differences are rarely substantial. They argue that clinical investigators should only insist on expanded participation for women (or minorities) when there is a "biologically plausible" reason to expect a differential response to treatment. In mandating the inclusion of women, they argue, Congress has confused notions of political representation with scientific concepts of representativeness.[38]

I can think of several objections to these criticisms. The first is that there *are* some clinically important biological differences between men and women: for example, in the lower rates and later age at which women develop heart disease.[39] The second is that some clinically relevant differences are arguably social rather than biological: the higher rates at which women use health services, for example, or the more advanced stages at which African Americans "present" for diagnosis and treatment of breast and cervical cancer.[40] Such social differences can affect judgments about the feasibility and effectiveness of treatment, and should be

---

38 Steven Piantadosi and Janet Wittes, "Politically Correct Clinical Trials," *Controlled Clinical Trials* 14 (1993), 562–567; "Directive to the Director of NIH from the Membership of the Society for Clinical Trials," *Controlled Clinical Trials* 14 (1993), 559; Institute of Medicine, Committee on the Ethical and Legal Issues Relating to the Inclusion of Women in Clinical Studies, *Women and Health Research: Ethical and Legal Issues of Including Women in Clinical Studies* (Washington, DC: National Academy Press, 1994), vol. I, pp. 84–107; Curtis L. Meinert, "The Inclusion of Women in Clinical Trials," *Science* 269 (August 11, 1995), 795–796. For a different view of the statistical issues, see Kent R. Bailey, "Generalizing the Results of Randomized Clinical Trials," *Controlled Clinical Trials* 15 (1994), 15–23. For related charges of unthinking, "unscientific" conduct in regards to the AIDS activists, see Paul D. Stolley and Tamar Lasky, "Shortcuts in Drug Evaluation," *Clinical Pharmacology and Therapeutics* 52 (July 1992), 1–3.

39 Jerry M. Gurwitz, Nananda F. Col, and Jerry Avorn, "Exclusion of the Elderly and Women from Clinical Trials in Acute Myocardial Infarction," *JAMA* 268 (September 16, 1992), 1417–1422. See the discussion in C. E. Davis, "Generalizing from Clinical Trials," *Controlled Clinical Trials* 15 (1994), 11–14.

40 Jeanne Mandelblatt, Howard Andrews, Jon Kerner, Ann Zauber, and William Burnett, "Determinants of Late Stage Diagnosis of Breast and Cervical Cancer: The Impact of Age, Race, Social Class and Hospital Type," *AJPH* 81 (May 1991), 646–649.

incorporated into planning for clinical trials. But let me concede the general point, that Congress has confused the notions of political representation and statistical requirements for representativeness. What then?

In a democratic society, statisticians and clinical researchers have not only a right but an obligation to explain why they think Congress's requirements are misconceived. As John Burnham has noted, scientists in recent decades have backed away from efforts earlier in the century to explain science to the public.[41] In the 1940s, statisticians had rejected an appeal from their colleague Walter Shewhart to begin explaining to the public why "a knowledge of statistical reasoning had become essential to the wise conduct of modern affairs." Such efforts need not be merely "propagandistic," as Shewhart's contemporaries supposed.[42] Surely, the debate over the measurement of treatment effects in women and minorities represents an opportunity to educate about the effects of sample size on the ability to detect differences in event rates in terms far more compelling than the elementary statistics classroom usually provides.

At the same time, however, therapeutic reformers would have to acknowledge that the science of statistics cannot unilaterally dictate a "right" and a "wrong" policy for publicly funded medical research. At best, statistical calculations can indicate the consequences of the new congressional policy.

The consequences clinical researchers fear most are institutional: that a "quota" approach to designing clinical trials will overwhelm the limited resources available for such studies. Trials capable of detecting subgroup differences might have to be as much as four times larger than at present. Researchers contend that the new requirements would damage, if not mortally wound, a valuable social enterprise: the randomized multicenter clinical trial.[43]

Arguments over public policies of any sort are often less neat and more heated than scientists of any stripe would prefer. Yet they share in common with more decorous scientific exchanges an interest in institutions that often transcends the narrower technical matters at issue. In accepting the contention that clinical trials

41 John Burnham, *How Superstition Won and Science Lost: Popularizing Science and Health in the United States* (New Brunswick, NJ: Rutgers University Press, 1987). See also Lasch's discussion of the press in "The Lost Art of Argument," in Christopher Lasch, *The Revolt of the Elites and the Betrayal of Democracy* (New York: W. W. Norton, 1995), pp. 161–175.

42 William G. Cochran, *Statistics: One Man's View,* n.d., unpublished manuscript, Accession 9449, William G. Cochran papers, Harvard University Archives. For a historical approach to statistics that similarly regards such activities as propagandistic, see my colleague Mary Poovey's "Figures of Arithmetic, Figures of Speech: The Discourse of Statistics in the 1830s," *Critical Inquiry* 19 (Winter 1993), 256–276.

43 See the example in Piantadosi and Wittes, "Politically Correct Clinical Trials" (n. 38), 564–656. Since the regulations issued by NIH do not require trials in most cases to have the high statistical "power" and correspondingly large sample sizes necessary to detect such differences, it remains unclear whether the law will prove as onerous as researchers fear. *Federal Register* 59 (March 28, 1994), 14512. For anxieties about the future of the clinical trials enterprise, see, in addition to the sources cited in n. 38, Curtis L. Meinert, "NIH Multicenter Investigator-Initiated Trials: An Endangered Species," *Controlled Clinical Trials* 9 (1988), 97–102.

have failed historically to produce knowledge about the effects of therapy on women, the Congress decided to require NIH and researchers to design studies that would redress the situation. The Congress may well be wrong in assessing the extent of the problem or mistaken about the remedy it chose. But in a democratic polity, the only way to redress the error is to persuade legislators that the social injury being done to one institution – the multicenter clinical trial – is greater than the social injury being done to the groups who feel excluded from clinical research.[44]

Similarly if, as statisticians suggest, the modifications to clinical trial procedures desired by AIDS activists entail "trade-offs" between "unwise and hasty adoption" of new treatments and the high human cost of "delay in making new treatments available to patients," who is best equipped to make those decisions?[45] Should the research experience and knowledge of statisticians outweigh the personal experience of AIDS patients and their advocates? Should patients have a consultative but not a determining voice? On what grounds could we come together to discuss such choices?

Earlier in this chapter, I suggested that clinical research is "intrinsically" a social process: an activity conducted in a manner similar to politics, by groups of individuals with differing beliefs and interests, who must somehow persuade one another to enter into a temporary and partial alliance, and who then either succeed or fail to persuade others to act in concert with them. That view of science reflects the prevailing paradigm in my discipline: the history and sociology of science.

The view is most open to criticism, I would argue, because it offers a reductive view of politics. The notion of politics employed in most contemporary work on the history and sociology of science rejects distinctions of either scale or substance, failing to discriminate between the manuverings of a half-dozen researchers in a handful of laboratories and the global changes of regime or party that affect the economic and social lives of millions, or between a leftist politics concerned with social justice and the politics of a party that endorses inequality as the means to a better society.

Contemporary theories of science as politics are reductive in another sense, directly pertinent to the issues of therapeutic reform. They presuppose a view of politics as a contest in which the citizen's primary interest is in knowing who wins and who loses whereas the social analyst's main job is to describe the inequalities of power that lead to that result. An alternative view of politics holds that we should judge our institutions by the kinds of citizens they fashion, by whether they create citizens capable of judging, of fairness or of charity. The value of a

44 One might also argue that the perception that trials exclude women or minorities damages the same valuable social enterprise about which researchers are concerned, i.e., the controlled clinical trial.

45 Byron W. Brown Jr., "Comment," *Journal of the American Statistical Association* 87 (June 1992), 570.

policy, according to this account, lies in how well it enables us to examine collectively our beliefs, our practices, and our actions.[46]

How then would we judge the value of an organon – an instrument for producing knowledge? In the past, therapeutic reformers have made many claims on behalf of randomized controlled trials. Controlled clinical trials would "eliminate bias" in clinical experiments; they would provide a "scientific" basis for assessing therapies; their use would put an end to therapeutic controversies; they would eliminate physicians' overconfidence and therapeutic excesses. Such claims were exaggerated, the products of a youthful methodological and ideological naiveté.

Nowadays, spokespersons for randomized trials are more guarded and precise: "no other method for studying the merits of clinical treatment regimens can approach the precision of estimating effects and the strength of inference permitted by RCTs."[47] Such a statement may be read in two ways. On the one hand, it may be regarded as a claim that randomized trials offer us an exact measure of the value of alternative medical treatments. On the other, it can be read in light of R. A. Fisher's views that randomized experiments permit us to specify how *uncertain* we are when we claim that a new treatment works better than an existing one.

The first reading places the randomized clinical trial in the service of the "politics of objectivity," as Ted Porter has termed it. Here, statistics is used to "reduce public choices to rules" while "grounding those rules in the impersonal laws of nature and of number."[48] The second reading enlists statistics as a critical theory, a tool for examining knowledge and calling authorities to account.[49] The social value of forcing physicians (and the rest of us) to articulate our uncertainties

---

46 See the discussions in Marc K. Landy, Marc J. Roberts, and Stephen R. Thomas, *The Environmental Protection Agency: Asking the Wrong Questions* (New York: Oxford University Press, 1990), pp. 7–9, 282–283; Manfred Stanley, "The Rhetoric of the Commons: Forum Discourse in Politics and Society," in Herbert W. Simons, ed., *The Rhetorical Turn: Invention and Persuasion in the Conduct of Inquiry* (Chicago: University of Chicago Press, 1990), pp. 242–245; Amy Guttman, *Democratic Education* (Princeton: Princeton University Press, 1987), pp. 70–107; Elkin, *City and Regime* (n. 2), pp. 146–200; Marks, *Ideas As Reforms* (n. 3), pp. 259–264. The starting point for such discussions in the twentieth-century is John Dewey's *The Public and Its Problems* [1927] (Chicago: Swallow Press, 1954), esp. pp. 202–212. On the foundations of this view of politics, see Martin Diamond, "Ethics and Politics: The American Way," in Robert H. Horowitz, ed., *The Moral Foundations of the American Republic,* 2nd ed. (Charlottesville: University Press of Virginia, 1982), pp. 39–72; Ronald Beiner, *Political Judgment* (Chicago: University of Chicago Press, 1983).

47 John C. Bailar III, "Introduction," in Stanley H. Shapiro and Thomas A. Louis, eds., *Clinical Trials: Issues and Approaches* (New York: Marcel Dekker, 1983), p. 1.

48 Theodore M. Porter, "Statistics and the Politics of Objectivity," *Revue de synthèse* 114 (January–March 1993), 88–101. The quoted passage is from Porter, "Objectivity As Standardization: The Rhetoric of Impersonality in Measurement, Statistics and Cost–Benefit Analysis," *Annals of Scholarship* 9 (1992), 49. See also the discussion of competing justifications of the clinical trial in Marks, *Ideas As Reforms* (n. 3), pp. 244–249.

49 For a clear and strong, yet insufficiently reflexive statement on science and uncertainty, see Iain Chalmers, "Scientific Inquiry and Authoritarianism in Perinatal Care and Education," *Birth* 10 (1983), 151–164. For an argument along lines similar to mine, see Ann Oakley, "Who's Afraid of the Randomized Controlled Trial? Some Dilemmas of the Scientific Method and 'Good' Research Practice," *Women and Health* 15 (1989), 25–59, esp. 49–53.

about the benefits of medical treatment should not be underestimated. But neither should the dangers of a dogmatic view that makes statisticians or other experts overconfident in what they know. Opting for one over the other is not only, as is often assumed, a matter of choosing between rival philosophies of statistical inference: bayesian or likelihood perspectives against frequentist interpretations of probability. It is also depends on how and where critically minded statisticians do their work – how willing they are to expose the limitations of their own expertise, and how public the forums in which they question existing knowledge and authority.[50]

Why and how do forums matter? The choice of forums affects both the scope and aims of political discussion. Contemporary discussions of therapeutic reform embody what political theorist Manfred Stanley terms the "liberal forum" model, whose purpose is to create elite consensus about policy decisions. Discussion in the liberal forum aims at illuminating "relative trade-offs between morally plausible and politically practical policy" alternatives.[51]

Contemporary proposals for therapeutic reform begin from a common premise: clinical decisions are impaired because physicians lack evidence about the effects of therapy and/or the intellectual tools needed to evaluate that evidence. Some reformers, accepting the existing social structure of individual clinical decision makers, concern themselves with improving the information available to physicians, along with clinicians' abilities to assess that information.[52] Others who contend that medicine's existing social structure is obsolete propose that we devise new institutions to arrive at and enforce clinical practice guidelines. Discussions of policy alternatives then take place in predictable terms. Who participates: practitioners, insurers, consumers, government officials? Who wins and who loses? How rigid or flexible should guidelines and enforcement be?[53]

50 For a moving example of professional activism and integrity, see Mark Harrington, "In Memoriam: David Byar As an AIDS Activist," *Controlled Clinical Trials* 16 (1995), 270–275.

51 Stanley, "The Rhetoric of the Commons" (n. 46), 243.

52 For examples of various strategies, see Jonathan Lomas, Murray Enkin, Geoffrey Anderson, et al., "Opinion Leaders vs. Audit and Feedback to Implement Practice Guidelines: Delivery after Previous Caesarean Section," *JAMA* 265 (May 1, 1991), 2202–2207; Jerry Avorn and Stephen B. Soumerai, "Improving Drug Therapy Decisions through Educational Outreach: A Randomized Controlled Trial of Academically Based 'Detailing,' " *NEJM* 308 (June 16, 1983), 1457–1463; Douglas G. Altman and J. Martin Bland, "Improving Doctors' Understanding of Statistics," *Journal of the Royal Statistical Society*, ser. A, 154 (1991), 223–248; Lachlan Forrow, William C. Taylor, and Robert M. Arnold, "Absolutely Relative: How Research Results Are Summarized Can Affect Treatment Decisions," *American Journal of Medicine* 92 (February 1992), 121–129.

53 Jane Sisk, "Improving the Use of Research-Based Policy Making: Effective Care in Pregnancy and Child Birth in the United States," *Milbank Quarterly* 71 (1993), 477–496; Ayres, "The Use and Abuse of Medical Practice Guidelines" (n. 20), 436–438; William W. Parmley, "Practice Guidelines and Cookbook Medicine: Who Are the Cooks?," *Journal of the American College of Cardiology* 24 (August 1994), 567–568; Barbara K. Redman, "Clinical Practice Guidelines As Tools of Public Policy: Conflicts of Purpose, Issues of Autonomy, and Justice," *Journal of Clinical Ethics* 303–309; Colleen M. Grogan, Roger D. Feldman, John A. Nyman, and Janet Shapiro, "How Will We Use Clinical Guidelines? The Experience of Medicare Carriers," *Journal of Health Politics, Policy and Law* 19 (Spring 1994), 7–26; Lomas et al., "Making Clinical Policy Explicit" (n. 52), 11–25.

Such discussions leave the objects of policy unexamined and the institutional structures of medicine untransformed. A democratic forum, as Stanley terms it, would focus on "civic education" in which the premises of both policies and institutions would be publicly explored. Before choosing among policies, Stanley argues, we need to examine the institutions that give rise to those policies. What do they accomplish? Why do they exist?[54] In the case of medicine, this means coming to understand the premises on which both therapeutic practice and therapeutic reform operate.

Both therapeutic practice and therapeutic reform aim at improving the outcomes of medical treatment. But what do we want from medical treatment? The question seems foolishly naive, if not perversely so. Surely therapy's purpose is to cure disease and save lives. Yet a descent into the realm of medical practice reveals a variety of measures used to judge therapeutic outcomes – the relief of symptoms, indicators of physiological or biochemical processes, functional status – with each measure embedded in a mangle of disciplinary practices, scientific conjectures, and professional experience.[55] Therapeutic reformers offer their own preferred measure, the mortality rate, which since the sixteenth century has served as the quantitative coinage through by which we measure medical success. The choice among outcome measures, it is frequently asserted, is a technical matter – a question of relative convenience, reliability, and objectivity.[56] But is the choice only technical?

In the current era, medical advances determine not only whether we live or die but, increasingly, how we will live and die.[57] Ordinary citizens, those who are potential patients and the friends and relatives of such patients, have as much to

54 Stanley, "The Rhetoric of the Commons" (n. 46); Landy et al. (n. 46); Marks, *Ideas As Reforms* (n. 3), pp. 258–263. For a sustained example of critical and historical institutional analysis in this spirit, see Elkin, *City and Regime* (n. 2).
55 Milton Packer, "How Should We Judge the Efficacy of Drug Therapy in Patients with Chronic Congestive Heart Failure? The Insights of Six Blind Men," *Journal of the American College of Cardiology* 9 (February 1987), 433–438. I appropriate the phrase "mangle of practice" from Andy Pickering, hopefully without doing violence to his concerns. See "Objectivity and the Mangle of Practice," *Annals of Scholarship* 8 (1991), 409–424.
56 On the introduction and use of mortality rates prior to 1800, see Andrea Alice Rusnock, *The Quantification of Things Human: Medicine and Political Arithmetic in Enlightenment England and France* (Ph.D. thesis, Princeton University, 1990); Anne M. Fagot, "Probabilities and Causes: On Life Tables, Causes of Death, and Etiological Diagnoses," in Jaakko Hintikka, David Gruender, and Evardro Agazzi, eds., *Proceedings of the Pisa Conference on the History and Philosophy of Science* (Dordecht: D. Reidel, 1980), vol. II, pp. 41–104. For contemporary discussions of outcome measures, see M. L. Terrin, "Efficient Use of Endpoints in Clinical Trials: A Clinical Perspective," *Statistics in Medicine* 9 (January–February 1990), 155–160; Claire Bombardier, Peter Tugwell, Alexandra Sinclair, Caroline Dok, Geoff Anderson, and W. Watson Buchanan, "Preference for Endpoint Measures in Clinical Trials: Results of Structure Workshops," *Journal of Rheumatology* 9 (September–October 1982), 798–801; J. Wittes, E. Lakatos, and J. Probstfield, "Surrogate Endpoints in Clinical Trials: Cardiovascular Diseases," *Statistics in Medicine* 8 (April 1989), 415–426.
57 Alonzo Plough, *Borrowed Time: Artificial Organs and the Politics of Extending Life* (Philadelphia: Temple University Press, 1986).

say on these aspects of medical goods as any expert. As presently designed, however, our institutions give citizens little voice in these matters. Theirs is the consumer's choice: pick a brand or shop around.[58]

Our present difficulties are both conceptual and institutional. It is not simply a matter of redesigning the institutions that allocate medical goods or reexamining the principles on which we subsidize their distribution.[59] It is also a question of establishing institutions in which our traditional concepts of the benefits of medicine can be deliberated.

Why deliberated? First, because in numerous instances professional and lay concepts of the benefits to be gained by increasing our technological capacities in medicine are at odds.[60] These differences need to be articulated and explored, preferably in a context where the professionals do not hold the upper hand. Second, because there is no Archimedean point from which the benefits of new technological capacities can be calculated, once and for all. Different communities, with different traditions, will value these benefits differently.[61] Third, because most of us have yet to examine what we think about these matters, much less to discuss our thoughts with others. We have, at best, opinions, grounded in fears and hopes. Deliberation involves scrutiny of opinions, in the light of experience and reason as well as hopes and fears.

Our technocratic culture places a high premium on making decisions and, especially in the medical realm, on making the "right" decisions. Yet unless we create institutions that enable us to reflect on our decisions and to communicate those reflections to one another, we do not have an independent means to judge the "rightness" of these decisions. Judging decisions is a historical task, in the sense that our experience of past and present decisions provides us with a means to assess our future choices.[62]

---

58 The choices some consumers face are even more limited than that. See, for example, Rudolf Klein, "Models of Man and Models of Policy: Reflections on *Exit, Voice and Loyalty* Ten Years Later," *Milbank Memorial Fund Quarterly* 58 (Summer 1980), 426–428. See also Dewey, *The Public and Its Problems* (n. 46), p. 208–212.

59 See Victor Fuchs, *Who Shall Live? Health Economics and Social Choice* (New York: Basic Books, 1974), pp. 143–151; Lawrence D. Brown, "The Scope and Limits of Equality As a Normative Guide to Federal Health Care Policy," *Public Policy* 26 (Fall 1978), 482–532.

60 Barbara J. McNeil, R. Weichselbaum, and S. G. Pauker, "Fallacy of the Five Year Survival Rate in Lung Cancer," *NEJM* 299 (1978), 1397–1401; "Correspondence: Fallacy of the Five Year Survival Rate," *NEJM* 300 (1979), 927–928; Barbara J. McNeil, R. Weichselbaum, and S. G. Pauker, "Speech and Survival: Tradeoffs between Quantity and Quality of Life in Laryngeal Cancer," *NEJM* 305 (1981), 982–987.

61 Alasdair MacIntyre, "Patients As Agents," in S. F. Spicker and H. T. Engelhardt Jr., eds., *Philosophical Medical Ethics: Its Nature and Significance* (Dordrecht: D. Reidel, 1977), pp. 197–212.

62 Charles Taylor, "Social Theory As Practice," in *Philosophy and the Human Sciences: Philosophical Papers* (Cambridge: Cambridge University Press, 1985), vol. 2, pp. 91–115. Without a public forum for deliberating our interpretations and valuations of the present and past, we have no way of incorporating this experience into our collective decisions: it remains private (and often unarticulated, even to ourselves). See Michael J. Sandel, *Liberalism and the Limits of Justice* (Cambridge: Cambridge University Press, 1982), pp. 179–183.

I have no blueprint to offer for reforming therapeutic reform.[63] I write at a time when institutions for delivering and evaluating medical care in the United States are in the midst of an unprecedented historical realignment, with no one certain as to the future distribution of power and responsibility. Whatever the future holds for physicians, managers, patients, and citizens, we will still need to determine how the value of medical treatment should be judged and who shall do the judging. Here is where a knowledge of the history of therapeutic reform may prove useful.

My aim in this book has been to examine how therapeutic reformers in this century have conceived of their tasks and how they have gone about accomplishing them. I have also examined closely some episodes in recent history – the Diet-Heart study and the University Group Diabetes Program – in which reformers were unable to accomplish what they had hoped. Such historical scrutiny of science is sometimes viewed as antagonistic to science, especially when accompanied by a concluding chapter that argues the need for a public and democratic examination of the science of therapeutic reform. Yet history is hardly the only "critical" discipline, the only tool we need in thinking about the future of therapeutic reform. Statistics, too, is a critical discipline, no less capable of revising our assumptions and beliefs. In that sense, my argument concludes with an appeal for more, not less science in these matters. Only when we are all in a position to comprehend and evaluate the claims made by methodological reformers will we be in a position to make the best use of their advice. So long as we can only choose between deferring to their authority or ignoring their counsels, then we are left choosing between medical science and medical politics. And that is an unfortunate choice.

63 Various experiments – recent and ongoing – contain elements of what seems needed. The Oregon efforts at a public reassessment of priorities for Medicaid coverage and the Cochrane Collaboration, a cooperative venture of therapeutic reformers in organizing and making widely available the existing evidence on therapeutic practices in each clinical domain, both come to mind. On Oregon, see Martin A. Strosberg, Joshua M. Wiener, Robert Baker, and I. Alan Fein, *Rationing America's Medical Care: The Oregon Plan and Beyond* (Washington, DC: Brookings Institution, 1992). On the Cochrane Collaboration, see Iain Chalmers, "The Cochrane Collaboration: Preparing, Maintaining and Disseminating Systematic Reviews of the Effects of Health Care," *Ann NY Acad Sci* 703 (December 31, 1993), 156–163; Fred Mosteller, "The Prospect of Data-Based Medicine in the Light of ECPC," *Milbank Quarterly* 71 (1993), 523–532.

A NOTE ON SOURCES

The history of clinical medicine and research for the twentieth century is a new field. Until recently, scholars have concentrated their efforts on questions of social policy and professional politics, rather than on medical science. The reader will find references to the most useful historical work on clinical and laboratory research in the notes to each chapter. Published primary sources are best pursued through research in a combination of the *Index-Catalogue of the Library of the Surgeon General's Office* series 1–3 (Washington, DC: 1880–1932), and *Index Medicus*. Prior to 1895, the periodical literature is captured well in the *Index-Catalogue*; after that date, the researcher must turn to *Index Medicus* (1879–1899, 1902–1927, 1960–) and its various incarnations and competitors – *Bibliographia Medica* (1900–1902), *Quarterly Cumulative Index Medicus* (1927–1956), *Current List of Medical Literature* (1941–1959). Here, I have tried to provide an overview and guide to manuscript sources and repositories that may be of use to future researchers; a more comprehensive list of the manuscript collections and published materials used in writing this book is available in the notes.

For the history of drug evaluation and innovation prior to 1938, the weekly minutes of the American Medical Association's *Council on Pharmacy and Chemistry* are a unique source. Each week, council members received a mimeographed summary of reports on new drugs, along with the comments of other council members on the drugs, and on proposed council actions. The *Bulletin* contains valuable information about specific drugs, about council policies, and about the views of clinical researchers around the country who served as consultants to the council. It is an invaluable source for studying contemporary standards of pharmacology and clinical evaluation. Cumulated once or twice a year, the weekly reports were bound as the *Bulletin* of the Council on Pharmacy and Chemistry. The archives of the American Medical Association in Chicago has the only complete run of the *Bulletin,* which by the 1930s extends to several thousand pages a year. Partial runs donated by former council members may be found at some university libraries: the William Henry Welch Medical Library, The Johns Hopkins Medical Institutions, Baltimore, and the Agricultural Library, University of Wisconsin, Madison. Other copies reported in the *Union List of Serials* are either missing or were destroyed.

After 1938, the council's records are usefully supplemented by the records of the U.S. Food and Drug Administration (FDA), which keeps an unusually detailed record of materials regarding specific drugs and specific companies as well as more general issues concerning drug evaluation and regulation. The FDA's post-1938 records remain in the custody of the agency, and access must be requested through formal Freedom of Information (FOI) procedures. The FOI office facilitates scholarly access to the records, for requests made through the FDA Historian's Office, which has published an overview of the records and request procedures.[1]

In contrast to the AMA and FDA records, few drug manufacturers have made their records freely available to historical scholars. Although individual companies have on occasion made some records available to individual scholars, access is uncertain and in some cases restricted. The historian planning on using corporate drug records must be prepared for delay and disappointment. In some cases, substantial information on corporate research is available in the personal papers of academic consultants: the Vannevar Bush and Gregory Pincus papers in the Library of Congress contain ample material on Merck (Bush) and Ciba, G. H. Searle and Upjohn (Pincus), while the A. Newton Richards papers at the University of Pennsylvania archives contain extensive records of his collaboration with Merck. Whether the researcher interested in post-1960 corporate activities will be as lucky is doubtful: companies have increasingly tightened up on the management of papers provided consultants, advisors and directors.

Other government records of value include the records of the National Institutes of Health (RG 443), the Public Health Service (RG 90) and, for the World War II era, the Office of Scientific Development and Research (RG 227): all are on deposit at the National Archives. In addition, many recent NIH records remain in NIH custody, and access nominally requires an FOI request. The Historian's Office at NIH is helpful in identifying both records and record keepers. The records in question are all administrative records; at present, the National Archives does not keep the scientific papers and correspondence of individual NIH scientists. Some individuals have left their papers to the National Library of Medicine, others to university archives, and others have vanished.

The papers of individual researchers are invaluable for a study of this sort. Manuscript collections must be tracked through two guides: *National Union Catalog of Manuscript Collections* (1959–1993) and the on-line Research Libraries Integrated Network (RLIN), which has increasingly taken over the job of cataloging university manuscript collections. Many records, however, remain unlisted, and there is no substitute for contacting the associates, departments, and institutional repositories with which an individual was associated. The path taken by an

---

1 *A Guide to Resources on the History of the Food and Drug Administration* (Washington, DC: U.S. Food and Drug Administration, 1995).

individual's papers may be even more eccentric than the person's own career: the correspondence of cortisone researcher Philip Hench, for example, has ended up both at the Houston Academy of Medicine, Texas Medical Center Library, Houston, and in the Special Collections Department of the University of Virginia Libraries, Charlottesville, where Hench's brother was professor of English.

The historian studying twentieth-century clinical research is at the mercy of his historical subjects and the archival policies at the institutions at which they worked. Researchers, archivists, and administrators have long ago decided for the historian which records are, and are not, worth keeping.[2] Archivists in turn are ultimately dependent on the record-keeping habits of individual faculty members, and records concerning therapeutic research may be discarded even at institutions with substantial archival programs.

Among the collections I found particularly useful in this study were the archives at the Francis A. Countway Library of Medicine, Harvard Medical School, Boston; New York Hospital Archives, New York City; and the Alan Mason Chesney Archives, The Johns Hopkins Medical Institutions, Baltimore. Other significant institutional repositories include the archives of the National Academy of Sciences, Washington, DC, which contains the records of the Division of Medical Sciences of the National Research Council. The NRC committees were especially active in numerous areas of clinical research during and shortly after World War II. The Rockefeller Archive Center holds the papers of several non-Rockefeller philanthropies, including the Commonwealth Fund, active in medical research.[3] The American Philosophical Society has extensive papers from the initial generation of researchers at the Rockefeller Institute for Medical Research.[4] The National Library of Medicine manuscripts division collects papers not only of NIH scientists, but of nationally prominent researchers from around the country. The College of Physicians of Philadelphia has a collection of papers from prominent twentieth-century researchers who were members.[5]

Much of the record of post–World War II medical science remains in private hands. The records of statisticians working in medical research have been particularly hard to trace: pioneers like Donald Mainland and Joseph Berkson left no papers that I have been able to locate. Only a few among the key group of statisticians recruited by Harold Dorn to work at the National Institutes of Health have left papers in public repositories: Jerome Cornfield's papers (from relatively late in his career) are at the University of Iowa, and Nathan Mantel's papers were

---

2 For discussions of contemporary archival policies, see Nancy McCall and Lisa A. Mix, eds., *Designing Archival Programs to Advance Knowledge in the Health Fields* (Baltimore: Johns Hopkins University Press, 1995).

3 Emily J. Oakhill and Kenneth W. Rose, *A Guide to the Archives and Manuscripts at the Rockefeller Archive Center* (North Tarrytown, NY: Rockfeller Archive Center, 1989).

4 J. Stephen Catlett, ed., *A New Guide to the Collections of the American Philosophical Society* (Philadelphia: American Philosophical Society, 1987).

5 Rudolph Hirsch, ed., *A Catalog of the Manuscripts and Archives of the Library of the College of Physicians of Philadelphia* (Philadelphia: University of Pennsylvania Press, 1983).

deposited at the National Library of Medicine earlier this year (1995). Subsequent historians may wish to look in the records and correspondence of key training programs in statistics and biostatistics: for example, at Princeton University (John Tukey), University of North Carolina (Bernard Greenberg), and North Carolina State University (Gertrude Cox). The same holds true for clinical pharmacology and clinical research: only a few of the key individuals have left papers where historians can easily get at them. The historian of late twentieth-century medicine accordingly remains dependent on the goodwill and collegiality of individual scientists. As indicated in the acknowledgments, I have been especially fortunate in the help I have received from those I wrote about. Nonetheless, I am certain that there is much more to be said, and hopeful that the often ephemeral paperwork that historians rely on will make its way into welcoming hands where others can use it to tell the story better and more fully than I have done.

Some historians advocate making more extensive use of oral histories to supplement the imperfect archival record of twentieth-century medicine and medical science.[6] I have consulted the oral history collection at the National Library of Medicine, and conducted extensive interviews with my research subjects. However valuable these interviews are in coming to appreciate the perspectives and concerns of historical actors, I have found them of limited use when it came to writing up a narrative account.

6 See Saul Benison, "Oral History: A Personal View," in Edwin Clarke, ed., *Modern Methods in the History of Medicine* (London: Athlone Press, 1971), pp. 286–305; Paul Thompson, "Oral History and the History of Medicine: A Review," *Social History of Medicine* 4 (August 1991), 371–383.

INDEX